Advanced Systems for Improved Public Healthcare and Disease Prevention:

Emerging Research and Opportunities

Thierry Oscar Edoh
Technical University of Munich, Germany

A volume in the Advances in Healthcare Information Systems and Administration (AHISA) Book Series

IGI Global
DISSEMINATOR OF KNOWLEDGE

Published in the United States of America by
IGI Global
Medical Information Science Reference (an imprint of IGI Global)
701 E. Chocolate Avenue
Hershey PA, USA 17033
Tel: 717-533-8845
Fax: 717-533-8661
E-mail: cust@igi-global.com
Web site: http://www.igi-global.com

Library of Congress Cataloging-in-Publication Data

Names: Edoh, Thierry, 1968- author.
Title: Advanced systems for improved public healthcare and disease prevention : emerging research and opportunities / by Thierry Edoh.
Description: Hershey, PA : Medical Information Science Reference, [2018]
Identifiers: LCCN 2017045788| ISBN 9781522555285 (hardcover) | ISBN 9781522555292 (ebook)
Subjects: | MESH: Medical Informatics | Global Health | Delivery of Health Care
Classification: LCC R858 | NLM WA 26.5 | DDC 362.10285--dc23 LC record available at https://lccn.loc.gov/2017045788

This book is published in the IGI Global book series Advances in Healthcare Information Systems and Administration (AHISA) (ISSN: 2328-1243; eISSN: 2328-126X)

British Cataloguing in Publication Data
A Cataloguing in Publication record for this book is available from the British Library.

All work contributed to this book is new, previously-unpublished material.
The views expressed in this book are those of the authors, but not necessarily of the publisher.

For electronic access to this publication, please contact: eresources@igi-global.com.

Advances in Healthcare Information Systems and Administration (AHISA) Book Series

ISSN:2328-1243
EISSN:2328-126X

Editor-in-Chief: Anastasius Moumtzoglou, Hellenic Society for Quality & Safety in Healthcare and P. & A. Kyriakou Children's Hospital, Greece

MISSION

The **Advances in Healthcare Information Systems and Administration (AHISA) Book Series** aims to provide a channel for international researchers to progress the field of study on technology and its implications on healthcare and health information systems. With the growing focus on healthcare and the importance of enhancing this industry to tend to the expanding population, the book series seeks to accelerate the awareness of technological advancements of health information systems and expand awareness and implementation.

Driven by advancing technologies and their clinical applications, the emerging field of health information systems and informatics is still searching for coherent directing frameworks to advance health care and clinical practices and research. Conducting research in these areas is both promising and challenging due to a host of factors, including rapidly evolving technologies and their application complexity. At the same time, organizational issues, including technology adoption, diffusion and acceptance as well as cost benefits and cost effectiveness of advancing health information systems and informatics applications as innovative forms of investment in healthcare are gaining attention as well. **AHISA** addresses these concepts and critical issues.

COVERAGE

- IS in Healthcare
- Management of Emerging Health Care Technologies
- Rehabilitative Technologies
- Pharmaceutical and Home Healthcare Informatics
- Measurements and Impact of HISA on Public and Social Policy
- IT Applications in Physical Therapeutic Treatments
- Virtual health technologies
- Decision Support Systems
- Telemedicine
- Clinical Decision Support Design, Development and Implementation

IGI Global is currently accepting manuscripts for publication within this series. To submit a proposal for a volume in this series, please contact our Acquisition Editors at Acquisitions@igi-global.com or visit: http://www.igi-global.com/publish/.

The Advances in Healthcare Information Systems and Administration (AHISA) Book Series (ISSN 2328-1243) is published by IGI Global, 701 E. Chocolate Avenue, Hershey, PA 17033-1240, USA, www.igi-global.com. This series is composed of titles available for purchase individually; each title is edited to be contextually exclusive from any other title within the series. For pricing and ordering information please visit http://www.igi-global.com/book-series/advances-healthcare-information-systems-administration/37156. Postmaster: Send all address changes to above address.

Titles in this Series

For a list of additional titles in this series, please visit:
https://www.igi-global.com/book-series/advances-healthcare-information-systems-administration/37156

Big Data Management and the Internet of Things for Improved Health Systems
Brojo Kishore Mishra (C. V. Raman College of Engineering, India) and Raghvendra Kumar (LNCT Group of Colleges,India)
Medical Information Science Reference • ©2018 • 312pp • H/C (ISBN: 9781522552222) • US $255.00

Novel Applications of Virtual Communities in Healthcare Settings
Christo El Morr (York University, Canada)
Medical Information Science Reference • ©2018 • 247pp • H/C (ISBN: 9781522529583) • US $235.00

Handbook of Research on Data Science for Effective Healthcare Practice and Administration
Elham Akhond Zadeh Noughabi (University of Calgary, Canada) Bijan Raahemi (University of Ottawa, Canada) Amir Albadvi (Tarbiat Modares University, Iran) and Behrouz H. Far (University of Calgary, Canada)
Medical Information Science Reference • ©2017 • 545pp • H/C (ISBN: 9781522525158) • US $255.00

Patent Law and Intellectual Property in the Medical Field
Rashmi Aggarwal (Institute of Management Technology Ghaziabad, India) and Rajinder Kaur (Panjab University, India)
Medical Information Science Reference • ©2017 • 257pp • H/C (ISBN: 9781522524144) • US $200.00

Design, Development, and Integration of Reliable Electronic Healthcare Platforms
Anastasius Moumtzoglou (P&A Kyriakou Children's Hospital, Greece)
Medical Information Science Reference • ©2017 • 357pp • H/C (ISBN: 9781522517245) • US $205.00

For an entire list of titles in this series, please visit:
https://www.igi-global.com/book-series/advances-healthcare-information-systems-administration/37156

IGI Global
DISSEMINATOR OF KNOWLEDGE

701 East Chocolate Avenue, Hershey, PA 17033, USA
Tel: 717-533-8845 x100 • Fax: 717-533-8661
E-Mail: cust@igi-global.com • www.igi-global.com

To my princess, Yasmine Manuela Edoh, and my Mom, Colette Lea Alissoutin, I dedicate this first edition of this book.

Table of Contents

Foreword

Healthcare is an important service in great demand all over the world. Despite it is constantly improved, the problems to scale it to an ever-growing world population also seem to increase. The use of information and communication technologies (ICT) solutions in healthcare settings is an emerging trend to try to solve the current problems in the sector. This is the subject of this book.

Problems in healthcare supply seem to be very different in different parts of the world, especially in developing and developed countries. Whereas in developing countries there often is a lack of pharmaceutical products, of healthcare personnel, and of healthcare infrastructure, in developed countries problems origin from an over ageing population and increasing treatment costs. Also, information technology as an advanced technology is often assumed to be only applicable in industrial countries and cannot help with the demands of regions with a low degree of technological infrastructure. However, upon second look, it turns out that there are several challenges in healthcare which are quite similar in developing and developed countries, such as a lack of healthcare supply in rural regions of developed countries. Also, there are lightweight applications of ICT technology, which have the potential of major effects in all regions in the world, such as using cell phone technology for telehealthcare.

The book reports on several studies addressing quite diverse aspects of health care. The main common focus is on relations among developed and developing countries. Without going too much into the details, the book provides a broad overview of several aspects of health systems in several parts of the world, with a focus on Germany and Benin. It covers the use of ICT solutions in such diverse applications like pharmacovigilance, drug supply, and disease monitoring. Sometimes, solutions for common problems exist in developed countries, but they cannot simply be transferred to other contexts. In the healthcare sector technical solutions often work only if complemented by policy measures and vice versa. The book looks at both sides and considers technical solutions together with their social and political background aspects.

The book is also a very personal way of dealing with its subject. The author was born in Benin and now lives in Germany and thus has an intimate knowledge of the daily aspects of both worlds. Also, as a computer scientist doing research in the healthcare sector for many years, he knows both the technology and the application domain. He has actively taken part in all the studies reported in the book and can provide an authentic picture of their approach and achievements. The book should be considered as a snapshot of ongoing work in a highly relevant sector of modern life for a global society which is in a need for sustainable solutions.

Gunnar Teege
University of the German Federal Army of Munich, Germany

Preface

The challenges facing the global healthcare are on one hand the poor healthcare delivery services accessibility due to the poor organization, lack of information and communication technology systems, lack of diseases control and surveillance policies and systems, and non-existent health insurance in developing countries. On the other hand, developed countries also are facing limited access to the healthcare in rural areas, non-accommodation to patient needs, limited infection surveillance policies, high medical expenditures due to the faster growing elderly population, and too slow adoption of ICT systems in the healthcare systems. Particularly, the USA are facing high administration costs and inefficient health insurance system.

This book discusses the health care services delivery issues in global public healthcare system and proposes ICT based solutions for the improvement of health care services delivery and diseases prevention methodologies.

SUPPORTING TECHNOLOGY

Healthcare improvement and disease prevention relies on certain policies and technical support. The policies are defined by the Ministry of Health. The technology supports certain workflows and the health care professionals (HCP) along their daily tasks. In following, we briefly present certain technologies used to implement the advanced systems for improved public healthcare and diseases prevention.

Telemedicine

Health care provided at the remote using modern information and communication technologies, such as the internet, audio/video, computer, mobile devices (mHealth) and across geographic time, social and cultural challenges.

Telehealthcare

According to WHO, defined as "the integration of telecommunications systems into the practice of protecting and promoting health, and telemedicine is the incorporation of these systems into curative medicine" (Darkin & Cary, 2000).

Internet of Health Things (IoHT)

Integrates health objects with network connectivity from the digital and physical world. Furthermore. it combines personal health technologies and IoT and takes full advantages of IoT in expanding abilities to exchange useful data, enable improvements in context awareness, and the ability to initiate actions based on data that are collected and analyzed (Terry, 2016).

Istepanian, Hu, Philip, and Sungoor (2011) define the benefits of using the Internet of m-health Things (m-IoT) for non-invasive glucose level sensing. m-IoT puts together the functionalities of m-Health and IoT. mHealth (mobile Health) is health care services delivery supported by (smart) devices (i.e., smartphones, etc.).

Williams and McCauley (2016) define the *Healthcare Internet of Things* (IoHT) as:

The new embedded sensing capabilities of devices together with the availability of always being connected, to improve patient care whilst reducing costs.

Internet of Things (IoT)

The concept of IoT is back to 1999, where Kevin Ashton did the pioneering work linking to the new idea of using radio frequency identification (RFID) in the supply chain. Ashton (2009) writes:

"Internet of Things" started life as the title of a presentation I made at Procter & Gamble (P&G) in 1999. Linking the new idea of RFID in P&G's supply chain to the then-red-hot topic of the Internet was more than just a good way to get executive attention. It summed up an important insight—one that 10 years later after the Internet of Things has become the title of everything from an article in Scientific American to the name of a European Union conference, is still often misunderstood.

Please, look at Sheng et al. (2013) for more details about IoT Communication standards.

Crowd-Sensing

Crowd-sensing is a critical component of the Internet of Things (Liu, Shen, & Zhang, 2016). Crowdsourced data can be collected using participatory or opportunistic crowd sensing paradigms, where participants' smartphone sensors are used to collect information/data. Smartphone sensors or sensor systems are increasingly being used for measuring the quality of ambient air (Dutta, Gazi, Roy, & Chowdhury, 2016), temperature and particularly sensing bio-signals within an in- or outdoor crowd. Most traditional sensors (i.e., smartphone embedded sensors [Carpenter & Frontera, 2016]) are based on electrical working principles (Van Hoe et al., 2012), where they measure the quantity items using electrical means (Marika & Di, 2012). These sensors present limitations, that optical sensors overcome (Carpenter & Frontera, 2016).

Participatory vs. Opportunistic Sensing

Crowdsensing systems are either participatory or opportunistic. Participatory crowdsensing requires participants active involvement, participants perform computations and generate data as inputs for the systems, while in opportunistic requires fewer participants involvement, sensing is more autonomous, data are automatically generated without user involvement and computations are also automatically performed using participants' devices or available sensors (Chatzimilioudis, Konstantinidis, Laoudias, & Zeinalipour-yazti, 2012).

Energy Consumption

Traditional opportunistic crowdsensing and crowdsourcing data is energy-efficient but has poor real-time performance (Liu et al., 2016). Figure 1 presents the general mobile crowd sensing (MCS) framework, where participants open call, sense and collect data, aggregate analytics and send collected and transformed data to the data center. The MCS strategy consists of participatory, opportunistic and context-aware crowdsensing. Context-aware data sensing is triggered by pre-defined context (Liu et al., 2016; Chatzimilioudis et al., 2012).

Device-to-Device (D2D) Communication

Enables devices to communicate directly without interaction of base stations or access point. It is intended to exchange data utilizing various technologies

Figure 1. General mobile crowd sensing framework
Source: Liu et al. (2016) and Chatzimilioudis et al. (2012)

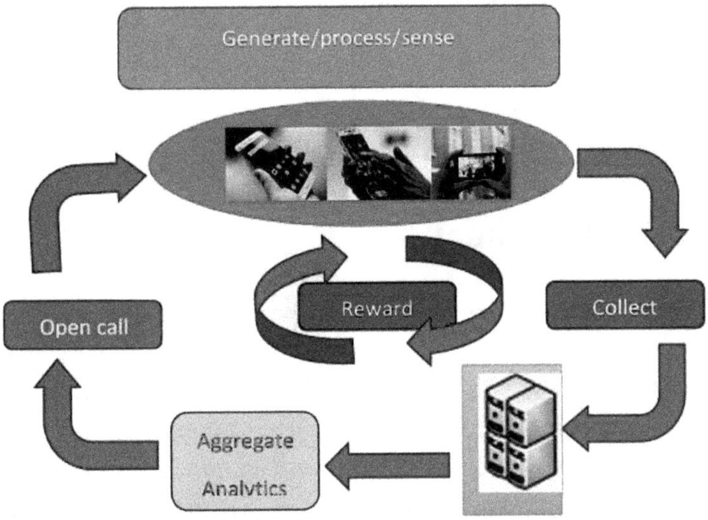

such as Ultra-wideband (UWB), Near Field Communications (NFC), ZigBee, Bluetooth, Wi-Fi-Direct or LTE Direct. The distance between the devices is relatively short and defined by the using protocol. The communication is technology dependent (Haus, Waqas, Ding, Li, & Member, 2016).

Machine-to-Machine (M2M) Communication

An autonomous communication, based on a cellular network such as GSM, LTE, etc., where the communication past through core networks via base stations or access points and M2M Server (application server). Compared with D2D, the communication is not direct, does not matter if the devices are approximate to one other. The distance between the devices is unlimited. Furthermore, the M2M communication is application oriented and technology independent (interoperability) (Haus et al., 2016).

Standard E-Commerce

A set of online business activities for selling and buying products services as well as transferring refers to an electronic commerce or E-commerce. The E-commerce is supported by the internet technology and Information and

Communication Technologies. There exist types of E-commerce: Business-to-Business, Business-to-Consumer (B2C), Business-to-Government (B2G), Consumer-to-Consumer (C2C), and mobile E-commerce (m-Commerce) (Andam, 2013).

TERMINOLOGY AND DEFINITIONS

Adherence to Treatment

WHO defines the adherence to treatment:

As the extent to which the patient's history of therapeutic drug-taking coincides with the prescribed treatment. Process-oriented or outcome-oriented are two methodologies and/or definitions that can be used to measure the adherence to treatment. While end-results of a treatment, e.g. cure rate, are the outcome-oriented indicator of success used to measure the adherence, Process-oriented indicators of success are used to measure the adherence by dealing with intermediate variables such as appointment-keeping or pill counts. (Scott & Mars, 2015)

According to WHO, improving adherence to treatment results in a much larger impact on overall global health than any other improvement of specific medical treatment (Hope, 1999). Our on-site study found out that non-adherence to treatment mostly in rural areas is due to the illiteracy, poor access to pharmaceutical and/or medical care, lack of health insurance or the high medical fees patients must pay.

Pharmacovigilance

Pharmacovigilance is the discipline for describing the process of monitoring and evaluating adverse drug reactions (ADR). All marketed drugs have side effects, which are described in the package leaflet. However, drugs can also present adverse reactions. A drug is a product whose purpose is to prevent, treat, or cure both physical and psychological diseases.

To prevent patients from the harm that can be caused by legal drugs, it is important to have an adequate mechanism for assessing and monitoring the adverse effects of the drugs, which the populations have used.

Adverse Drug Reactions (ADR)

John Murtagh defines ADR in Murtagh (2011) as:

'Any unwanted effect of treatment from the medical use of drugs that occurs at a usual therapeutic dose'. Almost every drug can cause an adverse reaction, which must be elicited in the history. Any substance that produces beneficial therapeutic effects may also produce unwanted, adverse or toxic effects. The severity of the reaction may range from a mild skin rash or nausea to sudden death from anaphylaxis. A study has shown that the incidence of adverse reactions increases from about 3% in patients 10–20 years of age to about 20% in patients 80–89 years of age.

Counterfeit Drugs

Counterfeit medications are a worldwide problem (Rudolf & Bernstein, 2004). Counterfeit drugs are fake drugs, which can be purchased at the black markets in the developing countries or through the internet in developed countries. They are illegal and dangerous for the health. A counterfeit drug is such contaminated drug or that containing the wrong, false dose, or no active ingredient.

Off-Label Drugs and Use

Prescribing a medication for a medical condition that is not described in the concerning drug label (package leaflet), which is approved by national regulatory bodies, is called "Off-Label" prescribing or off-label use of drugs. The theme of off-label use does neither imply improper nor illegal use of drugs. It may provide the only available treatment for "orphan" medical conditions, or for certain populations (children, pregnant women, very old patients; Blondon, Desmeules, & Besson, n.d.). The most common form of off-label-use involves prescribing available and marketed medicine, though, for indication (e.g., a disease or a symptom) that is not approved by the national regulatory bodies and not listed in healthcare authorities-required drug-labeling information. The theme "off-label use of drugs" can also be applied to the use of a marketed medication in a patient population (e.g., pediatric), dosage, or dosage form that does not have healthcare authority's approval (Wittich, Burkle, & Lanier, 2012). According to the definition Fukada,

Kohler, Boon, Austin, and Krahn (n.d.), the off-label-use does not consider the national aspect, while all German definitions include the national aspect of the concerning marketed pharmaceutical product. All health products which have no national market approval in Germany are classified as unlicensed-use.

Unlicensed drug use is common in all fields of medicine and may be encountered in therapeutic guidelines.

Disease Screening

Diseases Screening is a form of diseases prevention. It enables to detect diseases at an early stage in asymptomatic individuals at risk of certain medical conditions. Medical treatment could be provided to cure the affection.

Screening test differs from diagnostic test in many manners. Table 1 presents the differences between a screening test and a diagnostic test.

GOAL OF THIS BOOK

The key objectives of the present book are:

- To discuss how to improve the healthcare by using modern Information and Communication Technologies (ICT), methodologies, frameworks;
- To analyze the non-technical challenges and make recommendations;
- To initiate, among the scientific community, a discussion on proposed systems and on the global challenges;

Table 1. Screening test vs. diagnostic test

Pos.	Screening Test	Diagnostic Test
1	Done on asymptomatic individuals	Done on sick or ill individuals
2	Applied to groups, crowd	Applied to single patient
3	Results are arbitrary and final	Results are not final
4	Based on one criterion and cut-off	Based on evaluation of many symptoms and laboratory findings
5	Less accurate	More accurate
6	Less expensive	More expensive
7	Not a basis for treatment, but for prevention	It is used as basis for treatment
8	Initiated by a medical program	Initiated by the patient

- To encourage the reverse innovation, so that developed countries also learn from developing countries.

TARGET AUDIENCE

This book is written as a set of research work experiments and in-situ-tests results. It is presenting multidisciplinary themes in medical IT as well health in field of health informatics and thus, written for researchers on medical IT, health informatics, rural healthcare IT.

This book is mostly intended for the scientific interested in improving health care delivery services, increase access to health care services in both developing and developed countries. This book should also reach out healthcare professionals seeking for simples ITC system to improve their daily duty processes. ICT-professionals working at healthcare units may be concerned.

ETHICAL APPROVAL

For evaluation purposes, cohorts of participants were built in order to simulate, test, and evaluate the different systems proposed in this book. In collaboration with involved clinics and hospitals, we recruit patients using snowball approach. Each involved individual gives his consent so that their data can be collected, processed, and stored. The data were anonymously collected, processed, and stored. We also apply for ethical approval at the involved hospitals and clinics as well as at local municipal authorities.

OVERVIEW

- **Chapter 1, "Challenges Facing Healthcare Delivery Systems in Low-, Middle-, and High-Income Countries":** Challenges facing the global healthcare system worldwide have been discussed in this chapter. These challenges are categorized in (1) policies and (2) technological related challenges. Policies related challenges are organizational, infrastructural, and structural issues, which could only be improved by policy changes, re-structuration, politics will. The chapter presents certain solution approaches that show how ICT can solve the technical issues.

- **Chapter 2, "Scale the Agility in a Multidisciplinary Remote Care Services Delivery System":** Chapter 2 proposes a multidisciplinary remote care system to improve the global healthcare in tackling the challenges facing. This chapter analyzes issues that a multidisciplinary team in providing medical treatment to the multiple or single patient can face. The proposed approach, therefore, maps the care delivery process on an IT project development process using scale scrum development methodology to define a framework for efficient health care services delivery process.
- **Chapter 3, "Towards Secure Off-Label Drug Prescribing and Improved Drug Supply":** The developing countries are being faced severe drug-stock-out and high drug prices. Counterfeits drugs and additionally the use of off-label drugs are the direct consequences. Developed countries are facing another aspect of the off-label use drugs: the legal uncertainty among HCPs. Health insurance companies, Patient, and HCPs regularly face lawsuits due to conflicts relating to the refund of the medical costs in case of off-label-Use drugs or prescribing. This chapter proposes an ICT-based solution and makes recommendations to tackle the discussed challenges.
- **Chapter 4, "Challenges Facing Adverse Drug Reactions Reporting and Counterfeit Drugs Monitoring":** Adverse drug reactions are a significant factor of death in the global healthcare systems. FDA, for example, is assigned to the tasks to monitor adverse drug reaction in the USA. The chapter presents a picture of the pharmacovigilance in developed and developing countries, discusses the challenges and present a case study with solution approach to better protect the population against adverse drug reactions.
- **Chapter 5, "Novel Approach to Anticipate Emerging Infectious Diseases Spreading and Epidemics":** The recent Ebola epidemic in Africa with the enormous risk to be spread worldwide has shown the weakness of the existing infections surveillance and control policies and mechanisms. Studies have shown the limitation of the infections surveillance policies and systems that need to be improved. The chapter designs a solution approach to better monitor and control any infectious diseases outbreak. The presented system is tested in Africa and can be adapted to developed countries.

- **Chapter 6, "Early Detection Prediction and Prevention of Noncommunicable Diseases in People at High Risks of Communicable Diseases":** Traditional screening to predict and prevent diseases foresees that the patient should go to the physician and get screened. This mechanism in the in the age of IoT, globalization, and growing changes in the labor market has shown its limitations. Connecting the patient to the screening unit and physician presents more advantages and facilitate the data and information collection for an effective prediction of diseases outbreak and thus early prevention of the affection. The chapter discusses how to early detect and prevent diseases.

REFERENCES

Andam, Z. R. (2013). e-Commerce and e-Business. *E-ASEAN Task Force*, 1–47. Retrieved from http://www.kau.edu.sa/Files/830/Files/61164_Ecommerce and E Business.pdf

Ashton, K. (2009). That "Internet of Things" Thing. *RFiD Journal, 4986*. doi:10.1145/2967977

Blondon, K., Desmeules, J., Besson, M. et al. (n.d.). La prescription «off-label». *Revue Médicale Suisse, 4,* 1661.

Carpenter, A., & Frontera, A. (2016). Smart-watches: A potential challenger to the implantable loop recorder? *Europace, 18*(6), 791–793. doi:10.1093/europace/euv427 PMID:26847074

Chatzimilioudis, G., Konstantinidis, A., Laoudias, C., & Zeinalipour-yazti, D. (2012). *Crowdsourcing with Smartphones*. Academic Press.

Darkin, A. W., & Cary, M. A. (2000). *No Telemedicne and Teleheath Principles, Policies, Performances, and pitfalls*. Academic Press.

Dutta, J., Gazi, F., Roy, S., & Chowdhury, C. (2016). AirSense: Opportunistic crowd-sensing based air quality monitoring system for smart city. In 2016 IEEE SENSORS (pp. 1–3). IEEE. doi:10.1109/ICSENS.2016.7808730

Edoh, T. O. C., Kora, A. D., Pawar, P., Coulibaly, G. C., & Alahassa, B. R. U. (2016). Predicting telemedicine system user satisfaction in sub-Saharan Africa. *ICT Express*, *2*(4), 163–167. doi:10.1016/j.icte.2016.10.006

Fukada, Kohler, Boon, Austin, & Krahn. (n.d.). Prescribing gabapentin off label: Perspectives from psychiatry, pain and neurology specialists. *Can Pharm, 145*(6), 280–284.

Haus, M., Waqas, M., Ding, A. Y., Li, Y., & Member, S. (2016, December). Security and Privacy in Device-to-Device (D2D). *Communication Review*, 1–27. doi:10.1109/COMST.2017.2649687

Hope, K. R. (1999). *Corruption and Development in Africa* (K. R. Hope & B. C. Chikulo, Eds.). Basingstoke, UK: Palgrave Macmillan; doi:10.1057/9780333982440

Istepanian, R. S. H., Hu, S., Philip, N. Y., & Sungoor, A. (2011). The potential of Internet of m-health Things for non-invasive glucose level sensing. In *2011 Annual International Conference of the IEEE Engineering in Medicine and Biology Society* (pp. 5264–5266). IEEE. 10.1109/IEMBS.2011.6091302

Liu, J., Shen, H., & Zhang, X. (2016). A survey of mobile crowdsensing techniques: A critical component for the internet of things. *2016 25th International Conference on Computer Communications and Networks, ICCCN 2016*. 10.1109/ICCCN.2016.7568484

Marika, P., & Di, D. (2012). Article. *Sensors, Signal Processing & Applications, 5*(3).

Murtagh, J. (2011). *General practice*. McGraw-Hill Australia Pty Ltd. Retrieved from https://s3.amazonaws.com/academia.edu.documents/42614797/John_Murtaghs_General_Practice_5th_edition.pdf?AWSAccessKeyId=AKIAIWOWYYGZ2Y53UL3A&Expires=1506241968&Signature=7R0TegJCQKfadIuuYCosgMN%2BrAQ%3D&response-content-disposition=inline%3Bfilename%3DJoh

Rudolf, P. M., & Bernstein, I. B. G. (2004). Counterfeit Drugs. *The New England Journal of Medicine*, *350*(14), 1384–1386. doi:10.1056/NEJMp038231 PMID:15070787

Scott, R. E., & Mars, M. (2015). *Telehealth in the developing world: Current status and future prospects*. Academic Press.

Sheng, Z., Yang, S., Yu, Y., Vasilakos, A. V., McCann, J. A., & Leung, K. K. (2013, December). A Survey on the Ietf Protocol Suite for the Internet of Things: Standards, Challenges, and Opportunities. *IEEE Wireless Communications*, 91–98. 10.1109/MWC.2013.6704479

Terry, N. (2016). Will the Internet of Health Things Disrupt Healthcare? *SSRN Electronic Journal, 28–31*. doi:10.2139srn.2760447

Van Hoe, B., Lee, G., Bosman, E., Missinne, J., Kalathimekkad, S., Maskery, O., ... Van Steenberge, G. (2012). Ultra small integrated optical fiber sensing system. *Sensors (Switzerland)*, *12*(9), 12052–12069. doi:10.3390120912052

Williams, P. A. H., & McCauley, V. (2016). Always connected: The security challenges of the healthcare Internet of Things. In *2016 IEEE 3rd World Forum on Internet of Things (WF-IoT)* (pp. 30–35). IEEE. 10.1109/WF-IoT.2016.7845455

Wittich, C. M., Burkle, C. M., & Lanier, W. L. (2012). Ten common questions (and their answers) about off-label drug use. *Mayo Clinic Proceedings*, *87*(10), 982–990. doi:10.1016/j.mayocp.2012.04.017 PMID:22877654

Introduction

As this is the first edition of the book on *Advanced Systems for Improved Public Healthcare and Disease Prevention: Emerging Research and Opportunities*, interested readers will probably look for the contribution to Information and Communication Technology management literature. The principal objective of this edition is to present some emerging research and opportunities regarding the challenges facing the global healthcare system.

I'm working on an up-coming edition, where the implementation, deployment and test of the all in this present book discussed systems will be presented. Following aspects will be discussed:

- The global and detailed Architecture of each system;
- The technology supporting the implementation;
- The software development methodology like agile development or classical development methodology;
- The novelty of the system; and
- Overall, the contribution to IT management as well as health Informatics literature.

Thierry Oscar Edoh
Technical University of Munich, Germany
December 2017

Section 1

The Challenges Facing the Global Healthcare

Chapter 1
Challenges Facing Healthcare Delivery Systems in Low-, Middle-, and High-Income Countries

ABSTRACT

In the USA, there exist inequities in health delivery depending on whether you have healthcare insurance or not. People living in rural areas also are facing limited access to healthcare. The other high-income countries present, however, another picture. Healthcare insurance is mandatory and thus enables access to healthcare services. Nevertheless, these countries also face challenges such as the poor access to the healthcare services delivery in rural areas because of lack of general physicians. The cost burden is an important point that impacts the access to healthcare and care delivery to a certain group of individuals such as elderly people. The healthcare systems also are facing off-label-use challenges (see Chapter 5) that can also negatively impact the care delivery. In the low- and middle-income countries, the developing world, the poor access to healthcare services delivery is due to infrastructural, structural issues, and poor funding. Information exchanges and communication remain a challenge facing all public healthcare systems around the world, though at diverse level. This chapter aims at investigating the challenges facing the healthcare delivery systems around the world and proposing information and communication-technology-based solutions to tackle some challenges. The chapter further focuses on two case studies and generalizes the results and solution approaches to the other countries. For

DOI: 10.4018/978-1-5225-5528-5.ch001

these purposes, the Republic of Benin, representing the developing world, and the Federal Republic of Germany, representing the developed world, are selected as study cases.

INTRODUCTION

High-income countries own high organized and structured healthcare systems. Most of these countries use the health insurances to partially fund their healthcare systems. Though, there exist inequities in the healthcare delivery in the high-income countries, e.g. in the USA the access to adequate healthcare delivery depends on whether the individual has a health insurance or not. The rural regions have only a limited access to the healthcare (Brandeau, Sainfort, & Pierskalla, 2005)(Barkan, 2010). The western countries, except the USA, have national health insurance systems. The populations are mandatory insured and thus can easily access the healthcare delivery systems. Beyond this, the western public healthcare systems lack continuity and coordination of health care delivery, direct communication between the entities and doctors (A.C Greiner & Knebel, 2003). Although the challenges described in (A.C Greiner & Knebel, 2003) date back to 2003, the healthcare systems in the western countries are still facing these challenges [the result of the study we carried out in 2016/2017].

Despite, the joint funding systems of the governments and health insurances, the whole western public healthcare delivery system is facing challenges such as cost explosion, due essentially to the rapid aging of the western populations. The care delivery to elderly people is cost intensive since they are often affected by old related chronic disorders (Cognitive impairments). The medical treatment of disorders such as cognitive impairments, obesity, diabetes, heart diseases is cost intensive. A study in (Morgan et al., 2014) has shown the association between overweight (obesity) and the cost. An earlier study (Sturm, 2002) also demonstrated the correlation between the medical cost and the non-communicable diseases.

Beyond the financial challenges, the western countries public healthcare systems also face access to healthcare delivery like long waiting periods before visiting a doctor or long sitting in waiting room. For example, in Germany, most of the health insurances companies help their members to quickly get appointed by a medical doctor. The health insurance companies, therefore, provide their insured members with a portal for this purpose. An example of appointment portal can be seen here (https://www.dak.de/dak/leistungen/

arzttermine-online-1445166.html). The appointment issues represent a big challenge facing the public healthcare systems in the western countries. In an earlier 2005, the study had found out that the waits time to see a doctor is high in Europe (50% in the UK, more than 70% in Germany). The amounts were similar for visiting a specialist. Today, 12 years later the situation is likely to be different. The population is growing, more migrants are entering these countries, and the elderly population is fast growing. It is then becoming very hard to quickly get an appointment for medical purpose, particularly, the waits for specialists is longer as earlier.

During the case study in Germany, we met old people who were refused by medical doctors because they do not have the necessary capacity to take care of the new patient. Old people are looking for medical doctor practice close to their residence place.

The case study in Germany reveals that the German rural regions are facing a severe medical workforce shortage. By 2020 about 50.000 general physicians (GP) would be retired. This fact will negatively impact the care delivery in the rural regions, then the young doctors do not like to practice in rural regions because of the low income and lack of carrier possibility. Unfortunately, most old people are living in rural areas, and thus facing poor access to the healthcare services. This situation is common to all western countries and is more severe in USA (A.C Greiner & Knebel, 2003).

In the developing countries, in the recent years, the burden of diseases is rapidly increasing. Most people living in developing countries are facing the poor access to healthcare services delivery. Unlikely high-income countries, the poor access to care services is because of poor medical infrastructure. The rural and urban slums lack care units. The rare care units in rural regions lack expert medical specialists or most health professionals working there are undertrained (Thierry Oscar Edoh, 2010a). Additionally, the socioeconomic and cultural factors are decisive in how regularly a patient can visit a doctor (attend a health center in person). The patients are often hospitalized instead of being ambulatory or remotely treated, because of their remote residence, and thus occupy unnecessarily hospital beds and cause unnecessary costs.

According to the World Bank, most people in developing countries are living on less than one dollar a day. Therefore, beyond the poor state of most healthcare facilities, the economic situation, and poverty in the developing countries are part of the leading causes of poor healthcare services accessibility. Patient living on less than one dollar a day would prefer to buy foodstuff instead of visiting a doctor, even in the case of chronic diseases [survey results].

Most investigations carried out by the WHO have reportedly indicated poverty, lack of political will, poor national economy and not least the poor organization as the main deficiencies that underlie the enormous problems, particularly in the public health systems in Sub-Saharan Africa (SSA) countries. A study (Adeya & Cavanaugh, 2007) carried out by USAID in Benin stated that the main problem of the poor healthcare accessibility is due to severe lack of medical care facilities, particularly in urban slums and rural regions and additionally the lack of specialists due to brain drain. Similar conclusions have been made in studies conducted in other developing countries. A review conducted in (Harrison, Cohen, & Walton, 2015) indicates that unsafe and poor quality care such as infection, medication error or misuse and lack of patient safety skills is a problem in developing countries in Southeast Asia. Another study on maternal health care (Srivastava, Bilal, Preety, & Sanghita, 2015) had concluded that in the developing countries safe deliveries remain a major challenge and barriers to utilization of institutional deliveries pose also a major challenge for healthcare programs.

A particularity of the health system in the Sub-Saharan-African countries is the wide absence of Information and Communication Technology (ICT) systems. The weak ICT system landscape in the public healthcare systems and its poor usage are discussed in (T.O. Edoh & Teege, 2010)(Thierry Oscar Edoh, 2010a). In nearly all cases, patient data processing is carried out manually using paper documents. Other ICT systems applications, such as data mining or communication platforms are also mostly absenting in the African health sector. Medical statistics are scarcely conducted. A group of researchers has examined the Kenyan health system and noticed a "Digital Divide" in African countries. Even for South Africa, an earlier Study (Mars, Seebregts, & Rockefeller Foundation, 2008) pointed out major obstacles for a successful introduction of ICT in the health sector. In (Scott & Mars, 2015), the authors discussed Healthcare services issues and analyze the needs of the developing world accordingly. Some of these issues are poverty, communicable diseases, maternal and child health, violence and conflict and workforce shortages.

Launching Information and Communication Technology systems into the public healthcare in the developing countries presents certain challenges with regards to the technology level and the existing infrastructure. The Health Information System Program (HISP) project(Scott & Mars, 2015) thus worked for more than 10 years to develop and launch the District Health Information Software (DHIS) system described in (J. J. Braa & Hedberg, 2002) and summarized in (Keeton, 2012).

In Ireland, there exists a Homecare system project named CASALA[1], which is designed and implemented for elderly people. This has shown how Homecare and Telemonitoring can increase access to the healthcare delivery system for old and disabled people. Telehealthcare system is launched in Ireland since they want to improve access to healthcare for isolated people. Certain reports (Sluizer, S., Cashman, 1984) (Khani, 2015) estimate that outpatients have to wait up to 2 hours before being examined by a medical doctor. The 2011 International IT and Connected Healthcare Solution Summit, taken place on 11th & 12th May 2011 in Dublin, has shown how Telehealthcare help to increase the healthcare services in Ireland.

Since Telehealthcare/Telemedicine is showing to improve healthcare services in developed countries like Ireland (e.g. eHealth ERA project), USA (Alaska, e. g. AFHCAN Project), Greenland (e.g. TEMS system[2]) particularly in isolated regions (Niclasen & Mulvad, 2010), (Haveman & Flim, 2007). Adapted Telemedicine/Telehealthcare Technologies and solutions could also be implemented to improve the poor access to healthcare services in Benin.

This study aims at investigating the different challenges facing the different public healthcare systems around the world as well as improving the healthcare services, increasing the access to healthcare services.

In (Thierry Oscar Edoh, 2010a) the causes underlying the poor access to healthcare services in the developing countries are investigated and analyzed. It is figured out that launching Telehealthcare into the public healthcare systems in the developing countries could be a solution to tackle the challenges mentioned above, so that expert medical specialists could remotely assist undertrained caregivers working in urban slums and/or rural healthcare centers in providing preventive, curative, promotional or rehabilitative healthcare services. A survey on mobile health (mHealth) adoption in developing countries has reported that the use of certain mHealth technologies shows improvements in healthcare processes and public health indicators (Chib, Velthoven, Car, & Helena, 2015).

This study is a case-study with a focus on two countries; the public healthcare system in Benin, a West African country and the public healthcare system in Germany, a western country. The study results such as solution approaches and recommendation that are implemented for Benin could be also adapted and implemented for all SSA countries as well as other developing countries with respect to cultural and traditional means as well as social, economic, and technology level. The public healthcare systems are similar in all SSA countries. The cultural and traditional means also do. The same for Germany.

STUDY METHODS AND DATA

The author conducted several studies as well as literature review with focus on challenges facing the public healthcare systems in low-, middle-, and high-income countries.

In early 2015 to the beginning of 2017, case studies have been conducted in Sub-Saharan African as well as in western countries. Additionally, an exhaustive and comprehensive literature reviews have been conducted to find out which challenges the public healthcare systems are facing, and which solutions approaches are already implemented as well as to evaluate the results of any implemented approach

Samples Selection

In the scope of the conducted studies, 17 western countries representing the western world, 2 countries representing the middle-income countries, 5 African developing countries were selected. Purposeful, we have selected literature that has discussed challenges facing these healthcare systems. Thus, 45 articles, 5 books, 3 compendiums, and a huge of web pages have been selected and reviewed. The selected documents are published between 2001 and 2017 in bases owning good impact factor such PubMed, Scopus, etc. The selected journals belong to IEEE Xplore, Elsevier, Health Affairs, NCBI Bookshelf, and some online journals. This period is chosen in order to best analyze the evolution of the challenge facing the public healthcare systems and evaluate the impacts of diverse implemented solutions approach.

The countries have been selected regarding the cultural, linguistic similarity as well as social and economic diversity (Income level, technology level). Table 1 presents the different selected countries.

The non-probability form of snowball sampling was used to select the literature with relevant and significant contents in the domain: challenges facing the public healthcare systems, usage of ICT in the healthcare systems. A core literature is first identified. The relevant references cited by the core articles/books are selected, where in turn the relevant references here also are selected and so on. Thus, a significant set of articles are selected, reviewed and categorized.

A Snowball is a low-cost research method and useful in specific cases (Acharya, Prakash, Saxena, & Nigam, 2013) like the current study where articles on challenges facing western healthcare systems relating to the poor

Table 1. Selected countries in scope of the study

Pos.	Countries	Income Category	Type of Study
1	Australia	High-Income	Literature research
2	Canada	High-Income	Literature research
3	Denmark	High-Income	Literature research
4	England	High-Income	Literature research
5	France	High-Income	Literature research
6	**Germany**	High-Income	Literature research **Case study**
7	Italy	High-Income	Literature research
8	The Netherlands	High-Income	Literature research
9	New Zealand	High-Income	Literature research
10	Norway	High-Income	Literature research
11	Japan	High-Income	Literature research
12	Israel	High-Income	Literature research
13	Singapore	High-Income	Literature research
14	Sweden	High-Income	Literature research
15	Switzerland	High-Income	Literature research
16	United States	High-Income	Literature research
17	China	Middle-Income	Literature research
18	India	Middle-Income	Literature research
19	**Benin**	Low-Income	Literature research **Case study**
20	Togo	Low-Income	Literature research
21	Ghana	Low-Income	Literature research
22	Ivory Coast	Low-Income	Literature research
23	Cameroon	Low-Income	Literature research

access to the care services in certain regions are scarcely published. The snowball sampling is a method to select a research population or material through contact (social, virtual, or reference/recommendation). According to MacNealy, cited in (Latham, 2007), snowball sampling is defined as follow:

Snowball sampling is used in those rare cases when the population of interest cannot be identified other than by someone who knows that a certain person has the necessary experience or characteristics to be included (MacNealy)

Different research populations have been also built to conduct interviews. The Respondent-Driven-Sampling (RDS) method was used to implement the cohort. We opted for this method because it best fits the research requirements which are to recruits key persons who in turn will randomly recruit the cohort members and report their personal network size. These requirements are well supported by the five (05) assumptions of RDS.

Table 2 and Table 3 present the structure of the research population. In African developing countries, 782 care consumers and 91 care professionals (care providers) have been interviewed. In Germany, 80 care consumers and 18 care professionals have been interviewed. The interviews have focused on: (i) waits for specialists, (ii) workforce shortage, (ii) accessibility to care services, (iv) Electronic Medical Records and ICT Use, (v) care expenditures and funding -health insurance -, care delivery to elderly suffering from chronic disorders, and at least the care delivery at rural regions.

Table 2. Selected countries and the research population (health consumer) structure

Country	#Elderly People (>= 60 Years Old)		#Adults (Between 20 and 59 Years Old)		#Young People (0 to 19 Years Old)		Total
	Female	Male	Female	Male	Female	Male	
Benin	47	51	55	48	37	39	337
Togo	26	30	15	18	12	13	114
Ghana	27	25	17	19	14	15	117
Ivory Coast	20	20	25	23	20	22	130
Cameroon	16	21	13	13	10	11	084
Germany	7	8	21	24	11	09	080

Table 3. Selected countries and the research population (health provider) structure

Country	#General Physician		#Specialists (e.g. Cardiologist, Diabetologist, etc.)		Total
	Female	Male	Female	Male	
Benin	15	12	8	5	40
Togo	5	8	3	2	18
Ghana	3	4	2	2	11
Ivory Coast	2	2	2	2	8
Cameroon	3	3	4	5	14
Germany	5	6	4	3	18

Study Data

We conducted quantitative and qualitative studies in different African countries. Thus, various prospective randomized studies in several African public healthcare systems have been performed. Health professionals, health bodies and patients from five (05) sub-Saharan African (SSA) countries (Thierry Oscar Edoh, 2010b), (Thierry Oscar Edoh & Teege, 2011) have been interviewed. Data have been collected from the research population consisting of elderly, adult, and young people (with respect to gender).

Surveys are also conducted using questionnaires (online and paper format) and 1:1 interview. The surveys are focused on:

1. Healthcare Accessibility
2. Quality of healthcare services and health costs
3. Use of traditional healthcare services

The collected data were evaluated in the light of socio-cultural influences, traditional manners, financial and familiar situation, as well as the education level the interviewees own.

A case study is also conducted in Germany with the objectives to compare the literature findings with the realities in the countries. A research population has been built and interviewed. A case study is defined as the *intensive study of a single unit with an aim to generalize across a larger set of units* (Gerring, 2004). The strategy behind the conducted case studies is to get significant results that can be applied to the other countries in same income category.

The country Benin, an African low-income country, is selected as a study subject to examine the challenges facing public healthcare systems in low- and middle-income countries. In Benin the information and communication systems, the structure, and the infrastructure consisting the healthcare system have been evaluated. Public, as well as private hospitals, clinics, district hospitals, rural health units, pharmacies, were involved in this study.

In Germany, the investigation has been focused on interviewing the healthcare consumers and providers to figure out the challenges in point of view of each actor in the system. Since the German public healthcare, like the healthcare systems in most western countries, is best structured and features better medical infrastructures such as several hospitals, clinics, doctor practices, several university-hospitals. This study, therefore, bas been focused on the health care services delivery, information and communication systems, and financial means only.

Additionally, literature reviews have been conducted on public healthcare systems, health care services delivery, and access to healthcare in Developing countries (Srivastava et al., 2015), in South Africa (Williamson, Heywood, Williamson, Stoops, & Heywood, 2015), (Mayosi et al., 2014), (Thierry Oscar Edoh, 2010b), (Adeya & Cavanaugh, 2007), (Joseph K. Rotich, Phd, Terry J. Hannan, Mbbs, Faye E. Smith, Ms, Wilson W. Odero, Md, Nguyen Vu, Md, Burke W. Mamlin, Md, Joseph J. Mamlin, & Robert M. Einterz, Md, William M. Tierney, 2003)(Joseph K. et al., 2003), (J. Braa & Hedberg, 2000), in Tanzania, Nigeria, Kenya, Morocco, and Algeria (WHO Africa 2011) (Development, Development, Hospital, & Hospital, 2015), (WHO, 2015 -http://www.who.int/features/2014/morocco-maternal-health/en/-) as well as western countries (see references).

The words "challenges", "facing", "healthcare", "low-income", "middle-income", and "high-income" have been used to find and select the documents for literature review. The selected documents have then been classified by publishing year and income-country category. Table 4 presents a part of the materials used for the literature research.

Table 4. A sample of select articles and books

Pos.	Description	Title	Publishing Year/Category
1	This chapter describes current and future challenges in the delivery of healthcare in poor an rich countries (Brandeau et al., 2005).	Healthcare Delivery: Current Problems And Future Challenges	2005/Book chapter
2	This blog describes the major issues the USA health system is facing (Binder, 2013).	The Five Biggest Problems in Health Care Today	2013/Web article
3	This book chapter presents the core competencies healthcare professionals should have to be able to address challenges facing the care systems. It, further, describes the challenges the western car systems (A.C Greiner & Knebel, 2003).	The Core Competencies Needed for Healthcare Professionals	2003/Book chapter
4	This chapter describes these challenges and examines the resulting implications for the education of health professionals and its reform (Ann C. Greiner & Knebel, 2003).	Chapter 2 Challenges Facing the Health System and Implications for Educational Reform	2003/Book chapter
5	To estimate the direct healthcare cost of being overweight or obese throughout pregnancy to the National Health Service in Wales (Morgan et al., 2014).	Obesity in pregnancy: a retrospective prevalence-based study on health service utilization and costs on the NHS	2014/Journal article
6	This paper compares the effects of obesity, overweight, smoking, and problem drinking on health care use and health status based on national survey data (Sturm, 2002).	The Effects of Obesity, Smoking, And Drinking On Medical Problems And Costs	2002/journal article

continued on following page

Table 4. Continued

Pos.	Description	Title	Publishing Year/Category
7	This paper reports on a 2005 survey of sicker adults in Australia, Canada, Germany, New Zealand, the United Kingdom, and the United States. Sizable shares of patients in all six countries report safety risks, poor care coordination, and deficiencies in care for chronic medical conditions.	Taking the Pulse of Health Care Systems: Experiences of Patients with Health Problems In Six Countries	2005/journal article
8	This book discusses the social and health issues in USA (Barkan, 2010)	Social Problems: Continuity and Change	2010/Book
9	This book the medical workforce shortage in Germany (Kopetsche, 2010).	Dem deutschen Gesundheitswesen gehen die Ärzte aus! (*Workforce shortage in Germany?)*	2010/Study report
10	This publication presents overviews of the healthcare systems of Australia, Canada, China, Denmark, England, France, Germany, India, Israel, Italy, Japan, the Netherlands, New Zealand, Norway, Singapore, Sweden, Switzerland, and the United States.	2015 International Profiles of Health Care Systems	2016/Study report
11	Countries around the globe are investing in health information and communications technologies (ICT) as critical tools for improving care for chronically ill patients (Adler-Milstein, Sarma, Woskie, & Jha, 2014)	A Comparison of How Four Countries Use Health IT To Support Care for People With Chronic medical Conditions	2014/Journal article
12	This paper presents the findings of a new scorecard designed to assess and monitor multiple domains of U.S. health system performance (Schoen, Davis, How, & Schoenbaum, 2006).	U.S. Health System Performance: A National Scorecard	2006/Journal article
13	This paper profiles the EMR systems in developing and developed countries (SIKHONDZE & LOUWRENCE ERASMUS, 2016)	Electronic Medical Records: A Developing and Developed Country Analysis	2016/ Proceedings
14	This paper assesses the state of health information technology (HIT) adoption and use in seven industrialized nations (Jha et al., 2008)	The use of health information technology in seven nations	2008/Journal articles
15	This article examines the major challenge for low- and middle-income countries in achieving broad coverage of health interventions and optimizing health outcomes (English, Irimu, Agweyu, Gathara, & Oliwa, 2016)	Building Learning Health Systems to Accelerate Research and Improve Outcomes of Clinical Care in Low- and Middle-Income Countries	2016/Journal article
16	This article describes the role of ICT in improving the patient-provider partnership in consumer health informatics (Abaidoo & Larweh, 2014).	Consumer Health Informatics: The Application of ICT in Improving Patient-Provider Partnership for a Better Health Care	2014/journal article

continued on following page

Table 4. Continued

Pos.	Description	Title	Publishing Year/Category
17	This paper highlights the importance of being able to access health information and how traditional media methods have been utilized to allow this within a developing country setting, highlighting the clear digital divide. The paper then addresses the impact of convergent communication technologies and mobile technologies in providing a means of addressing existing health care problems within a developing country setting. (Chhanabhai & Holt, 2010)	The Disparity Information and Communication Technology for Developing Countries has in the Delivery of Healthcare Information	2010/Journal article
18	This 2009 survey of primary care doctors in Australia, Canada, France, Germany, Italy, the Netherlands, New Zealand, Norway, Sweden, the United Kingdom, and the United States finds wide differences in practice systems, incentives, perceptions of access to care, use of health information technology (IT), and programs to improve quality (Schoen et al., 2009).	A Survey of Primary Care Physicians in Eleven Countries, Perspectives on Care, Costs, And Experiences	2004/Journal article
19	This article presents the German healthcare delivery system (Busse & Riesberg, 2004).	Health Care Systems in Transition	2012/Journal article
20	This presents the structures and infrastructures of UK (Scotland) healthcare system (Steele & Cylus, 2012)	United Kingdom (Scotland): health system review	
21	This report from The Commonwealth Fund Commission on a High-Performance Health System examines fragmentation in our healthcare delivery system and offers policy recommendations to stimulate greater organization—established mechanisms for working across providers and care settings (Anthony Shih, Karen Davis & Anne Gauthier, Rachel Nuzum, 2008).	Organizing the U.S. Healthcare Delivery System for High Performance	2008/Report
22	This book deeply presents the US healthcare system and its challenges(Knickman & Kovner, 2015)	Health Care Delivery in the United States	2015/Book
23	This web article describes the structures of German healthcare system and the care delivery (I. für Q. und W. im G. (IQWiG), 2017).	Das Deutsche Gesundheitssystem (*The German Healthcare System*)	2017/Web-article
24	This article describes, compares, and evaluates the healthcare systems of three western countries (Ridic, Gleason, & Ridic, 2012).	Comparisons of Health Care Systems in the United States, Germany, and Canada	2012/Journal article
25	This article presents the different challenges facing the European healthcare systems	https://www.united-europe.eu/news-and-opinions/what-others-write/europes-healthcare-systems-face-reform-to-meet-growing-challenges/	2015/Web-article

Study Limitations

The study has taken place in Africa and presented several limitations. There are very few healthcare systems related information available. The few collected data are mostly from an academic study carried out by non-African universities or international organization such as USAID. Electronic Medical Records system are most scarce or non-existent. The few patient data found are stored in papers and are uncompleted. We, therefore, conducted interviews to collect the missing information.

Regarding the western countries, we found few kinds of literature on the poor access to the healthcare services in the western rural regions. We, therefore, seek for this information on the internet and found several forums as well as magazine articles on the topics. Interviews with the healthcare professionals have been conducted in order to evaluate the information collected from the non-scientific sources.

STUDY RESULTS

The major challenges facing the public health systems in developing countries are limited economic resources, demographic structure (quickly growing population), big burden of diseases, rapid epidemiological changes, increased public demand for specialized treatment, brain drain of health professionals, lack of health insurance, poor access to healthcare, particularly severe in rural areas and in the urban slums.

Middle-income countries are facing high healthcare demand from aging population, medical cost coverage issues due to lack of funding system such as health insurance (Brandeau et al., 2005). The challenge facing here are like those facing in low-income countries.

The western counties present another picture. Their public healthcare systems have better performance; the medical costs are mostly covered by the health insurance or national health insurance.

The major challenges facing these healthcare systems are inequity in the health care services delivery and poor or limited access to healthcare in rural areas (for example, USA (Brandeau et al., 2005) recent investigations have confirmed these facts), medical workforces shortage in rural areas (for example in Germany (Kopetsche, 2010), in USA (Ann C. Greiner & Knebel,

2003)), too much unnecessary care (Binder, 2013), poor accommodation to patient needs (Ann C. Greiner & Knebel, 2003), high expenditures challenges.

Structure and Infrastructure of Public Health Care Systems

Low- and Middle-Income Countries

The public healthcare systems in the most developing countries are similar. In a previous study, we pointed out that the public healthcare systems in all sub-Saharan African (SSA) countries present similar structures, are facing the same infrastructural challenges (Thierry Oscar Edoh, 2010a). However, public healthcare systems in the Asian developing countries are more developed than the SSA ones. Though, the Asian developing countries face at diverse level similar infrastructural issues in their public health care systems.

African healthcare systems can be divided in three (03) healthcare services zones (Figure 1), where all countries within a health region have a similar public healthcare system, health care services deliveries issues, and economic situation.

Figure 1. Regions with similar public healthcare systems and healthcare deliveries

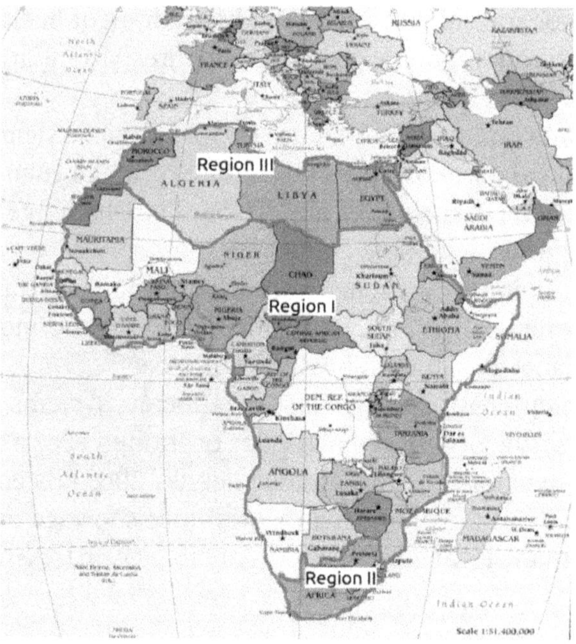

The public healthcare system and the quality of health care services deliveries in the countries located in the health region III are higher than those in the health region I. The access to health care and pharmaceutical care services in the region III health systems are near to those observed in developed countries. Beyond these aspects, the rural areas in the health region III are however facing similar issues like rural areas in the health region I and II (Thierry Oscar Edoh, 2010a).

The health region II presents a specific health care landscape. Different health care services delivery levels are fund within the same country (Thierry Oscar Edoh, 2010b).

The public healthcare systems in the SSA countries fall under the purview of the Ministry of Health (MOH) and aim at providing appropriate, qualitative healthcare services to the population even in the rural regions.

The public healthcare systems in the SSA countries are pyramid-shaped and dispose of three service levels:

1. **National Level:** Is assigned with the tasks to define the national health policies.
2. **Middle-Level:** Coordinates (at least theoretically) all activities defined at national level.
3. **The Municipality, City, and District Level:** Represent the decentralized unit. Medical facilities are subdivided into public hospitals and a network of public or private medical services. They are intended to assure good accessibility to the healthcare delivery facilities.

These healthcare systems are relied on two pillars, the public and the private healthcare sector. Both system parts are under the responsibility of the Ministry of Health (MoH).

Structure and Infrastructure of the Health Care System in the Republic of Benin

The public healthcare system in Benin, Benin as a study subject, will be described in order to give insight into the structures and infrastructural means in the SSA public healthcare systems.

The medical infrastructure in Benin presents a pyramid-shaped structure with five (05) levels (Maniatopoulos et al., 2009), which are, from the button to the top of the pyramid,

1. **County Hospital/ Health Center:** CSA (Centre de Santé d'Arrondissement),
2. **Communal Hospital/Health Center:** CSC (Centre de Santé Communal),
3. **District Hospital:** HZ (Hôpital de Zone),
4. **Department Hospital:** HD (Hôpital Departemental), and University Hospital: CNHU (Center National Hospitalier et Universitaire).

Figure 2 illustrates the different levels of the healthcare infrastructure in Benin. The facilities of the lowest level (CSA) just provide the primary healthcare delivery, such as a small surgery (injury) or consultation for malaria infection. The next level, CSC, offers a little more health services. Therefore, the amount of the beds in a CSC is about 13 beds and more personnel, and ambulance station - The third level, HZ, from below of the pyramid, can provide almost all conventional medical achievements and possesses a relatively good healthcare delivery system. The amount of the employees is higher than in a CSA and a CSC together and up to 200 beds are available in the category of hospital. The number of in-patient per year is clearly higher than in a CSA and a CSC combined. (30270 receptions per year comparing to 16996 receptions per year in the CNHU) (Adeya & Cavanaugh, 2007). These situations remain [our research results].

Figure 2. Structure of the healthcare system in Benin

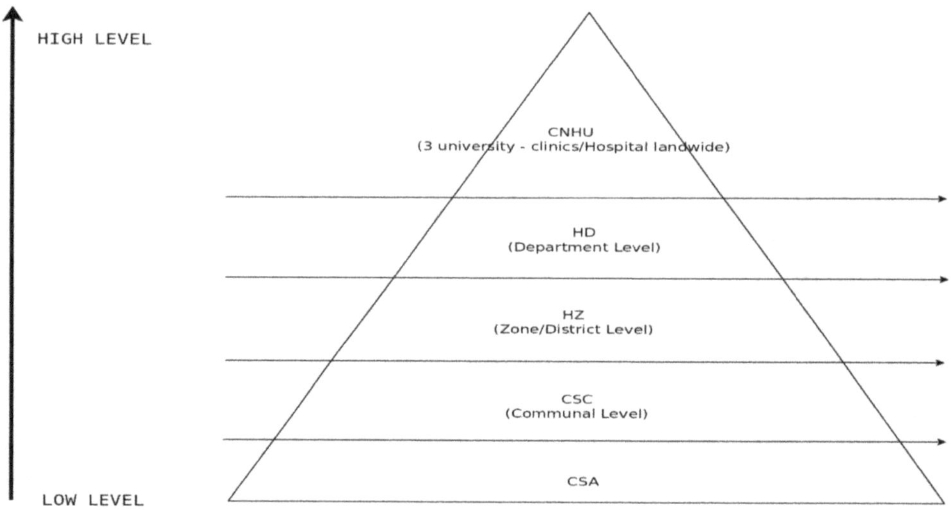

Table 5. Structure of the medical infrastructure in Benin

Facility Categories	Facilities per Department	Total of Facilities in Benin
CSA	46	425
CSC	08	075
HZ	03	027
CHD	01	005
CNHU *(Available only in Cotonou, Porto-Novo, and Parakou At national level: **[CNHU-HKM]**, **[CNHPP l'HOMEL]** **[CNHNP Jaquôt]**.)*	1	003
Facilities in medical private sector	> 400 *(In Cotonou only)*	2197 ***(legal & illegal)***

Each Hospital of type HD has a capacity of around 300 beds. University Hospital (CNHU) disposes of up to 600 beds. The difference between both healthcare facilities categories HD and CNHU is about the amount of personnel and the beds, and the size of the healthcare delivery services: for example, radiology or cardiology department is more important and more equipped in a CNHU than in an HD. CNHU has more care specialists and is a university clinic. In comparison with HD, research projects are carried out in CNHU. There are more beds in large cities and particularly in the south of the country. A Report of the ministry of health (MoH) in 2004 had issued the disparity between different health centers concerning a number of beds, care specialists and medical infrastructure. A survey conducted in 2014 in the scope of the present study, revealed that these disparity issues reported by the MoH in 2004 are not yet fixed. Table 5 summarizes the amount of existing medical facilities in the entire country as well as their density.

The institutional data exchange is illustrated in Figure 3. Figure 4 shows the patient booklet, where his data are stored. The communication and information exchange are mostly paper-based.

The public healthcare system in Benin, as all SSA countries care systems, is a publicly financed governmental responsibility.

In 2001, in Abuja (Nigeria) the NEPAD (New Partnership for Africa's Development) had recommended to the 53 African Countries to allocate at least 15% of total government expenditure to the health. They should steadily increase their budget allocation to meet the so-called Abuja 2001 target by 2015 (NEPAD, 2007). Unfortunately, Benin spends every year 7,5% of his

Figure 3. Data and Information's flow within SNIGS
Source USAID.

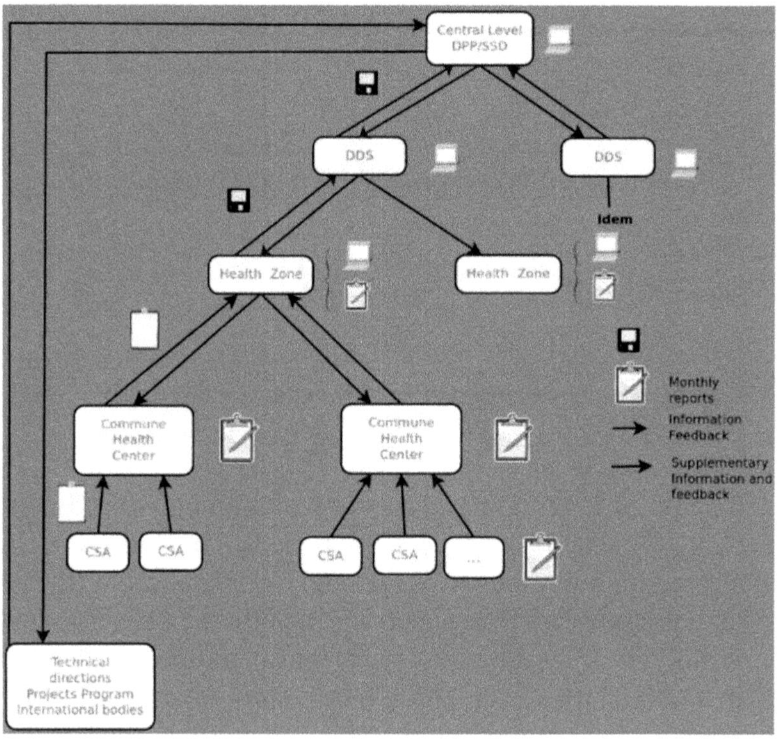

Figure 4. Booklet for Patient's data record

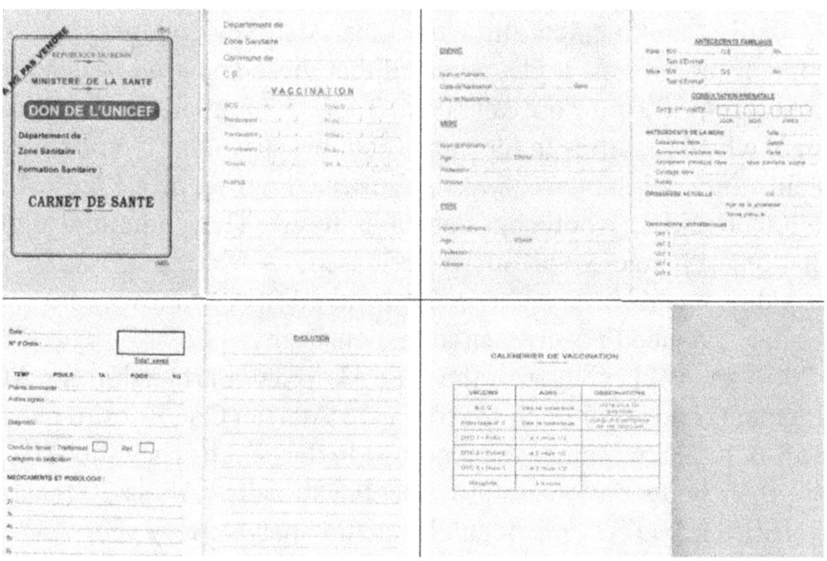

global national budget for its public health system[3]. In 2014 Benin spends accordingly 129 million dollars for the public health system. According to NEPAD Benin must allocate 258 million dollars to its public health system. A health insurance system is therefore needed to help to meet the in Abuja 2001 target of 15% of the national budget.

It's recommended to launch a health insurance where each inhabitant would pay 1000 Frs CFA (about $ 1,5) a month. The population of Benin is estimated to 10 million people. Such health insurance would bring each month about 15 million dollars. Launching the proposed health insurance could thus bring around 180 million dollars per year into health budget, i.e. 10,5% of the national budget. The system would then dispose around 310 million dollars per year, i.e. 18% of the national budget and can thus improve a lot of care services.

High-Income Countries

Unlike low- and middle-income countries, high-income countries have well-functioning healthcare systems and efficient funding systems[4]. However, the USA health funding system is commercial. There exists no national health insurance system like in Europe. The health insurance can be purchased at the private market (Ridic et al., 2012).

The European healthcare systems are similar and facing similar challenges. Since the European population is fast aging, the countries healthcare systems are facing high demand from the elderly people (Ridic et al., 2012).

Structure and Infrastructure of the Health Care System in the Republic of Germany

The structure and infrastructure of the German healthcare system will be outlined in this section since it is the study subject of the current study.

The German health system is decentralized, self-governed and supported by many factors such as health insurance companies, quality assurance institutions, the Ministry of Health, etc. The care system in Germany is based on three pillars: outpatient care, the hospital sector, and outpatient and inpatient rehabilitation facilities. The health insured citizens and employers pay some contributions that added to subsidies from tax revenues are used to funding the healthcare system. In comparison, the UK or Sweden healthcare are state health systems that are funding with taxes.

The federal Ministry of Health (MOH) defines the health policy, prepares laws, and sets up the administrative regulations which provide the framework for the activities of self-administration in the healthcare sector. The institutions and authorities dealing with health issues such as the federal Institute for Drugs and Medical Devices, the Federal Institute for Sera and Vaccines, the Federal Institute for Communicable and Non-Communicable Diseases (Robert Koch-Institute), the Federal Center for Health Education, and the German Institute for Medical Documentation and Information assist the federal MoH (I.-Q. und W. im G. (IQWiG), 2017)

A key feature of the healthcare delivery system in Germany is the clear institutional separation between (1) the public health services, (2) primary and secondary ambulatory care, and (3) hospital care, which has traditionally been confined to inpatient care. (Busse & Riesberg, 2004)

Germany is a federal state and thus composites of 16 states called ***Länder***. Each land defines on top of the federal healthcare policy its policy so that the healthcare services and their levels differ among the ***Länder*** (Busse & Riesberg, 2004)

The German healthcare system offers:

1. **Primary and Secondary Ambulatory Care:** Ambulatory healthcare is mainly provided by private for-profit providers, including physicians, dentists, pharmacists, physiotherapists, speech and language therapists, occupational therapists, pedologists, and technical professions. (Busse & Riesberg, 2004)
2. **Secondary and Tertiary Hospital Care:** German hospitals have traditionally concentrated on inpatient care; sectoral borders to ambulatory were strict. While acute hospitals in the hospital plan provide outpatient emergency care, only university hospitals have formal outpatient facilities. Day surgery and ambulatory pre- and post-hospital care have become other fields of increasing activity. Since 2004, hospitals have been granted additional competencies to provide care to outpatients that require highly specialized care on a regular basis. Also, participation in integrated care models offers new opportunities to become active in ambulatory care. (Busse & Riesberg, 2004)
3. **Social Care:** Social care is delivered by a broad variety of mainly private organizations that complement family and lay support for the elderly, children with special needs, mentally ill and the physically or mentally

handicapped. The Länder are responsible for planning (and guaranteeing the delivery) institutionalized care and schools for children with special needs. Most providers of institutional care belong to the six members of the Federal Alliance of Voluntary Welfare Organizations. (Busse & Riesberg, 2004)

4. **Pharmaceuticals:** Pharmaceutical policy seeks to balance targets of healthcare and industrial policy. Health care policy is primarily concerned with safeguarding quality and safety, improving health and containing costs for statutory health insurance (SHI). (Busse & Riesberg, 2004)
5. **Statutory Insurances:** The statutory long-term care insurance typically consists of the mandatory social long-term care insurance and the mandatory private long-term care insurance. (Busse & Riesberg, 2004)

Figure 9 summarizes the organization/structure of the German healthcare system and the key actors as well as the relation between them. This figure does not show the data exchange between the different care providers and care consumers. The study reveals a lack of automatic and electronic data exchange between the institutions. The extra-institution communication and

Figure 5. Type of data exchange and communication in German health system

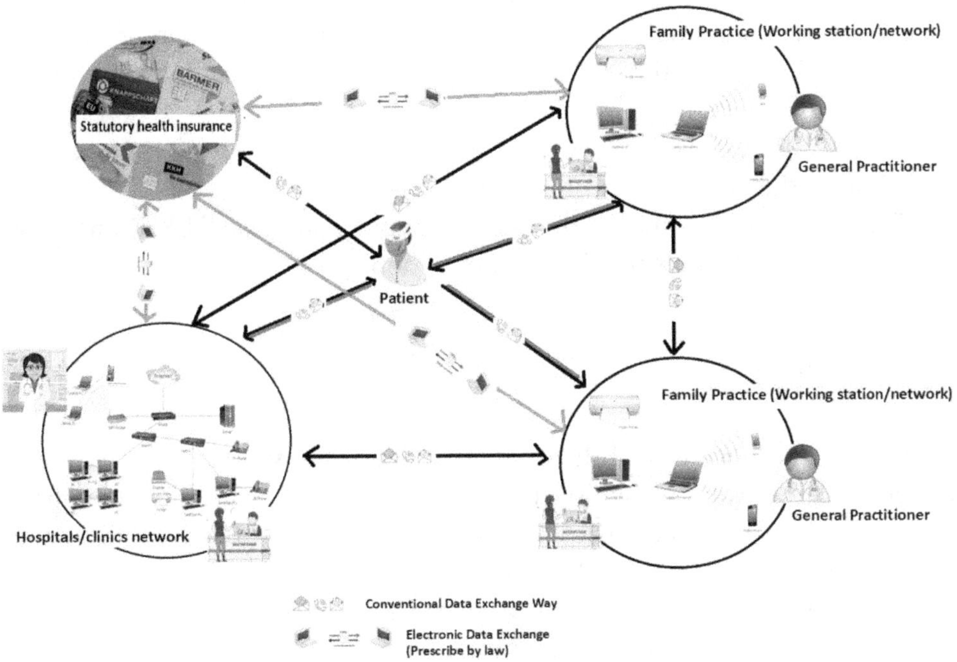

Figure 6. Example of paper-based medical records in German healthcare system

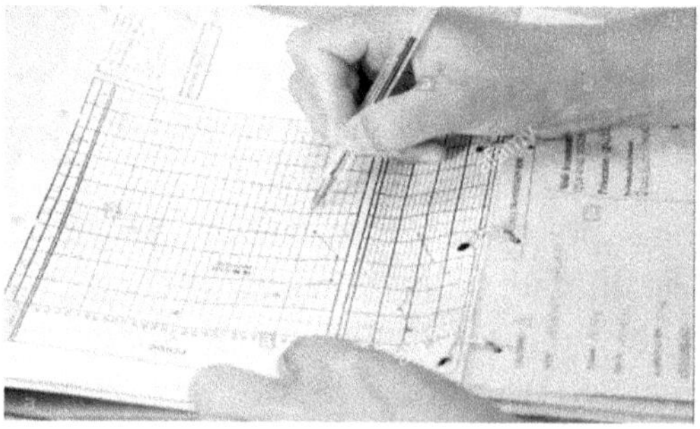

Example of Patient dossier still in use in some German hospitals and clinics.

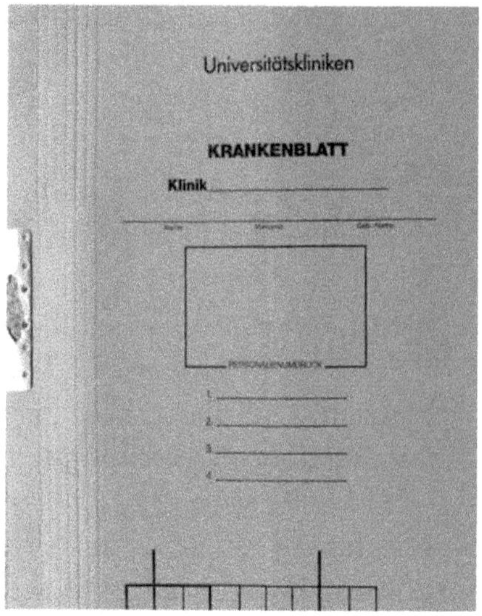

data exchange are mostly paper-based or through the patient self. The intra-institution communication is well organized and electronic based. In early 2012, Dr. S. Krolop gave a presentation on the topic where reveals the lack of electronic data exchange between the key actors in the German health system. A study (Biesdorf, Deetjen, & Möller, 2016) carried out in 2016 by Mckinsey & Company describes the present data exchange process and way in the German health and propose a digital health system where data is electronically exchanged.

Figure 5 illustrates the communication intra-and extra-institutional data exchange in the German health system.

Figure 6, Figure 7, and Figure 8 show some examples of EMR and paper base medical in the German healthcare system.

DISCUSSION

Comparing the German healthcare system (like most western countries) with the healthcare system in Benin (representing the low- and middle countries) points out that western countries' healthcare systems have better performance, efficient funding, which enables a better access to health services in western countries (excepted the United States of America, where each citizen must cover his medical costs) than in low- and middle-income countries. Additionally,

Figure 7. Example of Data collection and processing system (German nursing house)

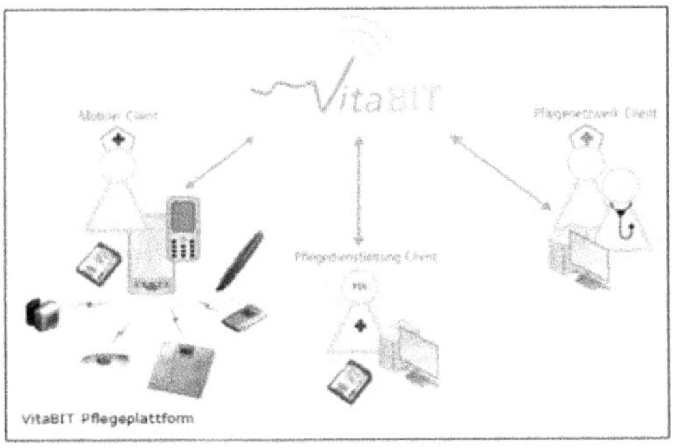

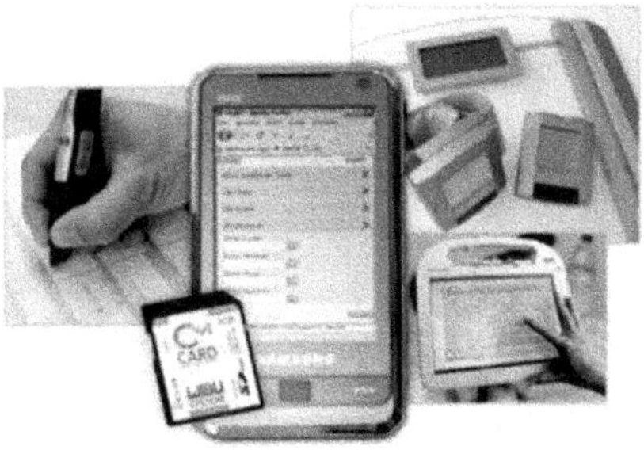

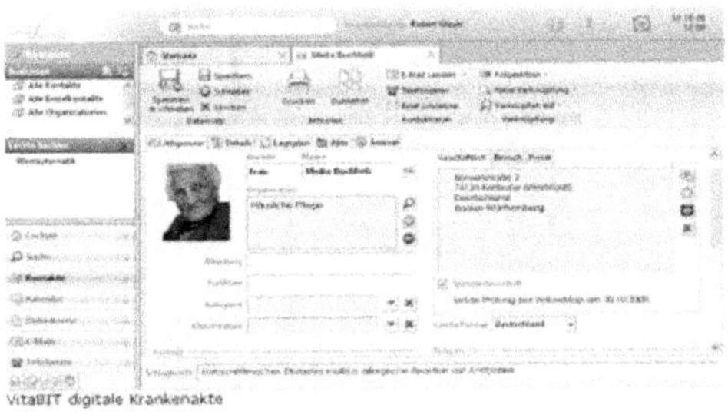

Example of electronic Medical Records in a connected system.

This system is provided by VitaBIT to manage patient data in the German Nursing Houses. Any physician with access right can access the system and read the patient dossier.

Surce http://www.vitabit.org/

Figure 8. Example of EMR in a German hospital

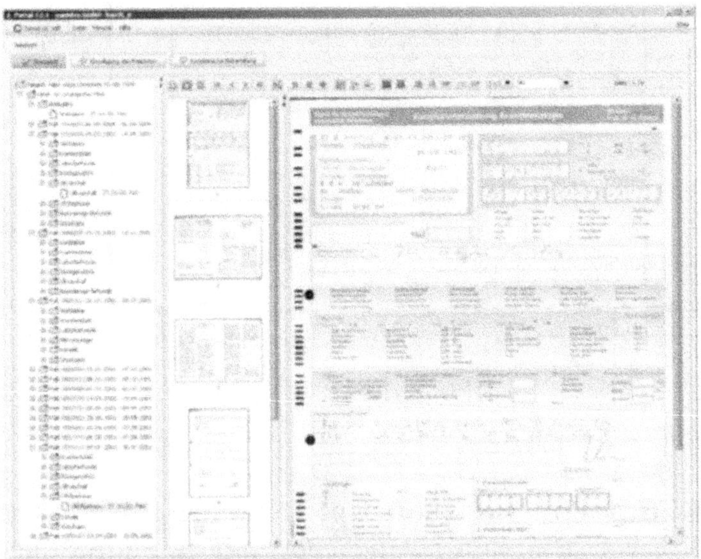

Example of Electronic Medical Records at a German Hospital

Source: http://www.smi.ukw.de/de/sap-klinische-verfahren/archivsysteme/digitales-krankenakten-und-belegarchiv.html

Figure 9. The organizational relationships of the key actors in the healthcare system
Source: Health Care Systems in Transition (Busse & Riesberg, 2004).

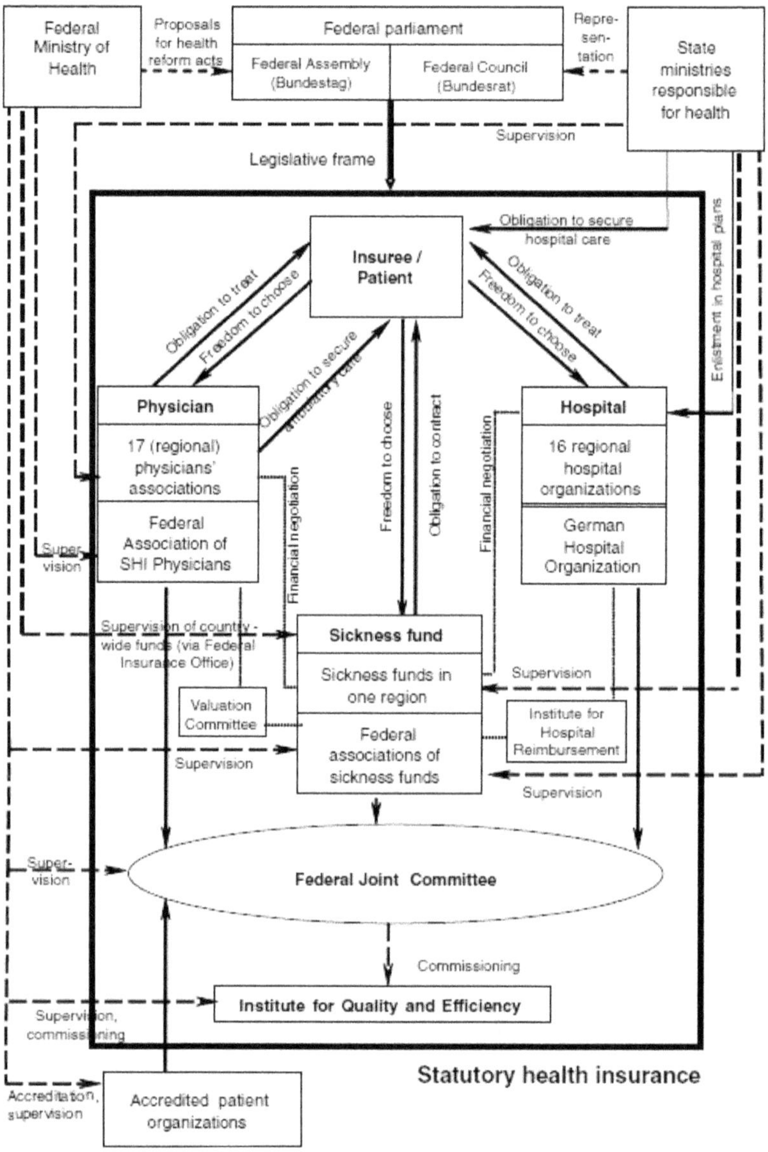

the western countries health systems are supported by best structured health care services delivery system with relative enough health infrastructures. Most developing countries healthcare systems present a pyramid-shaped structure. Unlike the developing countries, the literature research and surveys revealed that each inhabitant is living closer to a healthcare center (private GP practice, clinics, communal hospitals, university hospitals, etc.). In (Ridic et al., 2012) the authors show how the citizen in two western countries (German and Canada) are satisfied with their countries healthcare systems and policy.

Despite the good health structures and infrastructures in the developed world, the healthcare systems are also facing their own challenges. The next section will present the challenges facing the healthcare systems in low-, middles-, and high-income countries.

Challenges Facing the Health Care System

Table 6 presents a systematical overview of the challenges facing the different healthcare systems. Certain challenges are severe (S), middle (M), low (L), or non-existent (No) at some healthcare systems.

Table 6. Summary of the challenges facing the different public healthcare systems

Challenges Facing	Short Description	Income Countries			Observation
		Low	Middle	High	
		ICT			
Disparities in Access to Healthcare	Inequity in the access to healthcare delivery is noticed between urban and rural, between poor and rich, between insured and not insured	S	S	M	US Health system is more concerning than the other western countries' health system
Poor Pharmaceutical Care	Developing countries are facing poor access to the pharma care. The stocks often empty mostly in rural regions. It is difficult to purchase the medical prescription.	S	M	N	The developed countries do not face this challenge. They feature enough pharma industries. while developing countries import all the medicine from abroad.
Problems of counterfeit drugs	The counterfeit drugs issue is a global burden.	S	S	S	In the developing countries, counterfeit drugs are often selling in the drugstore, while in the developed countries, there exist special channels for the distribution
Personal Shortage	The healthcare delivery systems lack medical experts, nurses.	S	S	M	The developed countries face the personnel shortage issues mostly at the rural level. The urban area, however, faces this issue in nursing houses and nurse shortage. For example, most of the ´nurses working in Germany are from East Europe. In the developing world, workforce shortage is a matter challenge due to brain drain.

continued on following page

Table 6. Continued

Challenges Facing	Short Description	Income Countries			Observation
		Low	Middle	High	
Diseases Control and surveillance	Public healthcare systems worldwide are often facing serious diseases outbreaks despite the different diseases surveillance tools available in most health systems	S	S	L	Developing countries lack adequate surveillance tools and policies, while western countries are facing the limitation of the surveillance systems
Medical Data Processing and Communication Systems	The Hospital Information Exchange and Electronic Medical Records Systems are the central pieces of the medical data collection and processing mechanism. Most developing countries lack these tools. Developed countries are mostly using these tools, though are also facing challenges in exchanging electronically data between institutions	S	S	M	In developing countries, medical data processing is widely paper based
Waiting times	Long waiting times to access to specialized care is a challenge that is more facing western health systems than developing countries systems. The long waiting times are a consequence of a shortage of doctors and the possibility each western citizen must easily visit a doctor since they are national health insured.	M	M	S	Few people have access to health services in developing countries. The private health sector is not organized and developed like in western countries. So, the waiting time's challenge is less than in western countries.
Increasing obesity and other non-communicable diseases	According to WHO obesity and other communicable diseases are a big challenge facing the world health system.	S	S	S	This challenge is severe in all health systems around the world
Accommodation to Patient Needs Longer living (aging population)	The western population is fast aging; however, the healthcare system is not accommodated to their needs. The health system is more oriented and organized to tackle acute affection than chronic ones.	M	M	S	Developing countries population is younger than western ones and thus face few this kind of challenge
Continuous education	Developing countries doctors and other healthcare professionals lack continuing education. The health system lack of appropriate financial means for regular continuous education.	S	S	N	Western countries health systems offer more continuous education possibilities to the healthcare professionals. They work closely with researchers.

continued on following page

Table 6. Continued

Challenges Facing	Short Description	Income Countries			Observation
		Low	Middle	High	
Financial					
Funding and Health Insurances	The developing world health systems lack adequate medical costs funding systems because of lack of health insurances. Few people are health insured	S	S	M	Among western countries, the USA also face severe lack of medical costs funding, due to the structure and policies of the health systems relating to health insurances
High costs	Elderly people, repetitive medical treatments, lack of coordination regarding the treatment are factors of high costs facing all health systems	S	S	S	Health systems around the world are facing this challenge
Longer living (aging population)	Long living people are often subject to chronic diseases, which are factors of high costs	L	M	S	Western countries are more concerning
Increasing obesity and other non-communicable diseases	Obesity among the youth and non-communicable, chronic diseases, among the elderly population are factors of high medical expenditures.	M	M	S	Western countries are more concerning
Administrative					
Excessive bureaucracy	The structure and policies in the western countries health systems lead to high bureaucracy than in developing countries	M	M	S	Western countries are more concerning

continued on following page

The challenges are grouped by categories: (1) ICT, (2) administrative, and (3) financial.

1. **ICT:** Challenges in this category can be solved using Telehealthcare and/or information and communication technology
2. **Administrative:** Are categorized in this group those challenges, which require an organization and structure improvement
3. **Financial:** Need more investment to overcome the challenges in this group

Disparities in Access to Healthcare

In *low- and middle-income countries*, the differences in access to healthcare across the different population are the consequence of the structure described above and weak healthcare infrastructure. The medical facilities are often too far from the residential areas. Most rural regions lack municipal infrastructures such as streets, energy supply system, etc. The access to healthcare depends therefore on the place of residence of the patient. Thus, the rural population has poor access to healthcare in comparison to the urban population. In addition, the economic situation is an important factor in access to the healthcare. Due to the large distance between the places of residence and the pharmacies, pharmaceutical care remains also a major challenging problem that the public healthcare system is facing (Thierry Oscar Edoh & Teege, 2011).

As in most SSA countries, in Benin for example, 51% of the women are living relatively close to a hospital, more than 13% of the women live at least 30 kilometers far away from a hospital or a comparable facility, and the remainder has hard access to medical care (Klein, 2005). About 15% of healthcare delivery in Benin is provided by the private health sector. Most of the private health sector is in large cities. The quality of the services provided by the private sector is higher and more expensive than services provided by the public sector. This kind of facilities is only accessible for a part of the population, namely the rich population, Government members and their families. There exists also a "cheap private sector" in the healthcare system. This part of the private sector consists of small facilities with a maximum of three employees with elementary medicine background. It features only nurses who just provide basic healthcare delivery like prescription in case of non-complex malaria and/or small injuries. (Result of our recent survey)

Healthcare delivery in rural regions is quasi-non-existent. The causes are mainly the lack of medical infrastructure, missing of care specialists, health professionals, undertrained staff, insufficient funding of the public health system (health insurance policies are scarce).

Many annual reports carried out by WHO (World Health Organization) have reportedly indicated that healthcare systems in the Sub-Saharan African countries are in a poor state; however, these reports have never discussed the true causes leading to poor healthcare deliveries and the disparities in access to healthcare. Poverty is the most cited cause. However, poverty is only the peak of the iceberg. The low density of pharmacies and health centers in the entire country, the lack of health insurances the main causes of the disparities in the accessibility to healthcare.

In terms of healthcare delivery issues, the major challenges facing the public healthcare system in Benin are similar to those the Greenlandic health system has started fighting against in 2010 (Niclasen & Mulvad, 2010). However, Benin does not have the same telecommunication and city infrastructures like Greenland. Therefore, the main question to be addressed is whether the access to healthcare particularly in rural regions can be improved using Telehealthcare systems technologies inspired by the Telemedicine system implemented in Greenland[5] and adapt them to the technical and economic realities in Benin. Telemedicine or eHealth is understood as the use of information and telecommunications system to provide remote healthcare to the population. Telemedicine is usually assumed to mean curative practices. Telemedicine is playing an increasing role in health development, in education and training, in quality improvement and in the improvement of efficiency of healthcare services (J. J. Braa & Hedberg, 2002).

In the *high-income countries*, the rural populations are facing similar access to healthcare services issues. However, the causes here are different from those in low- and middle-income countries. In the US health system, for example, the access to the healthcare services is limited in rural regions. Further, it depends on whether one can pay the medical costs since the system is more commercial and each doctor can charge a medical treatment as he wants. (Schoen et al., 2006)(Ridic et al., 2012). Furthermore, the US healthcare faces a severe racial issue in the healthcare delivery system.

In (Barkan, 2010) the author state:

... studies find that African Americans are much less likely than whites to receive the procedures just listed. This is true when poor blacks are compared to poor whites and when middle-class blacks are compared to middle-class whites.

Regardless of the reason, the result is the same: African Americans are less likely to receive potentially life-saving cardiac procedures simply because they are black. Institutional discrimination in healthcare, then, is literally a matter of life and death.

The access challenges facing high-income countries health systems could be summarized to (i) long waiting time to have an arrangement with primary care doctors, (ii) difficult access to specialized care. A study (Schoen et al., 2009) carried out in 11 western countries, Germany included, has shown the access to healthcare services issues in these countries.

Primary care doctors' perceptions of access to specialized care varied significantly across countries. Dutch, Norwegian, and U.K. physicians were the least likely to report that patients had difficulty getting specialized diagnostic tests; Canadian, Italian, and New Zealand doctors were the most likely. (Schoen et al., 2009)

In (Schoen et al., 2005) the authors also figure out the waiting times as a challenge facing the healthcare delivery systems. The access challenges remain in Germany so that the statutory health insurance companies provide the patient with tools like web-pages to help them to quickly access specialized care.

Poor Pharmaceutical Care and Problems of Counterfeit Drugs

The developing countries are facing the poor access to pharma care. Thus, in large cities and particularly in the rural regions, it is often difficult to purchase all medicine on a prescription in one pharmacy. Often the patient must search in several pharmacies for the medicine and sometimes the patient cannot even afford to purchase all prescribed products.

The public healthcare systems in low- and middle-income countries are also suffering from counterfeit drugs, which can be purchased at any marketplace. Despite the various registered adverse, death cases, most people prefer to purchase those dangerous drugs, because they are cheaper than those at legal pharmacies, and are available anytime at the market (Thierry Oscar Edoh, 2010a).

A study (Nidhi, Indrajeet, Khushboo, Gauri, & Sen, 2011) carried in 2011 estimates that between 38% - 53% of antimalarial drugs sold in Asia and 30% of drugs sold in Kenya are counterfeit drugs. Developing world is severe facing the challenge. The study further estimates that in the developed world the counterfeit drug's sales increase by 15%annually. A Europol-report (Europol, 2015) in 2017 shows that the counterfeit drugs issue continuously increasing.

Medical Data Processing and Communication Systems

Data gathering and processing in the healthcare system of Benin remain largely paper-based. The paper-based data management systems about the living situation of people particularly in rural areas and slums, the rate of illiteracy and the poor organization of the healthcare centers impact negatively the quality of the medical data, the data security and thus the medical care. The patient data are recorded in a booklet (see Figure 4), which patients keep at home. Most of the patients, particularly in rural areas and urban slums, regularly lose their medical booklet. This influences negatively data protection/integrity and data security.

There exists no ICT based data processing system at the different healthcare units. This situation is more severe at all healthcare unit in the poor regions, rural regions, and slums. Patient medical data are recorded in a register. The information contained in such registers is incomplete and has no benefit for care delivery. During the study, many registers were found in a bad state under the table of the nurses or in a storehouse. Each patient must buy at each medical visit a booklet to record his data into it. The recorded data are temperature, name, address, weight, and size. At the end of the medical visit, the nurse records the prescription into the booklet. At the next visit, the nurse collects the booklet but does not use the information contained in it. Patient and health worker contribute together to data loss in the system. More than 1000 booklets were evaluated. The evaluated booklets contain no health history or any data useful for a care delivery.

Beyond the poor patient data processing, information exchange and communication within the healthcare system is mostly paper-based and takes long. The medical institutions have quasi-no IT infrastructure, particularly the medical facilities at the lowest level are poorly equipped.

Consequences of the situation described above are that 74% of reports and/or information within the system are wrong or contain incorrect data and are thus useless and can negatively affect the quality of the care delivery.

(…) Data quality is still a problem because reports are not free from errors. An internal evaluation of SNIGS conducted in 1999 revealed that the proportion of errors in the reports transmitted was not significant. However, considerable errors and distortions existed in some of the epidemiological data (for example, 74 percent of reports on new cases contained errors). (…) [USAID]

The Ministry of Health (MOH) indicated in its report in May 2007 that National Information System and Sanitary Management (SNIGS - Figure 3) has databases at the central, departmental and some health zones. Unfortunately, these digital databases cannot currently (in 2016/2017) be accessed through the Internet. There is a case definition for the data in it and standardized collection method. Following tasks are assigned to the actor within the system: (i) Epidemiological surveillance, quarterly meetings, (ii) Routine system (departmental team and sanitary zones) of annual meetings with the team SNIGS Central to validate the data and discuss the inconsistencies. The MOH has objectively declared that the annual meeting at the central level is insufficient and therefore has no effect on the expected improvement of data at the departmental level (Ministere de la santé, 2007) (Mathias et al., 2013).

The western countries use more Electronic Medical Records Systems (EMR) to collect and process the patient medical data (Williams, Austin, & Mha, 2008).

A study we carried out in Germany in 2016 has revealed that the EMR systems being used by private doctors are mixed: (i) paper-based and (ii) electronic. The most diagnostics are recorded in paper-based record systems. The hospitals are fully using electronic medical records. However, the information is only shared within the institution. Data exchange with another institution is mostly paper-based (see Figure 5).

In the scope of this study, we also analyzed 300 patient medical records (paper-based and electronic) with the objectives to compare the quality of the contents, the structure, and the limitations of the systems with those in developing the world. The (E)MRs we investigated were anonymized, thus any consents from the concerning were not needed. The (E)MRs contain significant information, which most are provided by the patient self. Beyond this information, the documents contain the full diagnostics. Unfortunately, the documents are not complete, then when the patient change the doctor, he leaves his medical record with the doctor, so that the new doctor lacks the previous data and can base on the reports of the patient.

Personnel Shortage

The workforce shortage a matter cause of the poor/limited access to healthcare delivery in some regions of the concerning country. So due to a brain drain from developing countries toward the developed countries, the low- and middle-income countries lack medical experts, general physician, nurse. The challenge is more severe in the rural areas than the urban areas, then the rural region has poor medical infrastructures.

As a developed country, Germany is facing an exodus from the rural regions to the urban areas. The workforce shortage is the direct consequence. The young medical doctors prefer to stay in the large cities where they can earn more. Thus, the health system faces a workforce shortage at the rural level. The study in points the case of Germany out (Kopetsche, 2010).

Diseases Control and Surveillance

The case of Ebola epidemic in Africa in recent years has shown the importance of pervasive screening. Infectious disease can quickly spread in a crowd such as in a supermarket, the market in Africa, festivities, dancing crowd, etc. It is therefore important to monitor crowds during their life-cycle collect and process the crowdsourced data to determine any risk of emerging infectious diseases. It is also important to collect data about infectious diseases through the health based on defined policies. The study we carried out in the African developing countries reveals a lack of policy and tools in the health systems to collect infections related data so that they can be analyzed. The recent Ebola outbreak in West-Africa leads the key actors in the different health systems to design and adopt diseases control and surveillance policies. However, these policies lack supporting materials such as ICT systems to collect, process, and share the information so that a quick decision would be taken.

The health systems in the western countries have, unlike developing world health systems, implemented policies and tools to control and monitor infectious diseases and antibiotics adverse among their populations (Paolotti et al., 2014)(Kinoshita, Tokumasu, Tanaka, Kramer, & Kawakami, 2017). The implemented policies and tools are, however, limited in collecting data from patients who do not visit a doctor and thus deliver their infections related data. In (Paolotti et al., 2014) the authors show this limitation and propose a web-based data collection system, that overcomes the limitation of existing surveillance methods and systems. A study (Heil et al., 2017) carried out in the Netherlands that can be generalized to all European countries reveals also that the method, policies, and the surveillance tool in the case of pertussis surveillance are less accurate.

Funding and Health Insurances

As described above, the western countries feature statutory (ex. Germany) or national (Sweden, UK) health insurances systems to cover the medical expenditures. Among the western countries, the USA are the only ones where health insurances are not mandatory and be insured depends on incomes, being rich or poor. Only retired and people over 65 years old are covered by national health insurance. Obama care is a response to this inequity.

In the developing countries, health insurances are quasi-non-existent. In Benin, for example, being health insured is a private concern. Some government employees benefit partially from national health insurance, which is only valid at the public health center. There exist health insurances companies, but the policies are too expensive for the common citizen *[Study results]*.

Accommodation to Patient Needs

The population is fast aging. This fact is less considered by the health system that is more designed for acute affections than chronic diseases, which are more available to elderly people. In European countries, the different health systems offer house nursing to old people and thus accommodate to needs of the old people suffering from chronic or age-related diseases. The western health system is not prepared to face these cases and involved in the prevention than a promotion of health. In (A.C Greiner & Knebel, 2003)the authors report cases about a 75-old woman in the USA who did get appropriate treatment. Her care has also suffered from bad communication. The authors conclude following:

.... In addition to the need for the health system to be more responsive to those with chronic medical conditions and more focused on prevention, the system has not done a good job in accommodating the diverse cultural needs and varying preferences of racial and ethnic groups. A recent IOM report that reviews a large body of research concludes that racial and ethnic minorities tend to receive lower-quality care than Caucasians, even when one accounts for differences in insurance status, income, age, and severity of medical condition...

The population in developing world is younger, thus, these health systems do face few elderly people suffering from chronic diseases.

During the literature research, no publication was found dealing with the subject. We, therefore, investigate the topic by surveying the healthcare professionals. We then found out that most people suffering from chronic diseases are treated ambulatory. No prevention policy or tool exist and further, the system lacks medical promotion regarding the subject.

Further Major Challenges

Energy Supply, Frauds and corruption (Hope, 1999) *and poor health insurance* are also major challenges, which the public health system is facing and suffering of. Poor health insurance is one of the underlying factor of frauds and corruption within the system.

Monitoring of and integrating *Traditional medicine and herbal treatment* into the public health system remains a challenge the health system is facing. On one hand, traditional medicine can become too dangerous, since most practitioners are illiterate and additionally perform mostly wrong medical diagnosis. On another hand, traditional medicine can well cure some diseases.

TELEHEALTHCARE AS SOLUTION APPROACHES?

This section presents solutions approach to the challenges discussed above. *To what extent can the Telehealthcare help?*

Tackling the challenges facing the public healthcare system regarding the healthcare services accessibility means to provide the health system with an adapted telemedicine solution that helps to overcome the accessibility and long waiting times challenges described above.

According to the definition (see *SUPPORTING TECHNOLOGY*), a standard telemedicine solution cannot tackle all challenges facing. For example, the definitions of telemedicine/telehealthcare do not issue about a personnel shortage in a healthcare system. Therefore, telemedicine solutions and systems must be adapted and extended with additional features to meet the needs and tackle the challenges facing.

Developing Countries: ICT Based Solution Approaches

The main challenges facing the healthcare here are: (i) poor access to health, more severe in rural areas, (ii) poor access to pharmaceutical care, (iii) lack of Electronic Medical Records systems, (iv) poor data management systems, (v) proliferation of counterfeit drugs, (vi) workforce shortage, and (vii) lack of continuous education.

As minor challenges, we can note (i) aging population, and (ii) poor accommodation to patient needs.

We, therefore, propose a remote healthcare system that combines the telemedicine, telehealth, eHealth, and mHealth technology with agile project organization and management paradigm. Compared to agile development, the proposed system disposes of a team as a pedestal for supporting the remote healthcare delivery systems using mobile phone technology. Following features are provided:

1. Diseases surveillance and monitoring using IoT/crowdsensing paradigm: Surveillance and monitoring of health have been recognized efficient and cost-effective
2. Electronic Medical Record (EMR): Improving the data collection, processing, and management as well as data exchange
3. Remote Diagnostic and Care Delivery: Bring the care service to patient
4. Continuous Education unit for care professionals
5. Patient Education
6. A subsystem to help traditional practitioners to perform adequate diagnostic and treatment: overcoming the personnel shortage issues
7. Pharmaceutical care delivery subsystem

The remote care system focusses on pervasive healthcare, health promotion, and prevention, patient education to increase diseases awareness among the population, improve the (continuous) training for health professionals, and improve the data collection and thus the quality of the data within the healthcare system. A remote care healthcare delivery solution has the potential to tackle the healthcare poor accessibility challenges facing the public healthcare delivery system.

A novelty in this system is to involve traditional practitioners in the system. Rural populations in developing countries are more confident of traditional medicine than modern medicine. While poor medical diagnosis is the big weakness of traditional medicine, there are diseases, which are best treated by traditional medicine. Since the rural population in those parts of the world are more confident of traditional medicine, therefore it's proposed to involve the traditional practitioners into the multidisciplinary health team and train them to perform a better medical diagnosis to provide the best care. Traditional practitioners will be coached and assisted by health professionals. It's further proposed a multimodal database to record information about traditional medicine and treatments. This would help to improve the traditional medicine, share information between health professionals and traditional practitioners, and between traditional practitioners and traditional practitioners. Because of the high illiteracy rate among the traditional practitioners a VoiceXML- based application (Speech Interface Languages) is proposed so that the practitioners can use it to record information into the multimodal database. The system provides also video interface to enable to record images and video materials into the database.

A further novelty of this approach is to adapt and use pervasive healthcare to improve access to healthcare tailored for a healthcare environment with a low degree of technical infrastructure in a poor state or non-existent.

Remote care specialists are required to be involved in the multidisciplinary remote healthcare system to assist nurses working at rural care units in providing care services. Care specialists from the private health sector could also be requested to participate in the system and help to minimize any eventual workload within the system. The remote care specialists are provided with MCSW systems, which they use in collaborating on a medical case. Patient-data can be shared through the MCSWS. The MCSWS enables video and voice conferencing communication. Most of the applications in use in the MCSWS are running on the mobile phone (from GSM to G3). Few desktop computer or laptops are in use in the system. The designed MCSWS provides a training feature for the undertrained nurses and doctors. All communications, in any case, are recorded and serve as training materials for the health professionals providing an assistance and treatment protocols. Because of the privacy-sensitive nature of health data, patient's personal data is erased from all training materials.

The global aims of the remote care system for the developing countries are:

- Increase the accessibility of healthcare services
- Increase the quality and continuity of care to patients
- Increase the focus on preventive medicine through early intervention involving traditional practitioners, village nursing, and NGOs
- Improve the Adherence to Treatment
- Reduce the overall cost of healthcare
- Improve education and training of caregivers;
- Provide services to remote areas in the case of natural calamities and disasters, and Remotely monitor chronic patients.

The proposed care system enables remote assistance to the undertrained caregivers, collaborating work between care professionals, delivery of remote healthcare to the patient at home, and educate the patient. The system consists of Telehealthcare system based on a network of medical centers, whereas at least one of the centers belonging to the network must be close to the patient's place of residence. It provides a (mobile) pervasive healthcare system for making healthcare available to the remote population at any time and in any

Figure 10. Structure of a Remote Care Delivery system

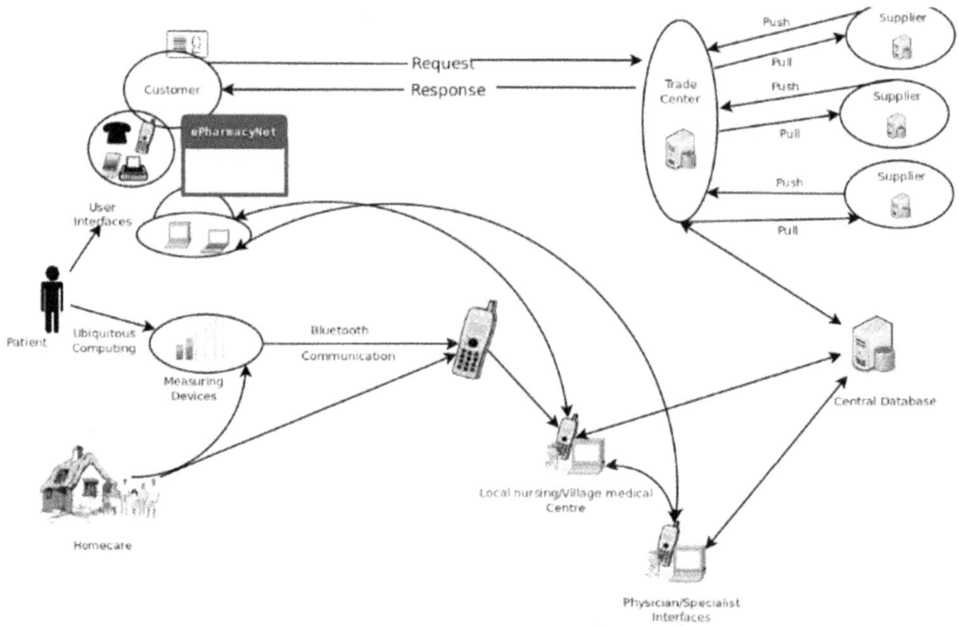

region of the country by removing locational/geographical, time and other restraints.

Figure 10 shows the high-level architecture of remote care delivery system. The payment, reminder (adherence to treatment) and MCSCW components are not shown in the overview architecture. The proposed remote care system consists of two subsystems:

1. **An Improved Drug Supply System (IDSS):** IDSS is an adapted mail-order-pharmacy (Thierry Oscar Edoh & Teege, 2011).
2. **A Remote Health Care Provision System (RCPS):** RCPS is a virtual Hospital network system providing a Hospital Information system, Enterprise Resource Planning and computer supported collaborative work system for hospitals-employees, medical doctors, nurses, enabling patient data management (data record system), tele-surveillance and remote healthcare delivery systems. Electronic health professionals and patient health cards, called eHealthCard, are also provided for accessing the system and enabling secure data processing and combating frauds.

Chronic patients can be provided with a wireless sensor network (i.e. Internet of Things) that will be sensing and delivering medical data such as bio signal to *RCPS*. Gateways, act as a proxy for the wireless sensor network system on the patient's mobile, which in turn acts as a proxy for the global pervasive care system. Gateways are interfaced on the patient's mobile phone and allow each sensor in the wireless sensor network to send/receive data to/from an application running on the patient mobile phone. An application transmits automatically all data from patient's mobile phone to the treating nurses/physicians.

In the case of home care, patient's family members can provide first aid if they are instructed (over the mobile phone) by a nurse or physician.

SOLUTION APPROACHES

A Multidisciplinary Health Care Team

Telehealth systems connect remote patient to doctors through ICT devices [Definition from WHO], though, regarding the religiously and/or traditionally conservative, populations could reject the system because of the lack of patient-to-doctor relationship, therefore, the concept foresees a multidisciplinary health team that in situ works with the patient and remotely works with the treating physician. The multidisciplinary team is an ad-hoc that is formed and committed to medical treatment tasks.

A multidisciplinary remote healthcare team consists of health professionals (doctors and nurses), NGOs workers (who played the role of social or community services, psychologist), pharmacists, and local communities. Table 7 summarizes the composition of the multidisciplinary team.

Challenges Facing the Implementation of a Standard Telemedicine Solution

Implementing a Telehealth system as described in (Scott & Mars, 2015) implies that ICT smart devices, reliable telecommunication infrastructure, simple or complex multimedia to video conferencing to virtual reality, and energy are available, the potential system users need basic to solid ICT knowledge and awareness of IT-security in term of data protection. The technology level and economic situation present several obstacles to implementing a standard

Table 7. Multidisciplinary team and assigned tasks

Team Members	Descriptions	Assigned Tasks	Infrastructure
Local Nursing/ Village Health Center health	Local Nursing or care units at village (rural) level are the central component in care delivery services within a multidisciplinary remote healthcare system. It is required that each health professional, working at these units, is proficient in the local language and dialects to communicate easily with the local population. Health professionals at this level work closely together with NGOs, community trained caregiver at many levels.	• Provide primary or specialized care • Oversee the patient-education for increasing diseases awareness, • Improve the disease prevention. • Inform individuals living around these care units about medical and health concerns • Visit the patient at home, train him on hygiene, prevention of infectious diseases, and first aid.	EMR Smartphone
Volunteer community trained Health Care Giver, NGOs, and Social Workers	Community trained caregiver and NGOs are mostly close to the population and work on voluntary base. They are present at the places lacking care units or health professionals. The healthcare professionals at the rural level are in turn assisted by the specialist at large hospitals.	• Provide first aid care to patients and organize patient transportation to a care unit in case of emergency • Assisted by health professionals at rural level in giving first aid to the patients. • Provide the patient with (all) needed medicine, then they know approximately the medical needs of each patient they are medically assisting • Conduct regular surveys to state on the medicine used in each care area.	Mobile Computer Supported Collaborative Work Systems (MCSWS) Mobile EMR
Trained Traditional Practitioners	Rural populations in developing countries are more confident of traditional medicine than modern medicine. While poor medical diagnosis is the big weakness of traditional medicine, there are diseases, which are best treated by traditional medicine. Since the rural population in those parts of the world are more confident of traditional medicine, therefore it's proposed to involve the traditional practitioners into the multidisciplinary health team and train them to perform a better medical diagnosis to provide the best care.	• Traditional practitioners will be coached and assisted by health professionals. • Perform diagnostics and treatment at areas lacking care units	Smartphone Desktop PC MCSW systems, video and voice conferencing ePharmacyNet
Pharmacist	Pharmacies at the healthcare units and pharmacies from private health sector are part of the multidisciplinary team.	• Provide medicine and other pharmaceutical products to remote patients • Help the patient to purchase drugs a remote pharmacy • Help the doctor to prescribe existing medicine	ePharmacyNet
Remote Care Specialists	Remote care specialists are remote physicians included in the team and who supervise all diagnostics and treatment.	• Assist nurses working at rural care units by providing care services. • Train the traditional practitioners to perform good diagnostics	MCSW systems, video and voice conferencing
Psychologists	The psychologists have the role of advisors and assistants within the team.	Assist, coach, and train the community caregiver, nurses, and traditional practitioners in daily work as well as the patients and their relatives during a medical treatment	

Table 8. List of obstacles to the implementation of a standard Telehealthcare system

Problems	Descriptions
(Tele) Communication	The infrastructure and the coverage of telecommunication systems (The Internet, telephone line, mobile phone system, etc.) are decisive for a well-functioning Telehealthcare system in the country. Telehealthcare requires a (large) bandwidth transmission system and a very high transmission quality for pictures (for example X-ray pictures, etc.) or video (video conference). This cannot be guaranteed today. Telephone connections must also be good. More than 90% of all regions in Benin are actually covered by mobile phone system (Thierry Oscar Edoh & Teege, 2011). However, internet penetration (33.1% in 2017) is not well established in the population. Even Telephone connections have not entirely covered the country yet for the use of Mobile Data services. Mobile SIM penetration in 2017 is 87.2%.
IT infrastructure for the system user and -operator	Standard notebook costs more than 500 dollars against 300 dollars in the high-income countries. Fortunately, in Benin like many developing countries, the number of mobile phone subscribers reached 9.63 million in 2013. In 2015, Benin accounts about 10 million of mobile phone subscribers for 9 million populations[6]. Our recent study conducted in 2014 showed that most people possess at least 2 to 3 mobile phones. Furthermore, GSM/2G, 3G mobile phones are more widespread than 4G capable mobile phones. Mobile phones are becoming ubiquitous.
Paying the medical fees	There is no electronic payment infrastructure compared to what exists in high-income. Most patients do not even have a bank account. Only a few people in the country possess a bank account and there exists no obligation for the inhabitants to register with the authorities. Doctor's fees must be paid before the physician treats the patient. How should the telemedicine services fees be paid in the case of a remote medical treatment? The issue can be solved by launching a mandatory health insurance for everyone, that will cover the most medical fees. Additionally, it is recommended to use the available mobile money solutions such as M-Pesa, MoneyGram, MTN Mobile money, etc.
Energy reliability	There is no reliable electricity supply for operating ICT equipment. ICT components must have automatic recovery functions which allow a restart after an electricity outage without damage to the system. There must be backup solutions to keep the system working when no electricity is available. This may be back up for electricity supply, such as a generator or solar power modules, or it may be a fallback mode based on paper and mobile phones.
Transportation in case of emergency	Unreliable transportation means and roads in the poor state are a factor underlying the poor access to healthcare too. Remote patients spend a lot of time to reach the next closer health center. Most of the time, they have to go more than 30 km and spend more than 3 hours to reach the next care unit. There is no transportation possibility available in remote areas due to the poor road-rail network. Ambulances for patient-transport are scarce in the whole country. Thus, in the case of emergency, remote patients are treated at home or delivered too late to the emergency center. Most of the time emergency-patients are carried to the hospital using public or private transportation. The drive takes long. Most of the patients are dying at the place of accident or during the transport.
Poor Health Insurance and underfunded Care System	There is no reliable health insurance system in the public health system in Benin. A survey conducted on the topic and discussion with the key persons had figured out a government health insurance in the public healthcare system. This health insurance is funded at 100% by the government for healthcare professionals and 20% for the other government employees. The remaining 80% are carried by themselves in the case of illness. Employees in the private sector or jobless have no health insurance. They must pay 100% of the medical fees. The healthcare problematic also underlies the poor healthcare accessibility.
Fraud and Corruption	Fraud and corruption are also factored leading to poor access to healthcare in developing countries (Mackey & Liang, 2012), particularly in Benin. They further adversely impact the infrastructures, financing, and social determinants of health. In Benin, each care unit at rural, district or national level possesses public pharmacy-infrastructures, which are intended to provide the patients with the basic medicine. Those pharmacies are often low in stock due to fraud occurring in the care units and/or because of poor planning. Caregivers sell the pharmaceutical products at black markets or use them for private concerns. Furthermore, patients are only provided with those products only if they bribe caregivers or have a relative working at the care units. This kind of corruption in any health sector, particularly in developing countries, can gravely and negatively impact the quality and the coverage of healthcare services. Price inflation or high medical fees could be the direct consequences and thus a barrier to access to healthcare delivery for resource-poor people.

Telehealth system. This leads us to adapt the designed system and select infrastructure so that to meet the obstacles (Table 8).

Remote Care System as Solution Approach

A wireless sensor network to provide pervasive mobile healthcare and wireless health monitoring services for chronic patients is designed and implemented. This is the class of the measuring devices connected to patient's mobile phone for transferring critical measuring values to the next hospital and inform the concerned members of the multidisciplinary remote healthcare system. The communication between the measuring station and mobile phone is a Bluetooth based communication and/or near field communication technology. Today most mobile phones feature this technology to communicate with other devices nearby using device-to-device (D2D) communication paradigm. The architecture of the proposed Telehealthcare system is Service Oriented.

The system features services responsible for a defined unique task such diagnostic service, education service, payment service, etc. which use diverse communication protocols to exchange data and information. Devices using the same communication protocol such as Bluetooth, Near Field Communication follow the D2D communication paradigm. Machine-to-Machine (M2M) communication paradigm is then performed for autonomous communication between machines.

System Interfaces

Smartphones are used as a gateway within the wireless sensors network placed at the patient to pervasively collect his bio-signals, which are partially processed and stored at the edge if the patient smartphone is not connected to the internet. The stored data are forwarded once the device is connected to the internet.

A remote system team's member can also use their smartphone to call (using D2D paradigm) the data stored on the patient smartphone and forward them to the system for further process. Figure 11 illustrates the data collection and forwarding to the remote care center.

The devices (tablet, laptop, fax-machine, land phone) as UI enables the user to access and interact with the application or platform (Figure 10).

Figure 11. Smartphone usage in data collecting, processing, and forwarding

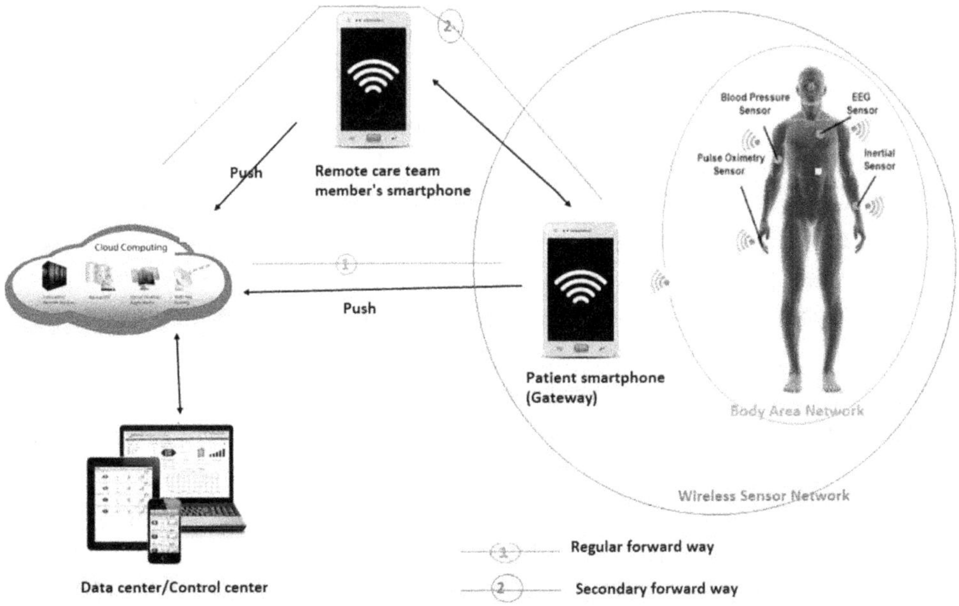

Figure 12. Electronic Medical Record form

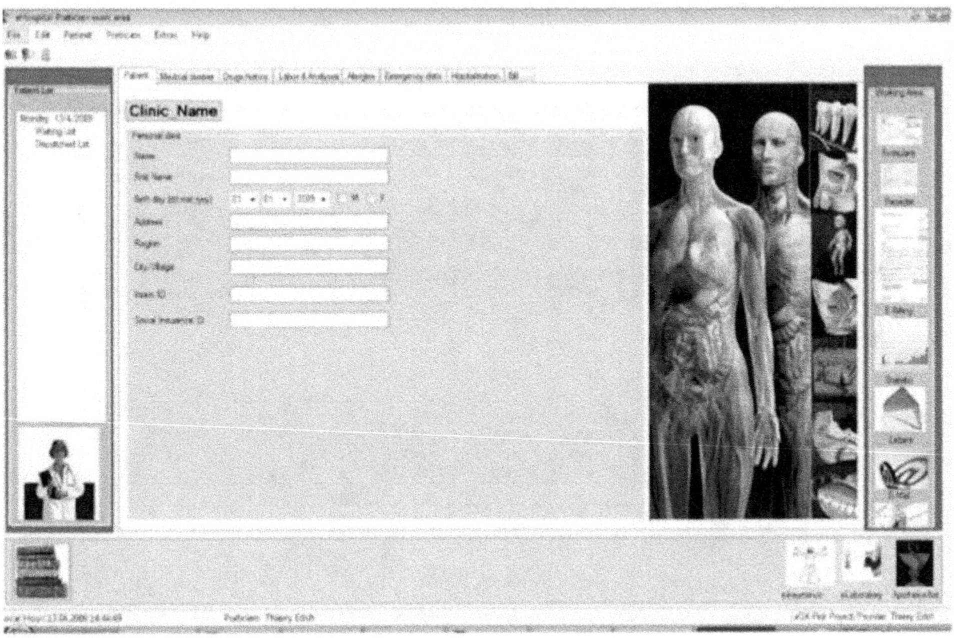

Graphical User Interfaces

A graphical user interface (GUI) is a purely textual user interface to a computer or computer program/application. A GUI enables interactions with an application where the client (in the case of server-client architecture) or the standalone application runs on a device (User interface). Web-browser, desktop GUI, and console are candidate GUI enabling interaction with the proposed system.

The remote care delivery application features a multimodal access interface, where the user can access and interact with the application through web-browser (Firefox, Microsoft edge/explorer, Google Chrome, etc.), an implemented desktop GUI (Text, voice), and console.

The application is a RESTful Web-Application accessible through web-browsers. The desktop variant of the is SOAP-web service based where the client on the desktop a dot-Net client using WCF (Windows Communication Foundation) technology to communicate with the java based server. The application has more than 150 user interfaces provided by all sub-components. The application is still in implementing; thus, the amount of GUI will certainly increase.

Figure 13. Appointment management form

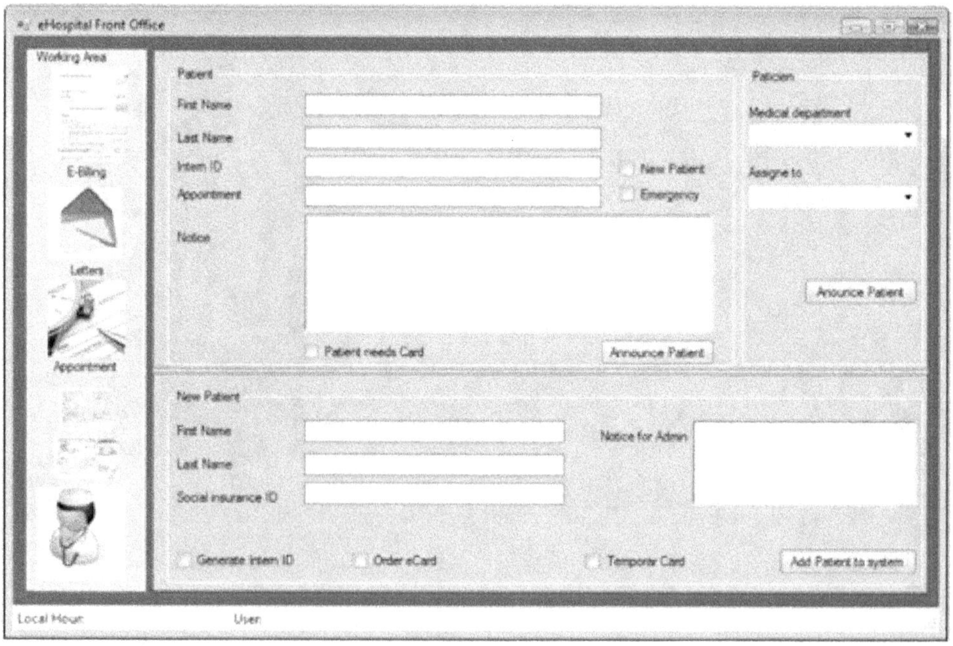

presents the form to access to patient medical records. Through this form, a remote physician can see the collected data at a remote chronic patient. The collected are pushed to the server in real-time or using the store and forward paradigm.

Figure 13 presents an appointment management form. This enables to register a new patient, to manage emergency cases, and to automatically request the concerning patient medical record from the server. New patients are patients who are not yet registered into the national central patient database.

Emergency patients are automatically assigned to an appropriate physician and his medical records are forwarded to the physician. In the case of

Figure 14. Medical electronic prescription form

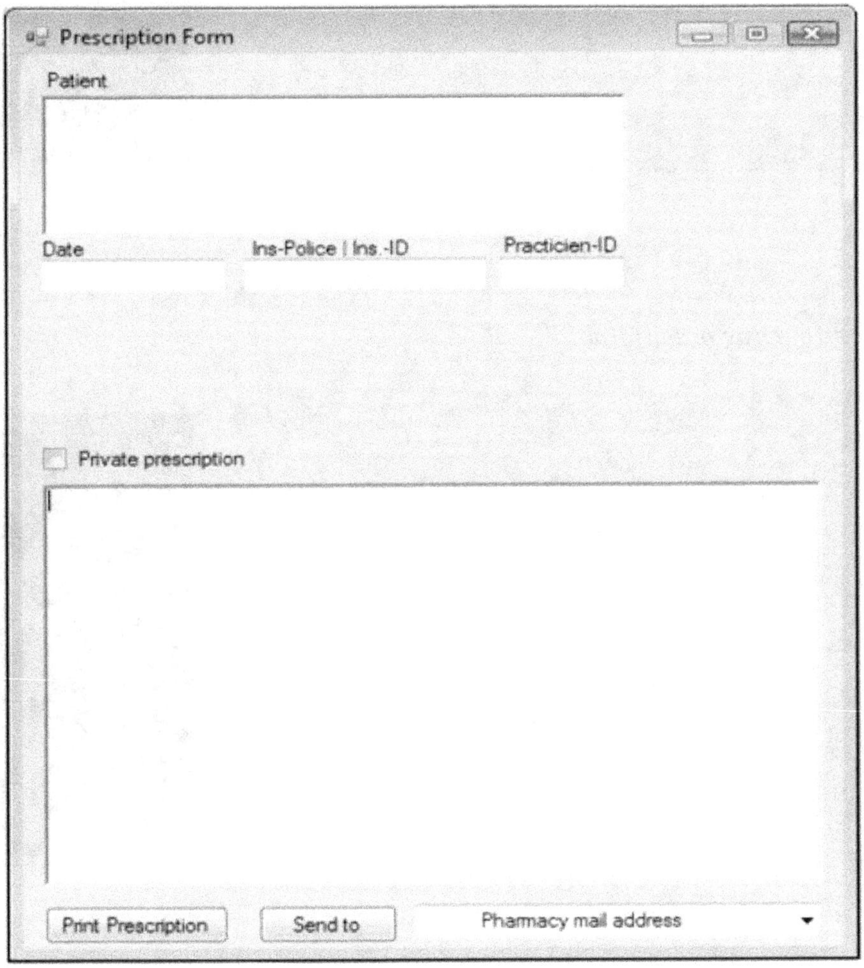

Figure 15. Drug search form

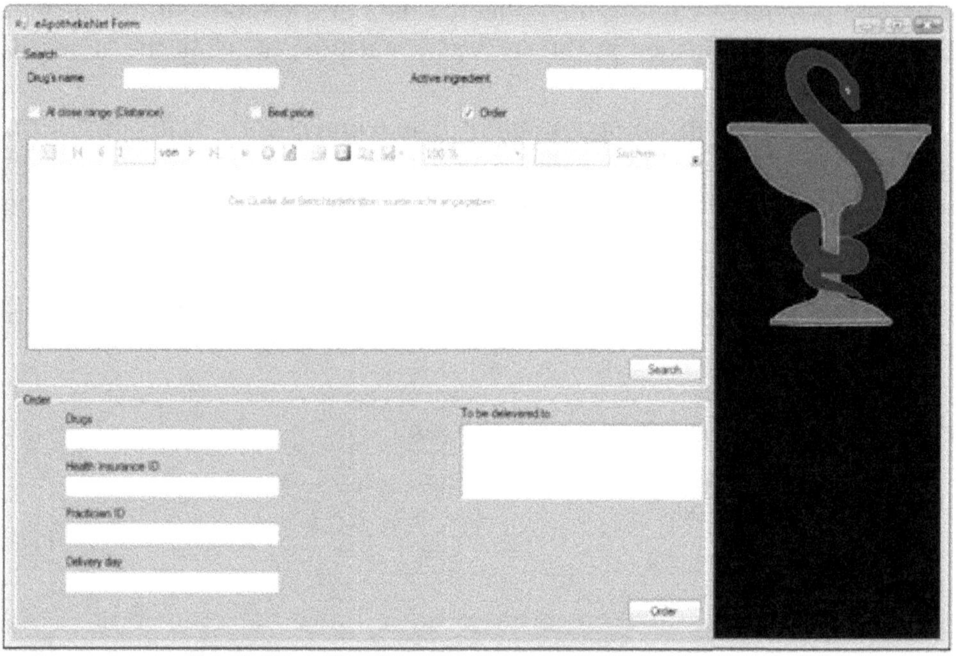

Figure 16. Drug order form

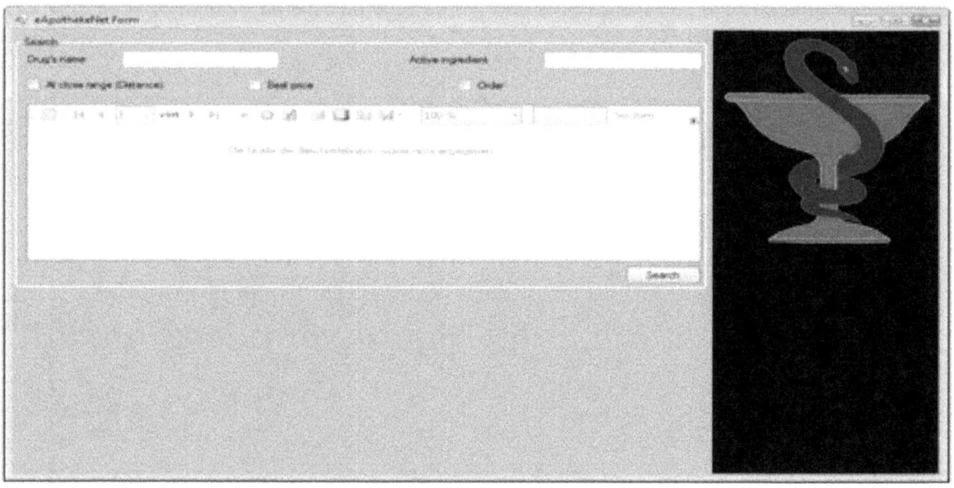

emergency, it is often difficult to collect the patient id to request his medical records. The system, therefore, provides a biometric identification feature, that enables the patient to identify himself using his fingerprint. The system collects the fingerprint and requests the corresponding ID which in turn is used to request the full medical records.

The treating physician can electronically prescribe medicine using this form. This form enables the physician to electronically order the prescribed products and the patient will be delivered at home.

To order the prescription, the system uses another sub-component, call IDSS, whose forms are presented in Figure 15 and Figure 16.

System Components

The system consists of the components described below; which, in turn, provide a set of functionalities.

Drug Supply System

A mail order pharmacy that enables to prevent the patient to go through several pharmacies before he could, if any, purchase the prescription. This component is deeply described in (Thierry Oscar Edoh, 2010a; Thierry Oscar Edoh & Teege, 2011)

eDignostic and eConsultation

Both components enable to remotely be visited by a doctor and perform a diagnostic. A remote physician could also use this component to assist a traditional practitioner in performing a diagnostic at a patient.

This component offers a special feature to overcome the language barriers in translating all information into local language so that the involved traditional practitioners can use the information too.

eDataManagement

Is a component for collecting, processing, persistent storing data. It provides a security mechanism to protect the data against any attack. The component consists of body areas networks, wireless sensors networks that are in charge to collect medical data and send to the eDataManagement server at the cloud. It furthermore collects data from other sources such diagnostic data, medication data, etc.

eHospitalNet

Is a network of involved health centers. It is a virtual Hospital-network Solution inspired by the network-centric operation healthcare discussed in (Maniatopoulos et al., 2009). Public Health Care Systems in developing countries, particularly Sub-Saharan Africa, are facing a set of technical, organizational, informational, personal, social, and financial issues. A network-centric operation healthcare seems, therefore, to be the optimal concept to meet the challenges these public health systems are facing

Logging Management

Each patient is advised to have an electronic health card secured with a personal identification number (PIN). This PIN system is intended for literate people. A picture-based password system, as shown in Figure 17, is used by illiterates as well as by elderly people to access the system. This solution approach consists of selecting pictures in certain order. Each selected picture corresponds to a digit from 0 to 9. An illiterate patient can then enter his PIN by selecting pictures in given order. Additionally, they can use the audio/ voice to enter their PIN. For example, an ID like "1234" will be given as "Monkey, Panther, Lion, Buffalo".

Figure 17. Picture-based PIN system

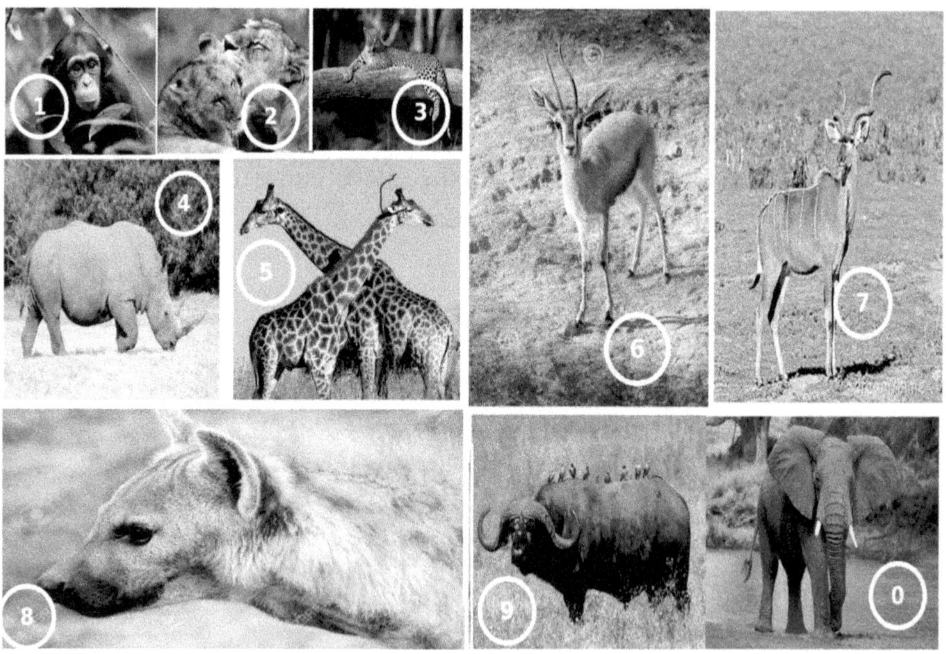

An alternative solution for illiterate patients is to employ the multidisciplinary health team to assist the patients during or for processing the call. Unfortunately, this may lead to security or privacy problems. Therefore, this person must be rigorously trained and should be always available. A family member could also play this role.

Measuring Module Unit

The measuring devices (Figure 18) are connected to patient's mobile phone via Bluetooth, and used for medical monitoring and surveillance. This component as already implemented in (T. O. C. Edoh, Atchome, Alahassa, & Pawar, 2016) and uses the ZigBee communication protocol. Using ZigBee enable to reduce the energy consumption. As already demonstrated above, energy supply presents a challenge for the public care system.

Central Database System

Is a central database for centralized medical data processing and promotes distributed data access for the patient's data. Distributed data access enables the storage approach which replicates gathered and recorded data at local

Figure 18. Measuring infrastructure for a pervasive computing (monitoring)

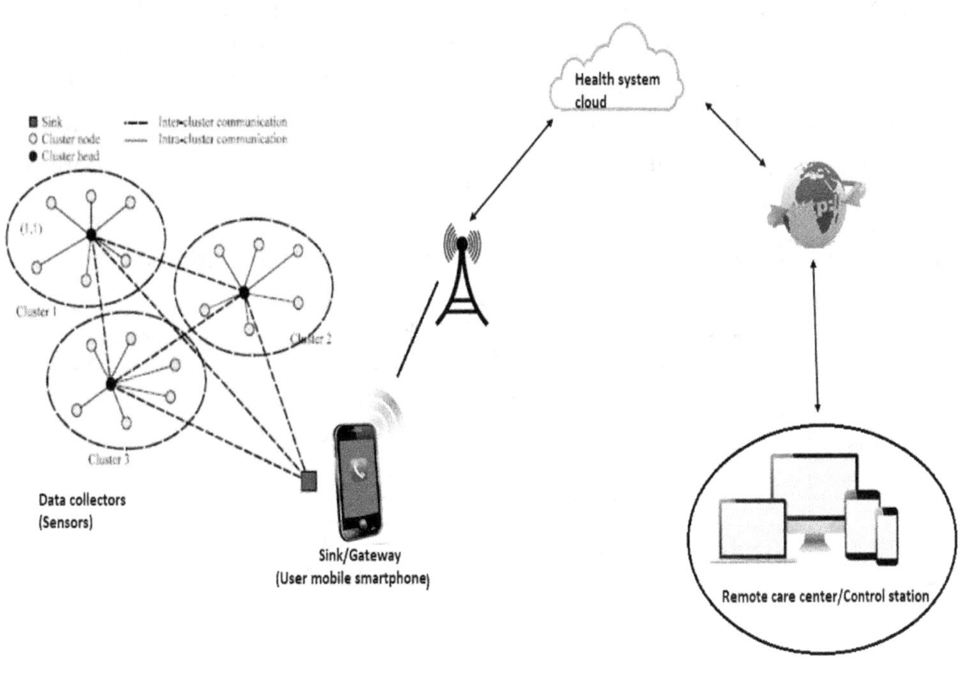

databases at different care units that are involved in the multidisciplinary remote healthcare system. This approach also allows the queries to be processed anywhere and at any time. The patient medical data is only replicated to the local database if the care unit requests at least once the data and configure the system to automatically replicate as soon as the patient dossier is updated in the central database.

Regarding the technical, connection issues that are facing, it is advantageous to keep patient's medical data updated at the local care unit, thus to assure the care delivery at any time.

Mobile Computer Supported Cooperative Work Unit

Computer-supported cooperative work (CSCW) is a generic theme covering and consisting of software tools, applications, and technology that supports a group of individuals working on projects at different sites. CSCW is based on the principle of group coordination and collaborative activities supported through computer systems. A Mobile Computer-Supported Cooperative Work (MCSCW) as a CSCW supported through the mobile computer and/or a mobile phone (Schrott & Gluckler, 2004) is implemented to support the communication in the remote care network.

Table 9 shows the technologies used to implement the remote care system's MCSCW. Only the existing and reliable technologies in the country such as mobile telephony and the internet, services such as SMS, MMS, Email, devices such as mobile phones of the first generation (GSM) and higher, notebook, tablet, and laptop are elements of the MCSCW. Those technologies and devices are accessible for all, reliable and cost-efficient. The mobile telephony covers more than 90% (Thierry Oscar Edoh, 2010b) of the country.

Table 9. A two-dimensional collaboration framework with used technology

	Communication	**Data and Information Sharing**	**Coordination/Instruction/Assistance**
Real Time/ Synchronous	• Mobile phone/ Line Phone • Video conferencing (Skype/Hangout)	• Electronic Whiteboards (electronic/presence) • Meeting facilitation (Trello & Slack)	Video conferencing (Skype/Hangout)
Asynchronous	• Email • SMS/MMS	• Document repositories • Team workspaces	• Email • SMS/MMS • Document repositories

Billing and Payment Unit

This functionality is the same as that was described in (Thierry Oscar Edoh & Teege, 2011). Additionally, external existing payment/money-Transfer services such M-Pesa, Mobile-Money, and PayPal are called using web service technology.

Diseases Spreading Prevention Unit

The risk of spreading diseases within (ad-hoc) crowds and the need to pervasively screen asymptomatic individuals to protect the population against emerging infectious disease request permanent crowd surveillance, particularly in high-risk regions. The case of Ebola epidemic in Africa in recent years has shown the need of pervasive screening. Infectious disease can quickly spread in a crowd such as in a supermarket, the market in Africa, festivities, dancing crowd, etc. It is therefore important to surveil crowds during their life-cycle collect and process the crowdsourced data to determine any risk of emerging infectious diseases.

We propose a smart health system that collects and transforms raw data into useful information, communicates with other smart devices and the people (e.g. emergency teams) to monitor outdoor (ad-hoc) crowd to prevent the spread of diseases. The proposed smart health system will integrate the physical and digital world (IoT/IoHT), where they interact with each other using object with network connectivity.

The smart health system, an Internet of Health Things, combines two paradigms: (i) crowdsensing and (i) Internet of Things. IoT is defined as a paradigm in which computing, and networking are embedded in objects, (Pena-Lopez et al.) and are equipped with embedded sensors, which in turn could be used to collect crowdsourcing data.

In the scope of this project, we foresee to use balloons and drones provided with fiber optic sensors and infrared cameras. The balloons and/or drones equipped with infrared cameras (IRC) and fiber Bragg grating sensors (FBGS) will permanent overfly cities in seeking for the (ad-hoc) crowd in order to collect crowdsourcing data such as temperature. Our system application would able to detect outdoor overcrowding (congestion) and thus contextually start collecting crowdsourcing data, which would be transformed into useful information. Fiber-optic sensing is an excellent solution to overcome the limitations of smartphones embedded sensors. (National Instruments, 2016). Furthermore, a pedestrian detection method in infrared images would be implemented for automatic crowd detection using the images produced by the IRC fixed on the balloon. A shape-based pedestrian detection method is presented in (Liu, Luo, & Yang, 2007) and a real-time pedestrian detection system that works on low-quality infrared videos is implemented in (Nanda & Davis, n.d.). A promising test was taken place and shows the feasibility of the planned system. In the upcoming research, the experiment and results will be presented and discussed.

System Functionalities

The following services and functionalities are offered in different types and manners: Patient-to-Physician/Nurse or Nurse-to-expert (physician) and Physician-to-Physician Service. Table 10 summarizes the main functionalities featured by the system.

Table 10. System functionalities

Functionalities	Descriptions
Teleconsultation, Telediagnostic and Emergency service	Synchronous and asynchronous teleconsultation is supported by the video conferencing component. Short Message Service (SMS) or Multimedia Messaging Service (MMS) technology are used for asynchronous consultation, where larges files can be sent too. Clinical findings, prescription, and recommendations are to the multidisciplinary team member closer to the patient and recorded into the patient electronic medical dossier.
Telemonitoring *(using Pervasive/Ubiquitous Computing)*	A study (Hersh, JA, PK, & Al., 2001) shows that Telemonitoring particularly homecare and pervasive computing, even in developed countries, can improve access to healthcare; increases satisfaction with delivered care, and may be cost-effective. Chronic patients can be monitored anywhere anytime using this functionality. Modern measuring instruments are connected to the patient's mobile phone. The patient's mobile phone will be used as a terminal that saves the received data into the central database using a Remote Procedure Call (RPC) for standard applications (low-level safety and security) and Restful Services for safety- and security-critical applications.
Data basis for Exchange of Experience	A database for medical intervention, treatments as well as experimental treatment procedures containing anonymous patient data and accessible for every physician presents the basis for exchange experiences. The data from the database would be integrated into a data warehouse, which, in turn, serves as a repository for data mining Business activities.
Patient Education and Continuous Education for the Medical Personnel	This functionality offers virtual seminars and learns room, scientific journals, webinars for continuous education. It further features a health relating information dissemination module intended for the patient education.
Adherence to Treatment Reminder	The reminder system is set at the start of any treatment so that it reminds the patient to take his treatment. It also reminds the caregiver to check whether the patient follows the treatment properly and visits the medical doctor for scheduled appointments. It is possible to include the patient relatives into this process so that they can also look at the patient and be sure that the patient regularly adheres to the treatment. The adherence workflow requires the medication parameter such as start and end date, time and time interval where the medicine should be taken. The system calls at the set time and requests the patient to take his medicine and notify the system about this. The patient will be reminded three times. The system would then call a patient's relative or the next health center or the treating doctor/nurse. The third person should bring the patient to adhere to the medication. Once the patient takes the medicine, he has to record this into the system (warehouse) so that at the end of the medication the treating doctor can analyze the recorded data and take accordingly a decision in the case of unsuccessful treatment.

Developed Countries: ICT Based Solution Approaches

The major challenges facing the health systems in the developed world are: (i) long waiting times to access specialized care, to visit a General Practitioner, (ii) limited access to healthcare services in rural areas, (iii) poor accommodation to patient needs (chronic diseases), (iv) less accurate diseases surveillance tools and policies, (v) lack of interconnection of all actors within a health system.

The minor challenges are poor access to certain drugs (ex. tropical infections) and workforce shortage.

SOLUTION APPROACHES

Poor Access to Scarcely Used Drugs for Non-Endemic Infections

To meet the minor challenges such as poor access to certain drugs, a reverse innovation approach can be applied herein using the Drug Supply Systems implemented for helping to purchase drugs in the developing countries.

Limited Access to Healthcare Services in Rural Areas

The proposed remote care system for developing countries can be also adapted to meet the limited access to healthcare in rural regions. The pervasive data collection unit can be used to pervasively screen the patient and thus collect significant data about infections. Traditional practitioners do not exist in the healthcare system of the developed countries. Therefore, the multidisciplinary team can be reduced to (i) Social/welfare worker, (ii) remote physician, (iii) nursing house, and (iv) mobile nurses

The global aims of the adapted remote care system are:

1. Improving the accessibility of primary healthcare services in rural regions
2. Reduce the overall cost of healthcare using telehealth
3. Launching ePrescrition to automatically collect pharmaceutical data
4. Enable the interconnection within a health system
5. Ubiquitous/Pervasive diseases surveillance
6. Reducing the waiting time to specialized care through telehealth (patient can be connected to remote specialist)

The medical workforce shortage issues can be partially solved using asynchronous telehealthcare solution, where the patient can asynchronously be examined by a doctor.

Poor Accommodation to Patient Needs and Chronic Diseases

Western countries are facing more migration issues than the other part of the world. We can notice the recent waves of refugees coming from Syria, Palestine, Africa, and others to Europe. Each ethnic group brings his cultural and economic problems to the host country. These cultural and economic issues impact the healthcare delivery system in the host country. In the USA, each citizen has to subscribe himself or through his employer a healthcare insurance. People older than 64 years benefit from a government health insurance. In this case, elderly refugees become a charge for the welfare fund. The young refugees or immigrants must pay for their own health. In Europe, we have another situation, where all legal immigration is included in the health insurance system, without contributing to fund the system. This fact reduces the financial resources in the healthcare system and thus impact negatively the care delivery in the system. Treatment für chronic is cost and time intensive. Due to the reducing financial resource, workforce shortage, lack efficient communication between the actors in the system, and lack of treatment policies regarding chronic diseases, elderly and in general chronic diseases patient do not receive appropriate treatment. In addition, the different cultural means present server limitation for the care delivery.

The Western countries populations are fast becoming elderly. Many elderly people are suffering from age relating chronic diseases, have cognitive decline. Elderly people living with age relating impairments have special needs. However, the healthcare systems in the developed countries are not prepared to face the above presented Issues.

To What Extent ICT/Telehealthcare Can Help to Solve the Challenge?

A Patient@Home (Homecare) and telehealth-based on well-defined treatment policies for chronic diseases have the potentiality to reduce the medical costs, provide appreciate treatment to the patient. The elderly people can stay at home as long as they are able to take care of themselves and use Patient@

Home solution. An electronic health system based on pervasive/ubiquitous computing could enable to permanently collect data on the chronic disease, analyze the data and provide an appropriate cost effective and efficient treatment at an opportune time to the patient. An EMR in a central database would facilitate a teamwork and the communication between the actors.

Diseases Surveillance Tools and Policies

The high-income countries have several policies and infrastructures for diseases surveillance. For example, Centers for Diseases Control and Prevention[7] (CDC) in the USA, European Center for Diseases Prevention and Control[8] in Europe. However, studies have shown that the current policies are limited. One of limitation of the current policies is due to the way the data are collected. For example, the patient reports to the physician any infection he is suffering from. Studies have shown that only a few patients go to the doctor and report an infection. This fact shows the weakness of the policies.

As a solution, we propose two ways: (i) incentive to encourage the population to report infections, (ii) a technical tool to opportunistically and participatory collect the information.

- **Incentive:** The government should declare the report of infections as mandatory. Though, it will difficult to control the population, so, an incentive system should be implemented.
- **Technical Tools:** Nowadays, almost everyone has a smartphone with internet access. We propose to implement a web-application the patient can use to report his infection. Once the infection is collected a public medical officer would visit the patient if he cannot attend the care unit. The officer will examine the patient and thus collect the necessary data and send it to the disease control unit.

Interconnected the Actors Within a Health System

There already exist in German significant ICT infrastructures and a good technical level. The country counts many IT specialists and several IT companies. All hospitals and clinics have launched since 2003 EMR systems and other data processing tools in their daily operations. However, the care units are not interconnected with each other to electronically exchange data and information.

A central database for patient medical data as well as a central data warehouse would centralize all medical with the possibility that each unit has his data and has the duty to replicate these data to the central database. Any authorized person can then access anywhere anytime the data. This is the way to interconnect the actors in the healthcare system.

EXPERIMENTS AND RESULTS

Access to Pharmaceutical Care Services

Problem Understanding

We collected various information during the test, both from interviews and conversations and from own experience. A major part concerned security aspects (see details in (Thierry Oscar Edoh & Teege, 2011)).

Feasibility

The mobile phone network provided a sufficient communication basis for the system. Network coverage existed in all test areas. The test showed that mobile phones are appropriate for processing an order, particularly in rural regions or regions without cyber cafés. The communication costs are reasonably low.

The test also confirmed the problems of delivery and payment, especially in rural regions. One specific problem occurred with cash payment on delivery. For security reasons, pharmacies prefer to hand out ordered medicine to a carrier only against prepayment. However, often the carrier had not enough cash. The alternative would have been to first collect the money from the customer and then fetch the medicine at the pharmacy. This may require additional tours by the carrier. The problem should disappear with an organized supplying service which is better trusted by the pharmacies.

Action Research

The test was conducted for about 2 weeks simultaneously in the test areas. During this time, a total of 434 volunteer patients used the system (Table 11). We interpret this as support for our hypothesis 95.6% of the test participants were villagers and many of them were women, predominantly mothers with

Table 11. Test participants and results

Participants	Genre	Large cities	Villages/Slum	Total
N=434	Females	6 (37,5%)	406 (97,13%)	412 (94,93%)
	Males	10 (62,5%)	12 (2,87%)	22 (5,07%)
Total		16 (100%)	418 (100%)	434 (100%)

small children from baby to children of 6 years of age. The highest participation was in test area I, as expected. However, the system was also used in the other two test areas and the participants were satisfied with the experience. We also succeeded in the purpose of the system implementation. Compared to the normal process, when the patients had to search and purchase the medicines by themselves, time and effort were substantially reduced.

Without the system, people, mainly in rural regions need one to three weeks to purchase a medicine. In addition, they must pay high transportation costs for traveling to several pharmacies. Using the system, the participants received the ordered medicine within two days. We thus reduced the time by up to 90%. Also, the transport expenses have been reduced.

Resistance

We encountered relatively few resistances to EpharmacyNet usage. The women accepted the system sooner than the male patients and appeared very satisfied with it. Some cases of refusal to use the system were due to a lack of trust. We address the general aspect of trust in "The trustee concept".

Access to Healthcare Care Services

Rapid Prototyping and Problem Understanding

For the test purpose, we implemented a prototype of the proposed system. We simulate a medical case and built a multidisciplinary team (MP). Each team member received a mobile smartphone. As communication platforms, we select Skype, WhatsApp, and Google Hangout.

We involved an experienced traditional practitioner. He can read and write. He also speaks and understands French.

Scenario 1

The rural population is informed about the test. The traditional practitioner (TP) can speak and understand the local tongue, so he communicates with the villagers in the local tongue.

The population visits the TP for any affection. The TP contact the head of the MP on one hand to define the tasks and in another to proceed with the diagnostics assisted by the (remote) care expert.

The MP defines and assigns to each member a task with exactly defined workflow.

Scenario 2

The patient uses his (smart)phone to contact directly the next care unit for a teleconsultation. The patient is requested to provide pictures and supplement materials to ease the diagnostics.

The MP is built and defines, in turn, the tasks and assigns them to the team members.

Data Gathering

We collected different data during the prior stages. The collected data helped to design the present prototype of the remote care delivery system. The collected data concern the care accessibility.

During the test, we collect again several data about the accessibility so that we can compare them with the previously collected data and perform a data analytics.

Feasibility

We used all selected instant message tools (Skype, WhatsApp, and Hangout) for simulating the mobile computer supported collaborative work. All the tools performed good results. We could send and receive large files, asynchronously and synchronously discuss. However, sending large files consumes many resources and take longer because of too small bandwidth in the entire country. We faced also high latency issues.

The test reveals that the organization must be accurate, the tasks must be good planned and assigned to the person with the needed competence. Additionally, a workflow is needed to be presented before starting the treatment.

Obviously, the TP involved in the test faced some understanding issues due to the weak knowledge of the French tongue. 1/3 of the instructions from the remote physician were wrongly implemented. This shows the limitation of the system and the need for an automated translator and medical dictionaries for each local tongue. Beyond this, 2/3 all written messages from the TP were incomprehensible. So, he was requested to only use the vocal message in his mother tongue.

We figure out that the TP could provide better diagnosis using this system and with the help of the remote physician. The treated patients (88%) have appreciated the treatment process as they were supported by a multidisciplinary team and can facile access to pharmaceutical products. 12% claim that a lot of people are involved in their treatment and thus fear to lose their intimacy and privacy, and a lot of people would know more than necessary on the healthy.

The test is still running. Till now, only 35 patients and 86 medical treatment are recorded into the system.

Action Research

The challenges facing, during the test, are collecting and analyzing. The prototype is improving regarding the results of the running analysis.

Our goal is to attend 5000 patients and about 15000 medical treatment cases and collect significant data so that we can perform a good action research.

FUTURE WORKS

Impact of Involving the Traditional Practitioners

The focus of our future work will be to investigate the impact of involving the traditional practitioners on (i) the quality of the healthcare delivery and (ii) workforce shortage. Since we are dealing with a multidisciplinary team, which work on a project (medical treatment), or one team member works on different projects at the same time, we could face many-to-one (many health caregivers, one patient) or many-to-many (many caregivers, many patients) relationship. So, it will be important to optimize the scaling problem that will be issued by the proposed system. The objective of the work will be to scale the agility in the care delivery process. We have in mind to use the scaling agile approach practiced in IT world.

Adherence to Treatment

The adherence to treatment is a matter pre-requisite for successful treatment. It is then important to investigate how the proposed system impacts the adherence to treatment.

Understanding Barriers (Tongue Issues)

Speech-based applications and systems (spoken dialogue and multimodal systems) are actually being implemented for a broad range of domains and applications such as medical applications, tourist guide systems, and so on (Bell, 2003)(Green, 2009). These kinds of systems or applications using speech as the principal mode of interaction will become increasingly prevalent (Fitzgerald, College, Net, & Firby, 2002).

To increase the usability of the proposed system, we would design and provide a multimodal interface and spoken dialogue interface to the users.

Interconnection of All Stakeholder in the German Care System

It is very hard to get authorized to test the proposed system for Germany. Patient data are specially protected by the law. We are in planning how to get the health-bodies to adhere to the project and let us perform the test. This test will be the focus of our future works.

CONCLUSION

In developing countries, the challenges facing public health systems are caused by the lack of organization, poor healthcare infrastructure, lack of qualified personnel, and weak funding (e.g. lack of adequate health insurance). These challenges could be addressed by information technology solutions; however, it is often not possible to implement solutions from developed countries without adapting them, because of the technology level in these countries and the cultural manner.

The developed countries have very good technologic infrastructures and structures to tackle the challenges facing their healthcare. Though, most of the solutions proposed need legal improvement that will lead to the implementation of the solution.

In this chapter, the author has proposed a virtual Hospital-network Solution that uses Telehealthcare and wireless sensor network technologies to provide pervasive/ubiquitous healthcare service to the population. It is aimed at enabling remote assistance to the undertrained caregivers, collaborating work between care professionals, delivery of remote healthcare to the patient at home, and educate the patient. The system additionally involves traditional practitioners and trains them to perform medical diagnostic.

In a prior study (Thierry Oscar Edoh & Teege, 2011), the access to pharmaceutical care was investigated. An E-commerce solution was proposed to overcome the issues. However, the implementation faced a set of obstacles for launching a standard E-commerce system. The obstacles were then analyzed, and workaround solutions were elaborated so that an adapted E-commerce system can be implemented.

A practical test has shown that the adapted E-commerce system has the potential to improve the pharmaceutical care delivery in the entire country no matter where the patient is living or resides. The adapted E-commerce system therefore extended to a multidisciplinary remote healthcare system to improve and increase the access to healthcare services.

The proposed solution approaches are based on ICT networking technology, which in turn needs a high and stable internet connection and reliable network services, high latency. However, the country is not yet entirely covered with mobile internet and, thus, mobile data services cannot be used everywhere. Though, since SMS and MMS are well implemented, everywhere available, and stable, the authors combine both mobile internet, where it is available, and mobile phone services to provide the telehealthcare to the population.

Regarding the internet connection challenges facing, the upcoming experimental will focus on the use of LI-WI to overcome the challenges.

Further, a novel Internet of Things technology to improve the efficiency of data collection from sensors to a collector in a low-power lossy network (i.e., the sensor network) will be implemented. A de-verticalized middleware to expose the different data and services with a unique interface, on top of which vertical application can also be created.

REFERENCES

AAID. (2015). *The Impact of Access to Quality Healthcare in Africa Research findings on Health Insurance Fund supported programs.* Retrieved from http://aiid.org/website/wp-content/uploads/2015/12/The-Impact-of-Access-to-Quality-Healthcare-in-Africa-Research-findings-on-Health-Insurance-Fund-supported-programs.pdf

Abaidoo, B., & Larweh, B. T. (2014). Consumer Health Informatics. *The Application of ICT in Improving Patient-Provider Partnership for a Better Health Care, 6*(2), 1–9. doi:10.5210/ojphi.v6i2.4903 PMID:25422724

Acharya, A. S., Prakash, A., Saxena, P., & Nigam, A. (2013). *Sampling: Why and How of it?* Academic Press.

Adeya, G., & Cavanaugh, K. (2007). Rapid Assessment of the Health System in Benin, April 2006. U.S. Agency for International Development.

Adler-Milstein, J., Sarma, N., Woskie, L. R., & Jha, A. K. (2014). A Comparison Of How Four Countries Use Health IT To Support Care For People With Chronic Conditions. *Health Affairs, 33*(9), 1559–1566. doi:10.1377/hlthaff.2014.0424 PMID:25201660

Africa, W. R. O. for. (2011). African Health Monitor. *Serial Publication of the World Health Organization Regional Office for Africa, 6136*(14). Retrieved from https://www.aho.afro.who.int/sites/default/files/ahm/issues/27/ahm-issue-14.pdf

Barkan, S. (2010). *Social Problems: Continuity and Change. Flat World Education*. Retrieved from http://catalog.flatworldknowledge.com/bookhub/reader/3064?e=barkansoc_1.0-ch02_s05

Bell, L. (2003). *Linguistic Adaptations in Spoken Human – Computer Dialogues Empirical Studies of User Behavior*. Academic Press.

Biesdorf, S., Deetjen, U., & Möller, M. (2016). *Eine Vision für ein digitales Gesundheits system in Deutschland.* McKinsey & Company.

Binder, L. (2013). *The Five Biggest Problems In Health Care Today.* Forbes.com.

Braa, J., & Hedberg, C. (2000). *Developing district-based Health Care Information Systems: The South African experience*. Iris.

Braa, J. J., & Hedberg, C. (2002). The struggle for district-based health information systems in South Africa. *The Information Society*, *18*(2), 113–127. doi:10.1080/01972240290075048

Brandeau, M., Sainfort, F., & Pierskalla, W. (2005). Health Care Delivery: Current Problems and Future Challenges. *Operations Research for Health Care*, 1–14. doi:10.1007/1-4020-8066-2_1

Busse, R., & Riesberg, A. (2004). Health Care Systems in Transition. *Copenhagen. WHO Regional Office for Europe on Behalf of the European Observatory on Health Systems and Policies*, *6*(9), 1–242.

Chhanabhai, P. N., & Holt, A. (2010). The Disparity Information and Communication Technology Developing Countries has in the Delivery of Healthcare Information. *The Open Medical Informatics Journal*, *4*, 195–201. doi:10.2174/1874431101004010195 PMID:21594006

Chib, A., Velthoven, M. H. Van, Car, J., & Helena, M. (2015). mHealth Adoption in Low-Resource Environments: A Review of the Use of Mobile Healthcare in Developing Countries. *Journal of Health Communication, 20*, 4–34. 10.1080/10810730.2013.864735

Edoh, T. O. (2010a). *ICT-Systeme zur Verbesserung der Gesundheitsversorg ung in den Gesundheitssystemen der afrikanischen Entwicklungsl änder. Fallstudien: Benin*. Universität der Bundeswehr. Retrieved from https://athene-forschung.unibw.de/doc/88986/88986.pdf

Edoh, T. O. (2010b). *ICT-Systeme zur Verbesserung der Gesundheitsversorgung in den Gesundheitssystemen der afrikanischen Entwicklungsländer.* Universität der Bundeswehr München: Athene-Forschung. Retrieved from https://athene-forschung.unibw.de/node?id=88986

Edoh, T. O., & Teege, G. (2010). EPharmacyNet: An approach to improve the pharmaceutical care delivery in developing countries-study case - BENIN. In *IHI'10 - Proceedings of the 1st ACM International Health Informatics Symposium* (pp. 859–863). 10.1145/1882992.1883125

Edoh, T. O., & Teege, G. (2011). Using information technology for an improved pharmaceutical care delivery in developing countries. Study case: Benin. *Journal of Medical Systems*, *35*(5), 1123–1134. doi:10.100710916-011-9717-y PMID:21519942

Edoh, T. O. C., Atchome, A., Alahassa, B. R. U., & Pawar, P. (2016). Evaluation of a Multi-Tier Heterogeneous Sensor Network for Patient Monitoring – The Case of Benin. In *MMHealth '16 Proceedings of the 2016 ACM Workshop on Multimedia for Personal Health and Health Care* (pp. 23–29). Amsterdam, The Netherlands: ACM Digital Library. 10.1145/2985766.2985772

English, M., Irimu, G., Agweyu, A., Gathara, D., & Oliwa, J. (2016). Building Learning Health Systems to Accelerate Research and Improve Outcomes of Clinical Care in Low- and Middle-Income Countries. *PLoS Med, 13*(4), 1–8. 10.1371/journal.pmed.1001991

Europol. (2015). *Situation Report on Counterfeiting in the European Union.* Retrieved from https://euipo.europa.eu/ohimportal/documents/11370/80606/2015+Situation+Report+on+Counterfeiting+in+the+EU

Fitzgerald, W., & Firby, R. J. (2002). Dialogue-based human-computer interfaces and active language understanding. *International Journal of Cognitive Technology, 1*(2), 275–286. doi:10.1075/ijct.1.2.04fit

Gerring, J. (2004). What Is a Case Study and What Is It Good for? *The American Political Science Review, 98*(2), 341–354. doi:10.1017/S0003055404001182

Green, A. (2009). *Designing and Evaluating Human-Robot Communication Doctoral Thesis in.* Academic Press.

Greiner, A., & Knebel, E. (2003). *Health Professions Education: A Bridge to Quality.* Academic Press. 10.17226/10681

Greiner, A. C., & Knebel, E. (2003). *Health Professions Education. Health Professions Education: A Bridge to Quality.* Washington, DC: National Academies Press; doi:10.17226/10681

Harrison, R., Cohen, S. A. W., & Walton, M. (2015, May). Patient safety and quality of care in developing countries in Southeast Asia : A systematic literature review Patient safety and quality of care in developing countries in Southeast Asia : a systematic literature review. *International Journal for Quality in Health Care*, 1–15. 10.1093/intqhc/mzv041

Haveman, H., & Flim, C. (2007). eHealth strategy and implementation activities in the Netherlands. *Report in the Framework of the eHealth*, 1–20. Retrieved from http://ehealth-strategies.eu/database/documents/Netherlands_eHealth-ERA_country_report.pdf

Heil, J., ter Waarbeek, H. L. G., Hoebe, C. J. P. A., Jacobs, P. H. A., van Dam, D. W., Trienekens, T. A. M., ... Dukers-Muijrers, N. H. T. M. (2017). Pertussis surveillance and control: Exploring variations and delays in testing, laboratory diagnostics and public health service notifications, the Netherlands, 2010 to 2013. *Eurosurveillance*, *22*(28), 1–8. doi:10.2807/1560-7917.ES.2017.22.28.30571 PMID:28749331

Hersh, W. R. (2001). Telemedicine for the Medicare Population. Rockville, MD: Agency for Healthcare Research and Quality (US).

Hope, K. R. (1999). *Corruption and Development in Africa* (K. R. Hope & B. C. Chikulo, Eds.). Basingstoke, UK: Palgrave Macmillan; doi:10.1057/9780333982440

IQWiG. (2017a). *Gesundheitsversorgung in Deutschland*. Retrieved from https://www.gesundheitsinformation.de/das-deutsche-gesundheitssystem.2698.de.html?part=einleitung-co

IQWiG. (2017b). *Gesundheitsversorgung in Deutschland*. Retrieved from www.gesundheitinformation.de

Jha, A. K., Doolan, D., Grandt, D., Scott, T., Bates, D. W., Technology, I., … Service, H. (2008). *The use of health information technology in seven nations*. Academic Press. 10.1016/j.ijmedinf.2008.06.007

Keeton, C. (2012). *Measuring the impact of e-health*. Academic Press. 10.2471/BLT.12.020512

Khani, R. (2015). *Improving Waiting Time and Patients' Experience in a Medical Retina Clinic*. Dublin, Ireland: Royal College of Surgeons in Ireland.

Kinoshita, T., Tokumasu, H., Tanaka, S., Kramer, A., & Kawakami, K. (2017). Policy implementation for methicillin-resistant *Staphylococcus aureus* in seven European countries: A comparative analysis from 1999 to 2015. *Journal of Market Access & Health Policy*, *5*(1), 1351293. doi:10.1080/20016689.2017.1351293 PMID:28804601

Klein, T. (2005). *Befindensweisen und therapeutische Wege in Dendougou, Benin* (Doctoral Thesis). Institut für Völkerkunde Universität zu Köln (University of Cologne).

Knickman, J. R., & Kovner, A. R. (2015). *Health Care Delivery in the United States*. Academic Press.

Kopetsche, D. T. (2010). *Dem deutschen Gesundheitswesen gehen die Ärzte aus!* Academic Press.

Latham, B. (2007). *Sampling: What is it?* Academic Press.

Liu, S., Luo, Y., & Yang, S. (2007). Shape-based pedestrian detection in infrared images. *Journal of Information Science and Engineering*, *23*(1), 271–283.

Mackey, T. K., & Liang, B. (2012). Combating healthcare corruption and fraud with improved global health governance. *BMC International Health and Human Rights*, *12*(1), 23. doi:10.1186/1472-698X-12-23 PMID:23088820

Maniatopoulos, G., Maniatopoulos, G., Mcloughlin, I., Mcloughlin, I., Wilson, R., Wilson, R., ... Martin, M. (2009). Developing Virtual Healthcare Systems in Complex Multi- Agency Service Settings: The OLDES Project. *Electronic Journal of E-Government*, *7*(2), 163–170.

Mars, M., Seebregts, C., & Rockefeller Foundation. (2008). Country Case Study for e-Health: South Africa. *E-Health Connections: Country Case Study Reports*, 1–46. Retrieved from http://ehealth-connection.org/files/resources/County Case Study for eHealth South Africa.pdf

Mathias, F., Amoussou, R. K., Acakpo, S. A., Zountcheme, S. A., Koukoui, N. R. Y., … Mama, R. S. (2013). *Annuaire des statistiques sanitaires annee 2013*. Retrieved from http://www.sante.gouv.bj/documents/Annuaire_2013.pdf

Mayosi, B. M., Ch, B., Phil, D., Benatar, S. R., Ch, B., & Med, D. S. (2014). Special report Health and Health Care in South Africa — 20 Years after Mandela. *The New England Journal of Medicine*.

Ministere de la santé, repiblique du B. (2007). *Evaluation du systeme national d ' information et de gestion sanitaires (SNIGS) du Benin*. Retrieved from http://www.who.int/healthmetrics/library/countries/HMN_BEN_Assess_Draft_2007_05_fr.pdf

Morgan, K. L., Rahman, M., Macey, S., Atkinson, M. D., Hill, R. A., Khanom, A., ... Brophy, S. T. (2014). Obesity in pregnancy: A retrospective prevalence-based study on health service utilisation and costs on the NHS. *BMJ Open*, *4*(2), e003983. doi:10.1136/bmjopen-2013-003983 PMID:24578535

Nanda, H., & Davis, L. (n.d.). Probabilistic template based pedestrian detection in infrared videos. In *Intelligent Vehicle Symposium* (Vol. 1, pp. 15–20). IEEE. 10.1109/IVS.2002.1187921

National Instruments. (2016). *Fundamentals of Fiber Bragg Grating (FBG) Optical Sensing*. Retrieved from http://www.ni.com/white-paper/11821/en/

NEPAD. (2007). *Africa Health Strategy: 2007 – 2015*. Retrieved from http://www.nepad.org/system/files/AFRICA_HEALTH_STRATEGY(health).pdf

Niclasen, B., & Mulvad, G. (2010). Health care and health care delivery in Greenland. *International Journal of Circumpolar Health*, *69*(5), 437–447. doi:10.3402/ijch.v69i5.17691 PMID:21118636

Nidhi, K., Indrajeet, S., Khushboo, M., Gauri, K., & Sen, D. J. (2011). Hydrotropy: A promising tool for solubility enhancement: A review. *International Journal of Drug Development and Research*, *3*(2), 26–33. doi:10.1002/jps

Paolotti, D., Carnahan, A., Colizza, V., Eames, K., Edmunds, J., Gomes, G., ... Vespignani, A. (2014). Web-based participatory surveillance of infectious diseases: The Influenzanet participatory surveillance experience. *Clinical Microbiology and Infection*, *20*(1), 17–21. doi:10.1111/1469-0691.12477 PMID:24350723

Ridic, G., Gleason, S., & Ridic, O. (2012). *Comparisons of Health Care Systems in the United States, Germany and Canada*. Academic Press. doi:10.5455/msm.2012.24.112-120.Comparisons

Rotich, J. K. (2003). Installing and Implementing a Computer-based Patient Record System in Sub-Saharan Africa: The Mosoriot Medical Record System. *Journal of the American Medical Informatics Association*, *10*(4), 295–303. doi:10.1197/jamia.M1301 PMID:12668697

Schoen, C., Davis, K., How, S. K. H., & Schoenbaum, S. C. (2006). *U.S. Health System Performance: A National Scorecard*. Academic Press. 10.1377/hlthaff.25.w457

Schoen, C., Osborn, R., Doty, M. M., Squires, D., Peugh, J., & Applebaum, S. (2009). A Survey Of Primary Care Physicians In Eleven Countries, 2009: Perspectives On Care, Costs, And Experiences. *Health Affairs*, *28*(6), w1171–w1183. doi:10.1377/hlthaff.28.6.w1171 PMID:19884491

Schoen, C., Osborn, R., Huynh, P. T., Doty, M., Zapert, K., Peugh, J., & Davis, K. (2005). Taking the pulse of health care systems: experiences of patients with health problems in six countries. *Health Affairs (Project Hope), Suppl Web*. 10.1377/hlthaff.w5.509

Schrott, G., & Gluckler, J. (2004). What makes mobile computer supported cooperative work mobile? Towards a better understanding of cooperative mobile interactions. *HCI Issues in Mobile Computing, 60*(5–6), 737–752.

Scott, R. E., & Mars, M. (2015). *Telehealth in the developing world: Current status and future prospects*. Academic Press.

Shih, A., & Davis, K. (2008). *Organizing the U. S. Health care Delivery System for High Performance*. Retrieved from www.commonwealthfund.org

Sikhondze, N. C., & Erasmus, L. (2016). Electronic medical records: A developing and developed country analysis. In *IAMOT 2016 Conference* (pp. 273–290). Academic Press.

Sluizer, S., & Cashman, P. (1984). XCP: An experimental tool for supporting office procedures. Proceedings. *IEEE-CS Press First International Conference on Office Automation*, 73–80.

Srivastava, A., Bilal, I. A., Preety, R., & Sanghita, B. (2015). Determinants of women's satisfaction with maternal health care : a review of literature from developing countries. *Biomed Central*, 1–12. 10.1186/s12884-015-0525-0

Steele, D., & Cylus, J. (2012). United Kingdom (Scotland) Health system review. *Health Systems in Transition, 14*(9), 1–150. PMID:23579054

Sturm, R. (2002). The effects of obesity, smoking, and drinking on medical problems and costs. *Health Affairs, 21*(2), 245–253. doi:10.1377/hlthaff.21.2.245 PMID:11900166

Williams, F., Austin, S., & Mha, B. (2008). The role of the electronic medical record (EMR) in care delivery development in developing countries: A systematic review. *Informatics in Primary Care, 16*, 139–145. doi:10.14236/jhi.v16i2.685 PMID:18713530

Williamson, L., Heywood, A. B., Williamson, L., Stoops, N., & Heywood, A. (2015). *Developing a District Health Information System in South Africa: A Social Process or Technical Solution? Studies in Health Technology and Informatics*. IOS Press. Retrieved from http://iospress.metapress.com/content/2mtquupfwbj5amyf/

ENDNOTES

1. www.casala.ie/www.netwellcentre.org
2. http://www.amdtelemedicine.com/success-stories/CustomerSuccess-Greenland.html
3. http://www.beninsante.bj/documents/DPP/CDMT_09_06_2010_FINAL.pdf
4. https://www.united-europe.eu/news-and-opinions/what-others-write/europes-healthcare-systems-face-reform-to-meet-growing-challenges/
5. http://www.itu.int/ITU-D/pdf/fg7/telegreen006.html
6. http://www.theglobaleconomy.com/Benin/Mobile_phone_subscribers/
7. https://www.cdc.gov/
8. https://ecdc.europa.eu/en

Chapter 2
Scale the Agility in a Multidisciplinary Remote Care Services Delivery System

ABSTRACT

The main objectives of healthcare systems are to provide healthcare services delivery to populations for health promotion, diseases prevention, and treatment. Healthcare systems can use the telemedicine paradigm or traditional direct care approach to deliver health services to the population. Healthcare delivery activities include simple activities, predictable (e.g., curing a small injury), as well as unpredictable, variable, and complex activities (e.g., heart disease treatment). Agile healthcare, learning from the agile software development methodology, seems to be an approach today to face the complexity of healthcare delivery. This chapter discusses how an agile paradigm can help to better coordinate healthcare delivery within the remote care system.

INTRODUCTION

Chapter 1 presented a multidisciplinary care team (MCT) as support for a proposed remote care delivery system. The MCT consists of healthcare and para-medical professionals as well as technical personnel. The MCT has to perform planned and unpredictable tasks every day. The more the team and project's tasks sizes increase the more performing the tasks becomes very

DOI: 10.4018/978-1-5225-5528-5.ch002

complex. Team members must regularly harmonize their work plans, have grooming meeting, coordinate each step of assigned tasks.

Medical treatment is a dynamic process, whose requirements can continually change according to the course of disease pattern or clinical pictures. This aspect of the healthcare delivery leads to the unpredictability and can render healthcare services delivery complex in certain cases. Therefore, physicians and entire medical treating team must quickly react to any change and change the course of the treatment accordingly. Precisely for this reason, adopting the agile methodology like Scrum in providing healthcare can present certain benefits and help to meet the high-level of complexity and uncertainty that can be faced.

Recently, the agile methodology is proposed as methodology approach for improving the healthcare services delivery. However, agile methodology is not yet implemented in the medical field (Fujita & Guizzi, 2015). In (Williams, 2017), the recognition that research in agile healthcare is limited. Sara Tolf et al., though, investigate in (Qin, Prybutok, Prybutok, & Wang, 2015) the agility approach in hospitals and point out five cornerstones that hospitals should build to optimally use the agile methodology in their care delivery systems. They state their finding as follows:

... Five organizational capacities were derived as necessary for hospitals to use the strategies optimally: transparent and transient inter-organizational links; market sensitivity and customer focus; management by support for self-organizing employees; organic structures that are elastic and responsive; flexible human and resource capacity for timely delivery...

The authors demonstrate how agile methodology can contribute to face uncertainty and flexibility in healthcare services delivery. We retain two matter points from the findings cited above: transparent and transient inter-organizational links and management by support for self-organizing employees. The mean "Self-organizing employees" implies flexible human and resource capacity for timely delivery. According to the authors, the transparent and transient inter-organizational links more focus on the interaction between an organization and its surrounding context where the key feature is to create relationships with the stakeholders in the external environment. This study indicates the increasing interest in developing or implementing agile healthcare to meet the increasing uncertainty, complexity of the healthcare services delivery, and the flexibility requested by a dynamic medical process.

The global healthcare system is facing low resources issues, e.g. understaffed care units, brain drain, workforce shortage. Developing countries are more affected than high-income countries. It is, therefore, important to implement an approach that can provide more valuable and efficient healthcare services to the population with fewer resources e.g. a small number of healthcare personnel, financial resources. Lean Methodology is an appropriate methodology supporting this approach. Lean methodology pursues the objectives to continuously improve its process so, to achieve the zero waste. Is an Improved healthcare services delivery process sufficient to meet or overcome uncertainty and flexibility in a dynamic system like medical treatment system? As indicated in (Fujita & Guizzi, 2015), the implementation of lean, so-called lean healthcare management, can increase or improve the healthcare performance, though, cannot handle the uncertainty and the flexibility issues healthcare services delivery can be faced. Giuseppe Converso et al. propose an agile logic in the chapter "A System Dynamics Model for Bed Management Strategy in Health Care Units" in the book, to overcome the high-level of complexity and uncertainty inherent to healthcare.

Agile healthcare is defined as a flexible managing approach to deliver healthcare to the populations and meet almost uncertainty that can be faced. It includes personalized care in term of Patient-center-care (PCC) and flexibility in the delivery of care services. PCC takes into consideration the patient's points. He defines the care and the physician implements it. The care is a target to the individual patient's needs (Tsuyuki & Krass, 2013). Table 1 summarizes the activities and characteristics of agile healthcare.

Eric King, from SolutionsIQ, and Victoria King, MD, report in an article entitled "*A Family Practice Transformation Based on Continual Learning and Adaptation*"[1] an interesting experience with agile healthcare at a family

Table 1. Summary of agile healthcare activities

Activity	Agile Healthcare Characteristics
Commissioning	Co-produced Patient/Person-centered
Delivery of care	Ability to deliver care to patient demand and expectation
Service design	Holistic methodology integrating healthcare providers, business process, commissioners, and patients
Organisation	Ability to synthesize new productive capabilities from expertise of people and physical facilities regardless of their internal or external location
Management	Emphasis on leadership (clinical and management), support, motivation, and trust specialized, skilled, and innovative employees

Source:(Williams, 2017).

medical practice. The patient-population visiting the family practice was consisting of young, middle-aged, and elderly patients. Developing and continually enhancing an exemplary standard of care are highly required by the patients. The five-years-experience with agile healthcare at the family practice has demonstrated the ability of this approach to meet at any time any issue generated by operated or occurred changes in term of employees' size, process and procedure. Clinical teams are divided into small groups regarding given medical skills; the medicals skills are determined to be the backlog item, as known in agile development methodology in fields of software. Agile methodology is shown to be adaptable to any organizational structures beyond the software development ones. This positive experience leads to the question of scaling the agility in the case, where the medical team cannot be divided into small teams as in the experience described above.

Scaling the agility in an organizational structure requires another framework as the framework used by traditional agile that is team oriented and vertical while the scaling agile is more horizontal and enterprise level oriented. Scale Agile Healthcare (SAH) is, therefore, an agile at the hospital/clinics level. In our context, it is agile at the multidisciplinary remote healthcare services delivery system that involves the underlying. multidisciplinary team.

We proposed a multidisciplinary healthcare team, in Chapter 1, that is aiming to deliver PCC, assists the patient, provides the healthcare service on demand (to patient demand and expectation). The team can be considered as an agile development team. The patient's health represents the product and the patient himself the customer. He can get provided with healthcare services on demand and according to his expectation. The question arises here is to what extent the patient expectation is to achieve and how to measure them? Beyond this, it matters to know which kind of team is providing the care service. In the case of the single team, a traditional agile approach can be applied here. The proposed team is multidisciplinary and thus, their multiple teams that would join their efforts together to deliver appropriate care services to the populations. Many scenarios would be considered in the scope of this study. The first scenario requests that a patient is treated by many medical and/or para-medical teams (multiple teams). The teams can also treat many patients from different care units at the same time. The team's size can quickly increase. The course of the treatment can negatively change and becomes very complex. Another scenario is that a team handles many similar medical cases. Both scenarios are scaling agility scenarios that pose some challenges to be met.

The primary goal of the chapter is to discuss scale agile healthcare in the context of remote care as described in Chapter 1. It further aims to define a framework for facilitating scaling agility within the proposed remote care system.

The remainder of this chapter is structured as follows: description of the patient-centered-care and focused-care following be the description of Agile methodology. We present our framework and evaluate.

Patient- or Person-Centered-Care (PCC) vs. Focused-Care (PFC)

Patient-Centered-Care (PCC) and Patient-Focused-Care (PFC), although different, are both important. Barbara Starfield, MD, MPH describes in (Starfield, 2011) both terms as patient-centered care as visit-based and person-focused accumulated-knowledge of people based. According to the summary presented in form of table (Table 1), the PFC shows more advantages like better recognition of health problem and needs overtimes and thus ease appropriate care in the context of the needs. The author further compares both approaches and the findings are presented the table (Table 2).

PCC is mostly initiated by the patient and thus called as care on-demand and with respect to the patient expectations. There exists no global or universal definition of term PCC. Though, most existing definitions emphasize certain core elements of what PCC is. Respecting the patient's choice and effective communication are the core elements in most definitions (Kitson, Marshall, Bassett, & Zeitz, 2013). Alison Kitson et al. conduct a narrative

Table 2. Person-Centered-Care vs. Person-Focused-Care by Barbara Starfield, MD, MPH

Patient-centered care	Person-focused care
Generally refers to interactions in visits	Refers to interrelationships over time
May be episode oriented	Considers episodes as part of life-course experiences with health
Generally centers around the management of diseases	Views diseases as interrelated phenomena
Generally views comorbidity as number of chronic diseases	Often considers morbidity as combinations of types of illnesses (multimorbidity)
Generally views body systems as distinct	Views body systems as interrelated
Uses coding systems that reflect professionally defined conditions	Uses coding systems that also allow for specification of people's health concerns
Is concerned primarily with the evolution of patients' diseases	Is concerned with the evolution of people's experienced health problems as well as with their diseases

review (Kitson et al., 2013) on PCC and point out significant themes and sub-themes. They summarize these findings in three groups of themes: (i) *Patient participation and involvement*, (ii) *Relationship between the patient and the health professional*, and (iii) *The context where care is delivered.* The first theme requires to respect patient choice and to involve him in the care delivery process and procedure. The literature review points out three sub-themes in the first theme:

- Patient participating as a respected and autonomous individual
- Care plan based on patient's individual needs
- Addressing a patient's physical and emotional needs

The second theme is subdivided into four sub-themes and is mostly concerning the communication between the patient and treating healthcare professionals.

- Genuine clinician-patient relationship
- Open communication of knowledge, personal expertise, and clinical expertise between the patient and the professional
- Health professionals have appropriate skills and knowledge
- A cohesive and co-operative team of professionals

The third and last theme is concerning the system issues that can be a barrier to PCC.

This review reveals that PCC is mostly concerning the patient's involvement in his care means. Furthermore, the PCC rests on the communication a good relationship between the patient's the treating personnel. Barbara Starfield reports in (Starfield, 2011) the same core elements on which PCC rests, These core elements are communication or interaction and adherence to the recommendation concerning the care.

In (Tsuyuki & Krass, 2013), Rosst Tsuyuki et al. state the vision of PCC as:

It is a professional obligation to take responsibility for and provide care targeted to the individual patient's needs.

The responsibility includes six points like respect for the patient, communication by good listening to the patient, empower the patient, informing the patient, and assisting the patient in reaching his goals. The authors in (Williams, 2017) point out the same/similar findings.

In the lights of the above, the requirements and assignments to the proposed multidisciplinary are more matches to the requirements of PCC than of PFC.

On the Weblog" Oneviewhealthcare.com" of May 15th, 2017, PCC is defined as:

.... Patient-centered care is the practice of caring for patients (and their families) in ways that are meaningful and valuable to the individual patient. It includes listening to, informing and involving patients in their care. The IOM (Institute of Medicine) defines patient-centered care as: 'Providing care that is respectful of, and responsive to, individual patient preferences, needs and values, and ensuring that patient values guide all clinical decisions.'

This definition above includes all findings and can be considered as a definition's approach.

Picker Institute is a nonprofit entity founded by Jean and Harvey Picker to develop a scientific approach to measure how successfully the healthcare system delivers patient-centered care. The Picker Institute, therefore, defines eight (8) principles of patient-centered care. Table 3 summarizes these 8 principles described on their home website. For more details, videos placed on the site can be watched.

Table 3. Picker's eight principles of patient-centered care

Pos.	Príncipe	Description
1	Respect for patients' values, preferences and expressed needs	Patients want to be kept informed regarding their medical condition and involved in decision-making. Patients indicate that they want hospital staff to recognize and treat them in an atmosphere that is focused on the patient as an individual with a presenting medical condition. • illness and medical treatment may have an impact on quality of life. Care should be provided in an atmosphere that is respectful of the individual patient and focused on quality-of-life issues. • Informed and shared decision-making is a central component of patient-centered care. • Provide the patient with dignity, respect, and sensitivity to his/her cultural values.
2	Coordination and integration of care	Patients, in focus groups, expressed feeling vulnerable and powerless in the face of illness. Proper coordination of care can ease those feelings. Patients identified three areas in which care coordination can reduce feelings of vulnerability: • Coordination and integration of clinical care • Coordination and integration of ancillary and support services • Coordination and integration of front-line patient care

continued on following page

Table 3. Continued

Pos.	Príncipe	Description
3	Information, communication, and education	Patients often express the fear that information is being withheld from them and that they are not being completely informed about their medical condition or prognosis. Based on patient interviews, hospitals can focus on three kinds of communication to reduce these fears: • Information on clinical status, progress, and prognosis • Information on processes of care • Information and education to facilitate autonomy, self-care and health promotion
4	Physical comfort	The level of physical comfort patients report has a tremendous impact on their experience. From the patient's perspective, physical care that comforts patients, especially when they are acutely ill, is one of the most elemental services that caregivers can provide. Three areas were reported as particularly important to patients: • Pain management • Assistance with activities and daily living needs • Hospital surroundings and environment kept in focus, including ensuring that the patient's needs for privacy are accommodated and that patient areas are kept clean and comfortable, with appropriate accessibility for visits by family and friends.
5	Emotional support and alleviation of fear and anxiety	Fear and anxiety associated with illness can be as debilitating as the physical effects. Caregivers should pay attention to: • Anxiety over clinical status, treatment, and prognosis • Anxiety over the impact of the illness on themselves and family • Anxiety over the financial impact of illness
6	Involvement of family and friends	Patients continually addressed the role of family and friends in the patient experience, often expressing concern about the impact illness has on family and friends. These principles of patient-centered care were identified as follows: • Accommodation, by clinicians and caregivers, of family and friends on whom the patient relies on social and emotional support • Respect for and recognition of the patient "advocate's" role in decision-making • Support for family members as caregivers • Recognition of the needs of family and friends
7	Continuity and transition	Patients often express considerable anxiety about their ability to care for themselves after discharge. Meeting patient needs in this area require staff to: • Provide understandable, detailed information regarding medications, physical limitations, dietary needs, etc. • Coordinate and plan ongoing treatment and services after discharge and ensure that patients and family understand this information • Provide information regarding access to clinical, social, physical and financial support on a continuing basis
8	Access to care	Patients need to know they can access care when it is needed. Attention must also be given to time spent waiting for admission or time between admission and allocation to a bed in a ward. Focusing mainly on ambulatory care, the following areas were of importance to the patient: • Access to the location of hospitals, clinics and physician offices • Availability of transportation • Ease of scheduling appointments • Availability of appointments when needed • Accessibility to specialists or specialty services when a referral is made • Clear instructions provided on when and how to get referrals

Source: http://pickerinstitute.org/about/picker-principles/.

We identify five principles having similarities with agile principles. This demonstrates how agile healthcare and patient-centered care are tied to each other. We will discuss this similarity in the next section.

STANDARD AGILE VS. SCALE AGILE

This section compares the traditional Agile (team-oriented) and Scale Agile (Enterprise oriented) methodologies and their applications in the medical field (Agile Healthcare).

In the Computer Science, especially in the software development, there are a lot of methodologies and project organization and management tools intended for better software development operations. It is worth to emphasize two groups of software development methodology: (i) the classical and (ii) the agile methodology. The classical or old and conventional methodologies comprise the Waterfall-model, V-model, spiral-model, Iterative-model, Prototype-model. The agile methodologies are Incremental-model, RAD model, lean, scrum, XP, Kanban.

In the recent years, engineers are using more the agile software development methodology and project organization and management (POM) in the health IT development. The conventional medical IT development follows the classic way defined by FDA (US Food and Drug Administration) or CE (European Conformity). There are existed many norms to be followed during the development and marketing process. For medical devices and software produced for the European market, EN 62304 and directives like:

- Directive 90/385/EEC regarding active implantable medical devices
- Directive 93/42/EEC regarding medical devices
- Directive 98/79/EC regarding in vitro diagnostic medical devices

are defined. These norms have defined medical product development processes that have to be strictly followed, otherwise, the marketing authorization will be denied. Agile methodology is not comprised and not recommended by these norms, though, the trend today is to apply this methodology in developing IT medical products.

It is a matter to notice that agile health-IT or medical-IT development process and methodology is different from agile healthcare. Agile Health-IT is the use of Information Technology System in healthcare systems to deliver healthcare services, while agile healthcare is adopting agile methodology and process in delivering care services.

This section and the entire chapter would focus on agile healthcare only.

Like software development processes, medical care services delivery processes and procedures are complex too and use appropriate techniques and processes for successfully diagnose and cure health issues in an individual.

A process is a set of repeatable actions for accomplishing tasks and generating added-value. In (Highsmith & Cockburn, 2001), Jim Highsmith et al. define the software development methodology as:

A software development methodology refers to the framework that is used to plan, manage, and control the process of developing an information system.

Bo Bergman et al. present in (Bergman, Neuhauser, & Provost, 2011) the five main processes in healthcare. These processes are like the software development processes. Ha°kan Aronsson et al. (Aronsson, Abrahamsson, & Spens, 2011) divide the care into three steps: (i) Diagnosis, (ii) treatment, and (ii) convalesce. The treatment phase can be composed of various iterations and/ or face many changes in the treatment plan due to complication in the course of the disease. We summarize in Table 4 the different activities consisting the healthcare and software development processes. Figure 1 presents the healthcare development life cycle as presented by Bo Bergman et al.

To understand how to use the agile methodology in delivering healthcare services, we like first to go through the agile and scale agile as well as project organization and management.

Table 4. Comparison of processes in healthcare with those in software development

Processes in Healthcare	Processes in Software Development
Keeping healthy	Project Initiation
Detecting health problems	Requirement
Diagnosing diseases	Analyzing
	Designing
Treating diseases	Implementing
	Deploying
	Testing
Providing for a Good End of Life	Maintenance

Source: (Bergman et al., 2011)/ Bo Bergman et al.
Source: (Highsmith & Cockburn, 2001)/Jim Highsmith et al.

Figure 1. Five main processes in healthcare
Source: (Bergman et al., 2011)/ Bo Bergman et al.

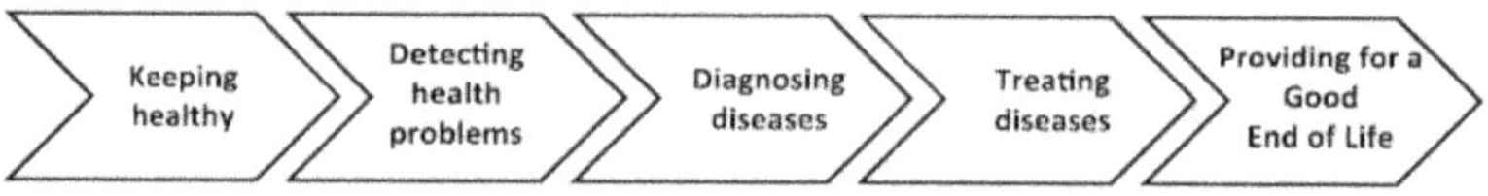

Figure 2. Care process according to Ha°kan Aronsson et al.
Source Ha°kan Aronsson et al. in (Aronsson et al., 2011).

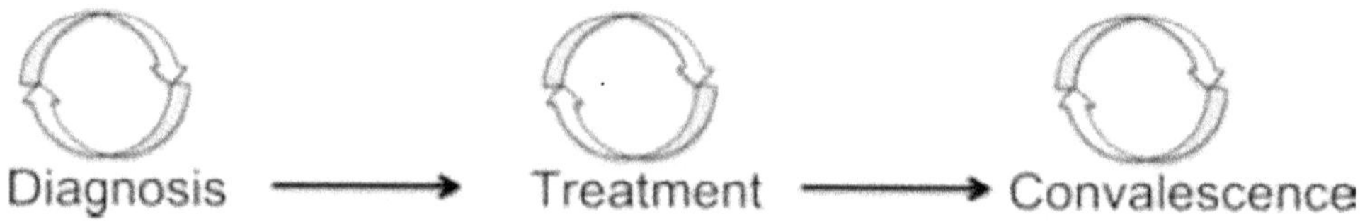

What Is Agile?

Agile development methodology is a type of incremental development, where the product or functionalities are subdivided into sub-products or sub-functionalities, which can be delivered on time and create added-functionalities. The main goals of the agile methodology are to reduce the cost and time to market. In (Highsmith & Cockburn, 2001), Jim Highsmith et al. define the agile methodology as;

Agile development combines creative teamwork with an intense focus on effectiveness and maneuverability.

The agile manifesto[2] has defined 12 principles for the agile development.

As described above, Scrum is an agile methodology and process for managing systems development. It is team oriented and self-organized. It reacts and tackles any change occurred during developing a system or solution. Scrum is iterative and projects developed using scrum are divided into sprints (Košinár, 2013). A sprint lasts from two (02) to four (04) weeks. Each sprint delivers a part of the final. This part can be used to create values.

Health care systems are, like other industries, structured and organized in the functional department with the chief objective to meet patient demands. This requires well-functioning processes. Each functional department is responsible for a group of patients (Aronsson et al., 2011).

Table 5. The 12 principles of standard agile development methodology

1	The highest priority of agile methodology is to satisfy the customer through the early and continuous delivery of valuable software.	7	Working software is the primary measure of progress.
2	Welcome changing requirements, even late in development. Agile processes harness change for the customer's competitive advantage.	8	Agile processes promote sustainable development. The sponsors, developers, and users should be able to maintain a constant pace indefinitely.
3	Deliver working software frequently, from a couple of weeks to a couple of months, with a preference to the shorter timescale.	9	Continuous attention to technical excellence and good design enhances agility.
4	Business people and developers must work together daily throughout the project.	10	Simplicity--the art of maximizing the amount of work not done--is essential.
5	Build projects around motivated individuals. Give them the environment and support they need, and trust them to get the job done.	11	The best architectures, requirements, and designs emerge from self-organizing teams.
6	The most efficient and effective method of conveying information to and within a development team is a face-to-face conversation.	12	At regular intervals, the team reflects on how to become more effective, then tunes and adjusts its behavior accordingly.

Source: Agile Alliance.

Agile development paradigm requires a development board on which different steps of the development are drawn. A backlog is defined, it contains a various item which represents the functionalities of the systems. The items are called "User stories" (US), that are moving from one stage to the next once the tasks at the stage are getting done. At a hospital there exist a case where the patient must go through different departments like the scrum user stories.

Imagine a patient undergoes a complex heart operation and must go through various medical stations. Such scenario is complex and susceptible to face several changes and uncertainty. An agile methodology will best help to meet, at any time, any change that can occur, since it works best in a situation like medical treatment with various uncertainty.

Scrum Tasks-Board

The scrum tasks board presents the work status of an agile team. The sprint backlog, the sprint duration, the ongoing tasks – user stories -, the impediments, Product-Owner review, sprint goals are displayed on the board. The board shows the progress of the tasks and of the team. A sprint is a development period or time interval (between 2 and 4 weeks) where a scrum team comments to certain tasks that should be done and delivered at the end of the sprint.

Figure 3. Example of a Trello tasks board

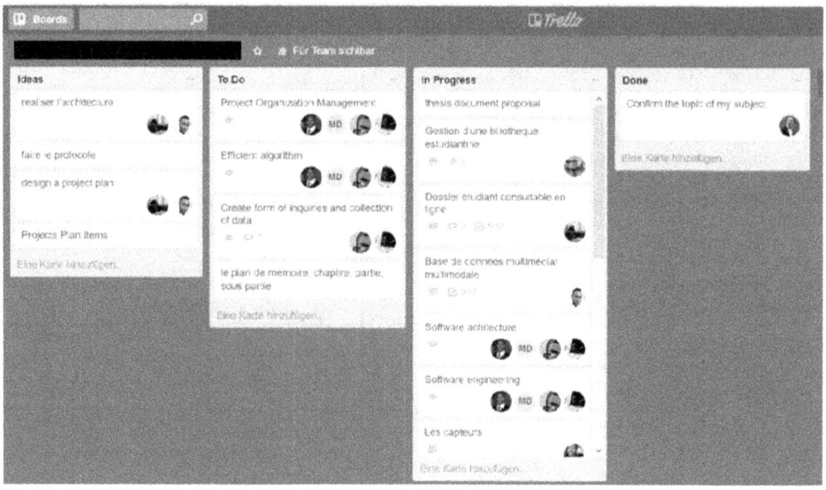

A scrum board can be physical or electronic. Team-members working on the same project at the same place could use the physical board and get their daily meeting on the board and update the board during the meeting. Team members working at geographically distributed places can use electronic tools like Jira and Trello to create their tasks board. Figure 3 shows the screenshot of an electronic tasks board created with Trello. This sample tasks board displays the ideas, the ToDos (the team backlog), the "In progress" Item (representing the different user stories in progress), and the "Done" (representing the implemented user stories). Each team can define the columns they need to track their work progress. The team is self-organized.

In medical filed and precisely in the case of the proposed remote care services system, team members can use electronic scrum board to bridge the geographical and different time zone issues and thus have their daily meeting online. The care units (hospitals or clinics) can follow the treatment progress. The patient's relatives as well as the patient himself, if he can, can also follow the progress and discuss with the team to get more informed.

The particularity of the proposed remote care system is to involve, especially in the developing countries, traditional practitioners (TP) into the system. However, most TP is an alphabet, therefore, it is a matter to implement an extension to these tools so that they can support voice features and thus permit TPs to participate as a full team member. We are working on implementing such a team tasks board so that TPs also can use it.

Scrum Team

The scrum team is assigned different tasks. The team consists of

1. A scrum master,
2. A product-Owner, and
3. The development teams.

Figure 4 illustrates the concept of the agile scrum and shows the relationship between the team members.

Scrum Master

The scrum master is the team member ensuring a smoothly process within the scrum team. He brings the rest of team to understand what scrum theory is and to adhere to it. He also assures that the team works without facing impediments. He assisted the team-members, prepares the board, serves the Product-Owner and the development team in certain tasks. He facilitates Scrum events as requested or needed. Table 6 summarizes the scrum master services to the other scrum team members and to the organization they are belonging to.

Table 6. Scum Master Services in software development manufacturing

Scrum Master Service To Development Team	Scrum Master Service to Product-Owner	Scrum Master Service to the Organization
• He coaches the Development Team in self-organization and cross-functionality as well as in organizational environments in which Scrum is not yet fully adopted and understood; • He helps the Team to create high-value products; • He removes impediments that can disturb the work's progress;	• He finds techniques for effective Product Backlog management; • He helps the Scrum Team understand the need for clear and concise Product Backlog items; • He facilitates to understand the product planning in an empirical environment; • He ensures the Product Owner to know how to arrange the Product Backlog to maximize value; • He facilitates understand and practice agility;	• He leads and coaches the organization in its Scrum adoption; • He plans Scrum implementations within the organization; • He helps employees and stakeholders to understand and enact Scrum and empirical product development; • He causes change that increases the productivity of the Scrum Team; and, • He works with other Scrum Masters to increase the effectiveness of the application of Scrum in the organization.

Source: Agile Alliance/Scrum guides (http://www.scrumguides.org/scrum-guide.html#team-sm)

Table 7. Scrum Master Service in agile healthcare

Medical Scrum Master Service to Medical Treating Team	Medical Scrum Master Service to Remote Medical Expert	Medical Scrum Master Service to the Care Unit
• Coaching the medical and para-medical treatment Team in self-organization and cross-functionality as well as in medical structures in which Scrum is not yet fully adopted and understood; • Helping the medical and para-medical Team to provide efficient care; • Removing impediments that can disturb the treatment's progress;	• Finding techniques for effective treatment activities Backlog management; • Helping the medical Team understand the need for clear and concise treatment detailed activities Backlog items; • Facilitating understand the medical treatment planning in an empirical environment; • Ensuring the medical expert knows how to arrange the medical activities Backlog to maximize value • Facilitating understand and practice agile healthcare	• Leading and coaching the care unit in its Scrum adoption; • Planning Scrum implementations within the care unit; • Helping healthcare professionals and stakeholders to understand and enact Scrum and empirical medical treatment; • Causing change that increases the productivity of the Scrum Team; and, • Working with other medical Scrum Masters to increase the effectiveness of the application of Scrum in the care unit.

Learning from the agile methodology in software development field, a scrum master in the multidisciplinary team in the proposed remote care delivery system should be multidisciplinary skilled, skilled in medical and para-medical treatment as well as in organization. He would have the ability to bring traditional practitioners and healthcare professionals together to work on a common project, e.g. treating a patient. He should provide several services to the care unit as an organization, healthcare professionals and para-medical personnel and traditional practitioners as a development team, and remote healthcare expert as product-owner. He should facilitate Scrum events as requested or needed to implement an agile healthcare.

Table 7 summarizes the services a medical scrum master should provide to other team members.

Product-Owner

The Product-Owner (PO) is representing the interests of the customer. He is responsible for the product and the deliveries. He performs, during a sprint, acceptance tests in testing the deliveries. At any time as well as during the sprint, the PO can proceed with changes at the functionalities and the team has to react and meet these changes.

In agile healthcare, the medical expert is acting as product-owner and can represent a medical committee and would be responsible for the entire medical treatment. He would define the treatment process and the different activities that will be performed. He would clearly identify and describe the items in the treatment backlog (items such as medication, medical exams, surgery if needed, etc.). He shares an understanding of the medical condition or diseases and treatment approach with the treating team. He would fix the priority of the treatment backlog items in order to maximize the medical outcome. Like performing acceptance test, the medical PO determines, through evaluation or medical examination, whether the treatment is successful.

Self-Organizing Team (Development Team)

The development team is a self-organizing and cross-functional team consisting of 5 to 7 team members. Big teams are subdivided into independent small teams that communicate with each other. Team members meet every day for a 5 minute-daily-meeting where each member reports his work's progress and impediments.

A medical team, playing the role of the development team, is in charge of performing the treatment defined by the medical committee represented by a medical PO. A traditional practitioner can constitute a team together with healthcare professional, nurse, NGOs, and others. Such a team can become big. In this case, the team can be subdivided into small teams fitting the scrum norm. The team should report at each daily meeting the progress and the issues facing and discuss with the medical PO as well as medical scrum master.

Scrum Meetings

Daily

The daily meeting is a 15-minute meeting where the entire scrum team, excluded the PO, discuss the work's progress. The PO can optionally take part to this meeting and thus reply to an eventual question from the development team. The scrum master organizes and manages the daily, asks during the meeting for impediments that he would resolve. The PO can make certain changes during the meeting.

Retrospectives

The retrospective meeting is one of the important meetings. During this meeting, the scrum team reviews the work, discuss different challenges the team has been faced and how to meet these challenges during the next sprint.

A retrospective meeting follows the objectives to summarize lessons learned during the sprint. The lessons learned could help to best implement the upcoming in avoiding and/or meet all challenges the team already experience with.

In agile healthcare, this meeting is very important. It would help to train the inexperienced healthcare personnel and the traditional practitioner. The lessons learned could constitute a knowledge database.

Grooming

The grooming meeting is the meeting where the representative of all scrum teams meeting work on the same project meet and discuss the implemented items. During the grooming meeting, coordinate the tasks for the future sprint. This meeting concerns only the POs and helps the POs in planning their backlog.

This meeting in agile healthcare will POs working on similar cases to meet and discuss the steps to follow to maximize the medical outcomes.

Estimation, Sprint Planning, Backlog Refinement

These meetings happened couple days before the sprint starts. At this meeting, the user stories are estimation to determine how long the implementation can take. This meeting is also used to plan and schedule the sprint and refine the backlog in clearing the unclear items so that each member understands what is requested.

What Is Scale Agile?

Scale agile is the Scrum of Scrum. Scaling agile problem occurs when there are multiple scrum teams working on the one same project and for the same product-owner (PO) or one many projects from multiple product owners. Each product-owner with his own product backlog (PB) representing their own Stakeholders. The main objective of scaling problem is to optimize the

Figure 4. Concept of agile healthcare

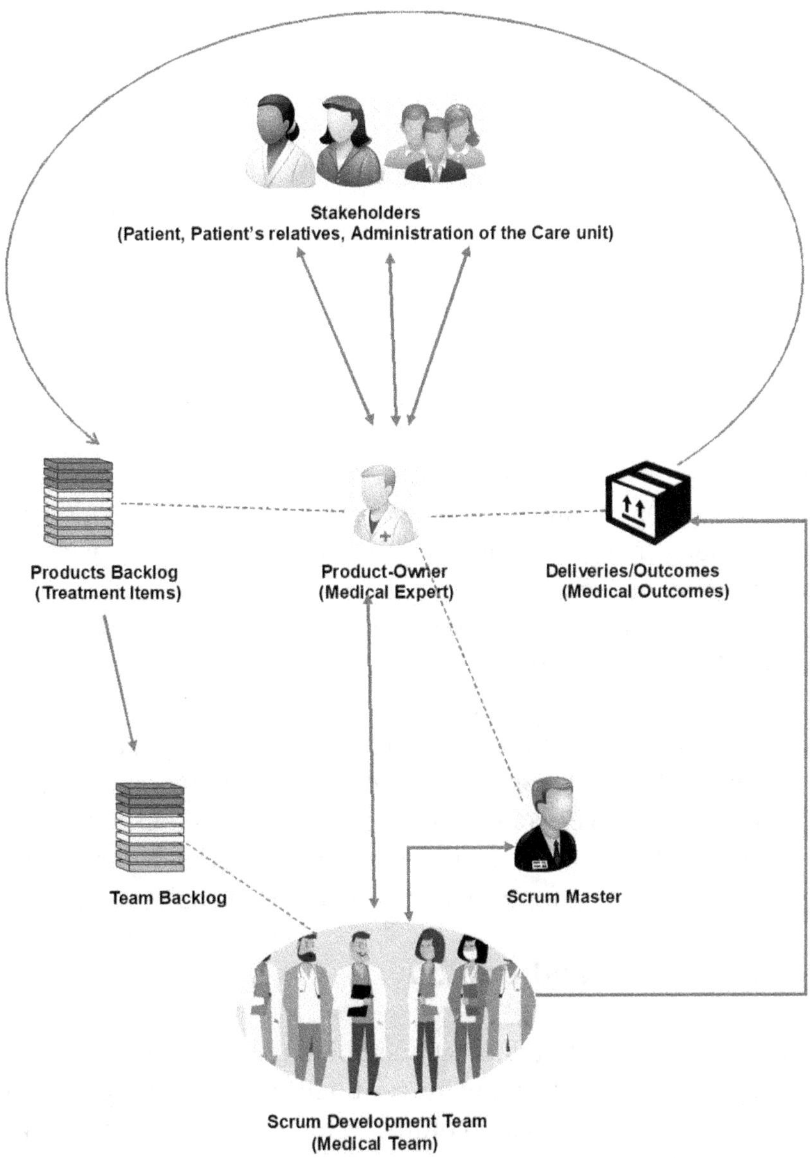

outcomes to the Stakeholders. The scaling problem, therefore, takes a lot of agility in different areas. The scaling problem well fits the medical response to an epidemic, where the care system is facing challenges generated by many Stakeholders, and many medical experts with different PBs. Another scenario generating a scaling is when a patient presents various medical conditions, for example, his is mentally ill, suffering from heart dysfunction, and also with diabetes type II. In the present case at least three (03) PO are needed with different PB, the Stakeholder is the same, but at least four (04) treatment tram is required. One team for heart diseases, one for psychology, another for psychiatric, a team for diabetes curing, a team for medical examination (Radiology, Computer tomography, etc.). These teams have to coordinate the treatment, report the health progress and ready for considering any ad-hoc change.

Scaling Problem

The scaling problem is actually facing challenges such as:

- Making Decision about the next steps and coordinate the team action.
- Figuring a global clinical picture in reviewing the various multifunctional teams' outcomes, from our example above different teams would work on the same medical outcomes.
- Assuring high communication among the teams in providing feedback about the outcomes to all the medical scrum teams involved in the medical treatment and the administration.
- Assuring that the teams do not confuse the treatment, and thus do not provide treatment intended for a patient A to another patient B.
- Assuring that is will possible to quickly build another functional team so to move the treatment from an existing team to the newly built team when the clinical picture changes – This case is quite frequent.

Agile Healthcare Methodology

The traditional medical treatment methodology consists of diagnosing, prescribing medicine, performing the treatment and examining the outcomes at the end of treatment. This kind of methodology is similar to the Waterfall Methodology. The waterfall methodology is a traditional non-agile software development methodology. The waterfall model is a sequential development methodology (Figure 5). The requirement is clearly defined and analyzed before starting the implementation. Each phase of the model must be completed before moving to the next phase. In (Balaji, 2012), S. Balaji et al. present the pros cons of waterfall methodology. They state that waterfall cannot meet and implement any change during the different phases of the model.

Figure 5. Waterfall Model Lifecycle

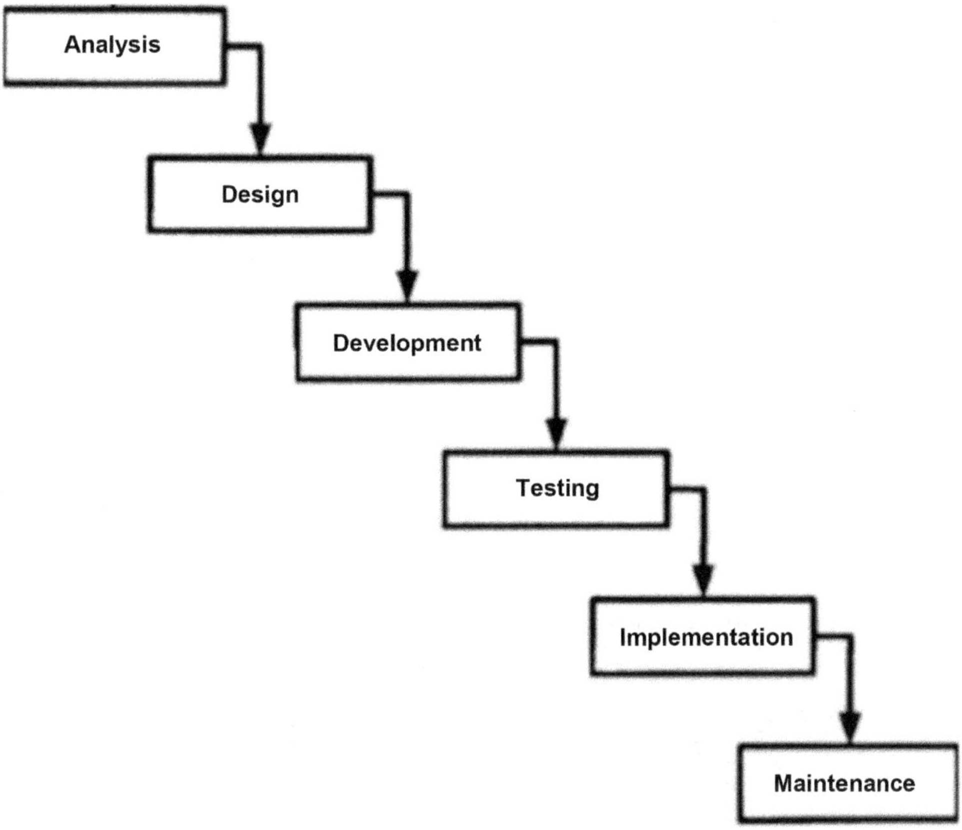

The problems with one phase are never solved completely during that phase and in fact, many problems regarding a particular phase arise after the phase is signed off, this result in the badly structured system.

If the client wants the requirement to be changed, it will not be implemented in the current development process. (S. Balaji et al.)

In the medical field, there are various uncertainty facing any medical treatment, especially if the treating team lack experiences with the medical condition it has to treat. Therefore, a waterfall like a methodology does not fit the situation since changes cannot be implemented during a current treatment. In agile healthcare, a medical treatment should have the ability to implement any change in the current treatment phase.

The agile healthcare methodology should be:

1. Visiting the medical doctor
2. Diagnosing the acute complains
3. Fixing a medical treatment plan
4. Building the different treating teams
5. Regular assuring the success of treatment, otherwise proceed with the necessary changes
6. Involving the patient and his relatives into the treatment process for assuring a patient-centered care
7. Assuring the communication among the teams
8. Repeat the steps 3 to 7 till the patient is successfully cured

Figure 6 illustrates a many-to-many relationship between Backlogs and Teams. There is also the case of many-to-one, many teams for one product-owner.

Figure 6. A many-to-many scaling problem illustration

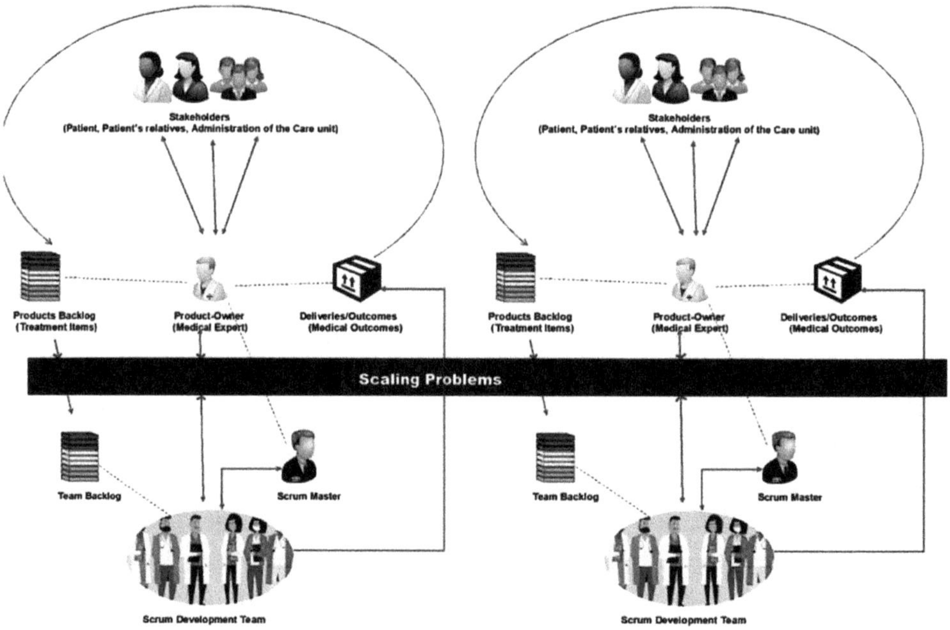

SIMILARITIES BETWEEN PATIENT-CENTERED CARE AND AGILE METHODOLOGY

The agile methodology enables to subdivide the final product into part-product that can be used to generate value. The final product is then incrementally implemented; thus, it needs continuity and transition between consecutive products.

Medical treatment requests also continuity and transition from a state to the next till the treatment get completed.

Both, PCC and agile development methodology presents here also a similarity.

Table 8 presents the similarities between agile methodology and patient-centered care.

Respect for Preferences

As Picker Institute recommends for PCC, the patient's values and preferences, as well as express needs, have to be respected during a medical treatment.

The agile manifesto also recommends taking into consideration any change the stakeholder expresses and insert it into the requirement for implementation. Thus, the stakeholder's preferences, values, and expressed needs are considered.

Both agile methodology and-and PCC are therefore similar to this point.

Table 8. Similarities between agile methodology and patient-centered care

Patient-Centered Care Principles	Agile Methodology
Respect for patients' values, preferences and expressed needs	Respect for Stakeholder requirements via the product-owner
Coordination and integration of care	Continuous integration of the deliveries into the existing system
Information, communication, and education	Communication with the client and among the development team
Involvement of family and friends	Involvement of the client during the development
Continuity and transition	Iteration till the entire is implemented

Coordination and Integration

Agile methodology requests continuous integration of deliveries. The integration required high coordination's tasks and analysis so that the new version of the product presents an added-value for the user.

In point of view of PCC, the care has to be coordinated and integrated into the existing care. The patient vulnerability should be coordinated and integrated into the care so that the patient gets a good feeling. It is known that the psychology and mental health can impact the body health positively or negatively. Therefore, the integration of the patient's feeling into the care will conduct to good outcomes.

Information, Communication, and Education

The patient needs more information on the progress of the treatment. It is important to communicate with patient and patient's relatives so that he knows his medical state. The patient also needs to be medically educated, know more about his medication.

In agile software development, Information and communication with the client/stakeholder as well as among the development team are very important so that all team member has all the time the same understanding of the product. The team members are regularly re-skilled/re-educated to meet the project's requirements.

The information, communication, and education are important for both, agile development and PCC.

Stakeholder Involvement

The agile manifesto recommends, like the Picker's principles, to involve the client/stakeholder into the development operation, where can express his changes or new needs that the team has to consider.

Patient's involvement in the care delivery process is a central point in the PCC. This allows the patient to express his needs and feelings that the medical has to consider for further care delivery

Continuity and Transition

The agile methodology enables to subdivide the final product into part-product that can be used to generate value. The final product is then incrementally implemented; thus, it needs continuity and transition between consecutive products.

Medical treatment requests also continuity and transition from a state to the next till the treatment get completed.

Both, PCC and agile development methodology presents here also a similarity.

ONGOING CASE STUDY

In the scope of the remote care delivery system proposed in Chapter 1, we conducted a case study to determine the impact of the agile healthcare on the system involving traditional practitioners (TPs).

The main goals of the ongoing case study are to compare the traditional medical treatment process and its outcomes with the agile healthcare process and outcomes. Furthermore, we pursued the objectives to investigate which methodology can ease the integration of TPs and the impacts on the training of the TPS, patient's education.

Purposely, we built two cohorts which are assigned to use one methodology and report their outcomes.

Case and Context

As the context of the first part of the ongoing evaluation, we choose the healthcare delivery system in the low- and middle-income countries only, since there exist no traditional practitioners in the high-income countries who can play the same role as the traditional practitioners are playing in the healthcare system in the low- and middle-income countries. In this context, we have the possibility to evaluate the impact of the different methodologies on the involvement of traditional practitioners into the healthcare services delivery systems and vice-versa.

The public healthcare services system in the Republic of Benin, a West African developing country, is subject to our case study. We select three rural areas where the healthcare services accessibility is very poor. These evaluation areas are optimally covered by GSM network (mobile telephony and internet).

The populations in these areas are most confident in traditional medicine than modern medicine systems. There are facing various challenges in access healthcare services, lack of pharmacies, modern care units, and medical workforce.

SAMPLING

Cohorts

We built two cohorts: (i) a cohort to conduct medical treatment using traditional medical methodology (a waterfall like a methodology) and (ii) a cohort using agile development like medical treatment methodology.

Each cohort is consisted of: (i) a medical expert, (ii) physicians and nurses, (ii) Psychologists, (iii) NGO-personnel, (iv) Pharmacists, and (v) traditional practitioners.

Additionally, we recruited patients suffering from malaria. Table 9 presents a detailed structure of the selected cohort's population.

- **Snowball Approach:** We recruited a medical expert, who in turn recruited certain physicians, who also recruited their colleagues and enrolled some patients. Thus, we selected 44 participants for the first part of the ongoing project's evaluation.

Table 9. Structure of the ongoing evaluation

Participants	Number of Participants		Total
	Cohort 1	Cohort 2	
Medical expert	1	1	02
Physicians (General Practitioner)	5	5	10
Psychologists	1	1	02
NGOs-Personnel	2	2	04
Pharmacists	1	1	02
Traditional Practitioners	3	3	06
Patients – Women	4	4	08
Patients -Men	3	3	06
Patients – young	2	2	04
Total	22	22	**44**

Methods and Materials

- **Qualitative Approach:** We are conducting a quantitative study in collecting data about the quality of the medical treatment completed by each cohort. To measure the quality of the treatment, we defined some criteria:
    - The treatment velocity
    - Relapse rate
    - Patient's satisfaction and evaluation of the treatment regarding
        - His involvement
        - The communication and information he received
        - Respect for values expressed needs
    - Impression of the traditional practitioner
    - Satisfaction of the medical expert
    - Team satisfaction

Data Gathering and Analysis

Each team report once a day their work's progress, as well as the impediments, facing. We asked them also to describe how they solve the impediments and if they face any change coming the expert or some person else.

During the first six treatment weeks, we asked the patients to evaluate their satisfaction regarding the methodology. It is well known that user satisfaction is subjective and can be biased. We, therefore, plan to interchange the team so that the one which uses agile in this evaluation phase will use the traditional methodology and vice-versa. The objective is to verify if the results we presently obtain are not biased and subjective.

Results

The data analysis points out that the velocity of the medical agile methodology is higher than the traditional one. The agile teams (two teams) have treated 7 of 9 patients quickly and successfully, while the traditional team has treated only 3 of 9 patients at the same time. Table 10 summarizes the results of the evaluation.

We figure out two relapses among the patients cured using the traditional methodology.

Table 10. Summary of the evaluation's results

Evaluation's Criteria	**Results**		
	Participants/Evaluation's Point	**Methodology**	
		Traditional	**Agile**
Velocity	Healing/cure Treatment	33,33%	77,77%
Relapse rate	Adult men	0%	0%
	Adult women	100% (total cured = 1 patient)	0%
	Young	100% (total cured = 1 patient)	0%
Patient's satisfaction	Adult men	66,66% (2 of 3) satisfied	33,33% (1 of 3) satisfied
	Adult women	25% (1 of 4) satisfied	75% (3 of 4) satisfied
	Young	Neutral	Neutral
Traditional practitioner impression	Methodology	0% satisfaction	66,66% satisfaction
Treating Teams	Physicians		
	Psychologists		
	NGOs-Personnel		
	Pharmacists		
Medical expert satisfaction	Collaboration with the team	Partially dissatisfied	Satisfied

At the end of the evaluation, we, additionally, asked the patients about their satisfaction regarding the treatment and the methodology. The young patients cannot express their satisfaction. The main reason was, the young were not really involved in the treatment process and procedure, instead of this, their parents were more involved. We did not collect or ask the parents about their satisfaction since we are only seeking for the feelings of the patients and not of their relatives. Women are more satisfied with the agile methodology than the men. Our investigation reveals that the women satisfaction is due to the communication and information as well as education possibility agile methodology offers. It seems that women like communication on the health more than men. We did not investigate this since the question is out of our evaluation's scope.

The traditional practitioners are more satisfied with the agile methodology than the traditional one. They appreciated the daily meeting, the inter-team communication, the role of the scrum master helping to resolve impediments as well as coaching the teams.

The remote medical expert was fully satisfied with the agile team because of the dynamism and the self-organization as well as the role of the scrum master in the team. Though, he states that complex operations have to be always discussed with him in order to assure the patient's safety and avoid death.

Base on collected data and a semi-structured survey, the traditional team members complain about impediments they have to solve by themselves, lack of communication among the team

This partial evaluation has demonstrated the potential of agile healthcare but also its limitation e.g. patient's safety.

CONCLUSION

Agile healthcare has a great potentiality to best provide care service to the patient. Though, it requires more training and enterprise intern political will from the manager board, since scaling agile can quickly become unclear for the manager.

It matters to emphasize agile healthcare is not applicable everywhere. It fit more situations where there exists more uncertainty.

In this chapter, the author provides the theoretical background of the agile development as well as of scale agile. Both methodologies are compared with each other. Further, the scaling issues have been discussed. The implementation of agile methodology in the medical field discussed. It has been shown how it makes sense to implement the agile heath care. The agile healthcare presents several advantages like flexibility in the treatment, more communication about cases, short reaction time and the treatment is more patient-centered.

This study introduces the notion of multimodal scrum board, which allows the scrum team members different ways to update the board. They can use their voice for example. The follow-up of this study will present the multimodal scrum board. The multimodal board is intended especially for illiterates like traditional practitioners, who can be involved in the healthcare supply chain in order to meet certain challenges as described in the previous chapter.

REFERENCES

Aronsson, H., Abrahamsson, M., & Spens, K. (2011). Developing lean and agile health care supply chains. *Supply Chain Management*, *16*(3), 176–183. doi:10.1108/13598541111127164

Balaji, S. (2012). *Waterfall vs v-model vs agile: A comparative study on SDLC*. Academic Press.

Bergman, B., Neuhauser, D., & Provost, L. (2011). Five main processes in healthcare: a citizen perspective. *BMJ Quality & Safety, 20*(S1), i41-2. 10.1136/bmjqs.2010.046409

Fujita, H., & Guizzi, G. (Eds.). (2015). *Intelligent Software Methodologies, Tools and Techniques* (Vol. 532). Cham: Springer International Publishing; doi:10.1007/978-3-319-22689-7

Highsmith, J., & Cockburn, A. (2001). Development: The Business of Innovation. *Science, 34*(9), 120–123. doi:10.1109/2.947100

Kitson, A., Marshall, A., Bassett, K., & Zeitz, K. (2013). What are the core elements of patient-centred care? A narrative review and synthesis of the literature from health policy, medicine and nursing. *Journal of Advanced Nursing, 69*(1), 4–15. doi:10.1111/j.1365-2648.2012.06064.x PMID:22709336

Košinár, M. (2013). Knowledge modeling of agile processes in healthcare systems development. *Lekar a Technika, 43*(4), 32–35. Retrieved from https://www.scopus.com/inward/record.uri?eid=2-s2.0-84923227828&partnerID=40&md5=cddef68cc45ad8c0651c117688f56452

Qin, H., Prybutok, G. L., Prybutok, V. R., & Wang, B. (2015). International Journal of Health Care Quality Assurance Article information. *International Journal of Health Care Quality Assurance, 28*(6), 574–594. doi:10.1108/IJHCQA-01-2014-0009 PMID:26156432

Starfield, B. (2011). Is patient-centered care the same as person-focused care? *The Permanente Journal, 15*(2), 63–69. doi:10.7812/TPP/10-148 PMID:21841928

Tsuyuki, R. T., & Krass, I. (2013). What is patient-centred care? / que sont les soins axes sur le patient? *Canadian Pharmacists Journal, 146*(4), 177–180. 10.1177/1715163513494591

Williams, S. J. (2017). *Improving Healthcare Operations*. Cham: Springer International Publishing. doi:10.1007/978-3-319-46913-3

ENDNOTES

1. https://www.scrumalliance.org/community/articles/2014/january/success-story-agility-in-healthcare
2. https://www.agilealliance.org/agile101/the-agile-manifesto/

Section 2

System for Improved Pharmaceutical Care

Chapter 3
Towards Secure Off-Label Drug Prescribing and Improved Drug Supply

ABSTRACT

Worldwide, among healthcare professionals an uncertainty as to what medical uses exactly fall under the theme of off-label-use is noticeable. The lack of a common definition complicates the comparison of methods of resolutions in different countries. A current ambiguity is shown to cause false patient education and invalid informed consent, hence leading to liability concerns. Due to several legal restrictions in Western countries, healthcare professionals are facing more legal actions (lawsuits) than their colleagues in developing countries. The health systems in the developing countries, particularly in Sub-Saharan Africa, are facing, in addition, severe drug supply issues. This chapter analyzes the issues from the viewpoint of the information and communication technology and proposes solution approaches.

INTRODUCTION

One of the problems in healthcare in developing countries is the bad accessibility of medicine in pharmacies for patients.

The insufficient supply of pharmaceutical products for the population is a major care delivery issue in the healthcare systems in the developing countries (Edoh & Teege, 2011). For the individual patient, a high time and effort are required to purchase all medicine prescribed by a physician.

DOI: 10.4018/978-1-5225-5528-5.ch003

A case study in a representative developing country, the Republic of Benin, had revealed that although the public pharmacies and dispensaries are relatively frequent, the supplied medicine or pharmaceutical products are very limited. The most supplied medicines are intended for common therapy such as malaria treatment. Patients are sometimes obliged to procure at the black market counterfeits (Edoh, 2010).

More than 90% of all private pharmacies are in few large cities of the country. The countries are facing low density of pharmacies and frequent drugs stock-out. In large cities as well as in rural regions, it is often difficult to purchase all medicines on a prescription in a single pharmacy, due to stock-out (Edoh & Teege, 2011).

The situations described above lead in several cases to the use of drugs off the label to overcome the lack of appropriate medicines.

Off-Label-use is worldwide a common practice that is not restricted (J., 2003). *In Canada and the United States, it is illegal to promote or advertise any medication for any indication other than that for which it was approved (F. Christine Fukada, et al. in* (Christine Fukada, MSc; Jillian Clare Kohler, PhD; Heather Boon, PhD; Zubin Austin, PhD; Murray Krahn, MD, MSc, n.d.)), while theoretically in high-income countries for example in Germany, no law prohibits a physician or other healthcare practitioner from prescribing an approved medication for other uses than their specific approved indications (off labeling use) (KVBW, 2012).

In developing countries, however, we do not find any stipulation that regulates the HCP liability.

Off-Label-Use is widely practiced in all areas of the medicine (estimated to 21% worldwide (Jansen, 2011)). In German, the Off-Label-Use is widely practiced and is generally, *"consider legal"* unless it violates some costs reimbursement regulations set by German healthcare insurances., specific ethical guidelines or safety regulations defined by the German Drugs Law (AMG).

Unfortunately, due to the legal uncertainty, the risk of financial ruin, insolvency and possible legal liability for the health practitioner in case of health damage, most of the health professionals do not accept having practiced it

The dissemination of off-label-use related information is authorized in the USA by American's regulation and largely accepted, while the European and South-African regulations are more restrictive. This fact generates, in European countries (e.g. Germany) and in Africa (e.g. South-Africa) an uncertainty among HCP (Jansen, 2011). The healthcare professionals could also face personal liability and be subjected to cost recourse process in case of prescribing off-label drugs or treatment.

In the developing world, most healthcare professionals (HCP) are not aware of being prescribing off-label drugs, medication, or treatment. South Africa has the most developed health delivery system in Africa (Edoh & Teege, 2011). However, the theme "Off-Label-Use" also receives here a little attention (Jansen, 2009). The literature research and survey have revealed that this fact is common to all African countries, furthermore, there exists no common and explicit definition of the theme of Off-Label-Use.

Due to a frequent drugs-stock-out in up to all African countries, off-label-use becomes a royal way for the medical treatment; for example in South Africa, cases are reported in (De Decker R, Gordon-Graham E, Seller N, 2009; "Off-label drug use," 2009). African HCPs act in most medical cases exactly like western pediatric psychotherapists. According to Prof. Dr. med. Jörg M. Fegert, Off-Label-Use and/or treatment are most frequently practiced in adolescent psychiatry (Prof. Dr. Lutz Goldbeck, Dr. Paul L. Plener, Prof. Dr. Franz Resch, n.d.) since most of the psychotherapy-drugs used in the children and adolescents therapy are only approved for adults use. Medical doctors use unapproved medicine and/or unapproved dosage for the adolescent psychotherapy due to the lack of approved drugs for that age group (adolescent psychiatric patients). Off-Label-Use and/or Treatment remains an important public health issue for infants, children, and adolescents because an overwhelming number of drugs still have no information in the labeling for use in pediatrics (Research, n.d.).

A legal uncertainty as to what medical uses exactly fall under the theme of off-label-use is regarding the lack of common and explicit definition noticeable among healthcare professionals for example in Germany, whereas, in the developing world, no legal uncertainty is noticed, due to the lack explicit regulation and control. Healthcare professionals, therefore, need drug information to assure the safety of treatment, however, legislative hurdles may hinder access to information, while at the same time broad dissemination of off-label information is considered a risk of circumventing marketing authorization. Though information dissemination regarding off-label-use is prohibited in European countries (Jansen, 2011) as well as in South Africa (Jansen, 2009). We lack studies regarding off-label-use in Africa; in (Thomas, 2014) the author reveals that of-label-use in children is little documented in Africa. The author further claims that he lacks documents or literature regarding studies on off-label-use in African children. Our review of literature confirms this fact. In (N. Krzy_zaniak* BPharm Sci

MPharm GradCertPharmMed Ph.D. Candidate, 2016) the authors conducted a literature review on off-label-use in neonatal and concluded that off-label in this category is limited published. We review a huge of articles and found no article, which presents a study on Off-Label-Use in African neonatal and in adults. To our knowledge and according to the exhaustive review of the literature we conducted, Sub-Sahara-African countries, except South Africa, have no regulation or stipulation.

PROBLEM ANALYSIS

Based on the collected data, we analyze, from the viewpoint of computer sciences, the different drug uses off-label and drugs supply the developing and developed countries are facing.

Drugs Supply Issues

The main aspect is missing information about where medicine is in stock. A second aspect is the patient's high expenditure for purchasing the medicine. Both aspects have a simple and standard ICT based solution: An E-commerce system. The drugs supply issues could be improved using E-commerce solution.

Table 1. Obstacles hindering the implementation of a standard E-commerce in developing countries

Problem	Descriptions
Internet Access	The internet penetration in 2017 is 33% Most rural regions are not covered so lacking of communication infrastructure. The Internet and even traditional phone lines are sparsely existent and only concentrated in the larger cities. The communication is considered as a major obstacle.
Illiteracy rate	A large percentage of people mostly living in rural areas are analphabets and can only use ICT equipment in a strongly limited manner.
Most pharmacies have no ICT equipment	The pharmacies own only billing application and database system. Only a few are present on the internet. Launching and using a standard E-commerce imply the acquisition of new ICT infrastructures. The ICT infrastructure acquisition cost can present an obstacle to launching the system.
Electricity Supply	There is no reliable electricity supply for operating ICT equipment. Most developing countries are regularly facing electricity shortages for several hours a day.
Delivery Service	There is no reliable delivery service. Postal transport is unreliable, too slow and too expensive.
Electronic Payment Infrastructure	There is no electronic payment infrastructure. Most patients do not even have a bank account.

However, a standard E-commerce cannot be launched into developing countries without adapt it to the local realities such traditional means, technology level, access to internet penetration, and the illiteracy rate. Table 1 summarizes the obstacles that could hinder the launch of standard E-commerce in developing countries.

Off-Label Drug Use

Off-label prescriptions must better serve patient needs than alternatives and must be supported by evidence or experience in order to guarantee patient safety and treatment efficacy. However, there is often little or no proven evidence of efficacy on much use of drugs for unapproved indications. A regulatory review of the benefits and risks of using the drug for unapproved indication has mostly not taken place. The lack of proven evidence of efficacy or reported experiences in dealing with off-label-use of certain drugs represents potential hazards for the patient with the legitimate desire for an effective treatment since the drugs are not sufficiently tested. Nevertheless, the use of medical products for unapproved indications is considered as an essential part of the therapies in oncology, neurology, and pediatrics. However, severe and very severe side effects that can lead to deaths due to drugs used for unapproved indications are reported. It is then important for the patient's safety and protection that drugs should only be used accordingly to the country's regulations and stipulation, which in turn would facilitate information dissemination regarding off-label-use and provide a system to collect proven evidence.

The proven evidence is therefore mandatory for a safe off-label-use practice. It's therefore important to define some solution approaches and techniques on the model of UK NHS Trust's guidance to thus assure safe off-label use in the German context. In (Christine Fukada, MSc; Jillian Clare Kohler, PhD; Heather Boon, PhD; Zubin Austin, PhD; Murray Krahn, MD, MSc, n.d.), the authors claim base on the results of the study the urgent need to educate Health Care Professionals (HCP) and disseminate information about off-label use. They assert following:

1. More widespread education for pharmacists, physicians, and other healthcare professionals on off-label issues such as the common use of non-traditional sources of information, including informal professional networks, is needed.

2. Better dissemination of evidence for off-label indications among prescribers is needed, particularly when clinical practice guidelines exist.
3. There is often a mismatch between scientific knowledge and practice and pharmaceutical product label claims, suggesting the importance of greater

The authors (Christine Fukada, MSc; Jillian Clare Kohler, Ph.D.; Heather Boon, Ph.D.; Zubin Austin, Ph.D.; Murray Krahn, MD, MSc, n.d.) found out that the off-label-use is idiosyncratic and based only on the experience of the physician. This clearly means that the off-label use of drugs does not rely on evidence. During our study, we find out the same behaviors by German and African HCPs whom we interviewed.

Our intention is to create large knowledge database, where any off-label use result can be stored. These stored empirical data have to be verified analyzed by a committee of a medical expert. Each HCP can access the database to input information or seek for information about similar off-label use cases.

This solution approach can be efficient if some legal obstacles get abrogated. Therefore, we recommend following:

Improving the Legal Circumstances to Assure Secure Off-Label-Use

The off-label-use reimbursement regulations (to prevent costs resources) should be valid for outpatient too.

Less liability for health professionals. The health system must produce more evidence and provide the health professionals with more information about off-label-drugs. In the case of health damage or death physicians shall not be liable because of off-label treatment, but because of wrong treatment. Off-label-use and approved treatment shall thus be co-equal regarding the Drugs law.

The pharmaceutical companies must be legally more involved in the Evidence capturing processes.

It shall be possible for the pharmaceutical companies to use the proven evidence' findings to extend drugs' indications without applying for a new mandatory marketing authorization. More collaboration between pharmaceutical companies and practitioners should be encouraged. Scientifically proven Evidence shall be accepted as clinical trials phase 2 and 3 and thus lead to indications extensions.

Define a clear refund politic for the off-label-use: Directives regarding costs recourse in the case of the off-label-drugs must be suppressed, thus practitioners should not anymore be subjected to costs recourse process. Also, all off-label-therapies' costs shall be case-based lump sum for the outpatient treatment too.

Ease the Drug Law Regarding the Extension of Indications

Improving the prescription policies is recommended

A sample of off-label policies of British NHS trusts shall serve as a model for guidance to healthcare professionals. Items shall be identified from the policies and tested for feasibility. Therefore, a survey with a web-based questionnaire will provide evidence for practicable management of off-label use among healthcare professionals, attorneys, and regulatory professionals.

Enabling Evidence gathering. Mandatory Reporting requirement for all off-label-use/-treatment: All off-label activities (with positive or negative results) must be mandatorily reported. This will lead to a high legislative certainty among the health professionals and less liability in the case of health damage must be provided for the health professionals. It is further important to prevent the health of any costs resources process after practicing an off-label-use/treatment. Soon those medical conditions listed above are met; it will be easy to capture more data about the off-label-use.

In the viewpoint of computer sciences, we propose some tools to ease the data capturing and data analysis.

METHODS AND MATERIALS

Sample Selection

Off-Label-Use Research Sample

We also built, in Germany as well as in Africa, two cohorts: (i) patient-cohort and (ii) healthcare professional's cohorts in each country. Data and information have been collected quantitatively and qualitatively analyzed. We compare the collected data from different cohorts with each other.

We reviewed 23 scientific papers selected using a snowball approach. Table 2 presents the selected research population selected in Germany. Table 3, Table 4, and Table 5 present the structure of the Beninese cohort involved in the Off-Label-Use study.

Drug Supply Research Samples

Table 6 presents the materials selected in the scope of the drugs supply study. We have found very few literature dealing with the topic. Only 5 scientific papers, which vaguely discuss the theme.

Table 2. German research population (Off-Label-Use)

Participants	Numbers	Contacted by
Organizations (Association of Statutory Health Insurance Physicians)	33	Letter, phone, Email
Hospitals (Rechts der Isar, University Hospital Cologne, etc.)	6	Paper-based questionnaire
General Practitioners (Bavaria)	12	Paper-based/online questionnaire
Medical associations	16	Paper-based questionnaire
In-patients/out-patients	00	-

Table 3. Beninese healthcare units (Off-Label-Use)

Participants	Numbers	Contacted by
Hospitals (public)	3	Paper-based questionnaire
Clinics (private sector)	2	Paper-based questionnaire

Table 4. Beninese health Care Professionals involved (Off-Label-Use)

Pos.	Professional Category of Involved Health Care Professional	Number
1	Cardiologists	8
2	ORL/ENT specialists	5
3	Pediatricians	2
4	General Practitioners (GP)	3
5	Pharmacists	2
6	Gynecologist	1

Table 5. Structure of involved patients in Benin (Off-Label-Use)

Pos.	Number of Patients Involved	Age Range
1	6 patients	< 10 y
2	10 patients	10 to 30 y
3	30 patients	31 to 60 y
4	04 Patients	> 60

Table 6. Selected prescriptions

Samples	Number
Prescriptions selected in Benin • In-patients (876) • Out-patients (124)	1000
Prescriptions selected in Germany • Out-patients (300)	300
Scientific papers selected	5

Study Data

We conducted a long-term study in carrying out several surveys (structural and semi-structural interview) in 2013/2014 in Germany and 2015/2016 in Africa. We designed online questionnaires (hosted on https://www.surveymonkey.de) and paper-based questionnaires.

We collect the study data in a semi-structured interview on off-label-use and drug supply in Germany and in Benin. We interviewed in- and out-patients, physicians, and others healthcare systems actors (Table 2, Table 3, Table 4, and Table 5). Furthermore, we combine cross-sectional and longitudinal studies approaches for investigating the causes of poor drug supply and poor access to pharmaceutical care in the developing countries, wherein a long-term study, we examine the correlation between the missing medicines and other parameters related to the patient such as age, income, gender, place of residence. We thus collected data about:

- Most missing medicines
- Categories/age/gender of patients facing this issue (poor access to pharmaceutical care)
- Income data
- Amount of off-label-prescribing and the frequency

- Why off-label-prescribing
- Which affections are mostly treated off-label
- What are the regulations and stipulations in use
- How information is disseminated on Off-Labe-Use

We presented and discussed a concept to improve the drug supply and secure the off-label-use with the hospitals and other health professionals. We thus collected significant data, information, and opinions that we analyze. The analysis helps to improve our concept.

RESULTS AND DATA ANALYSIS

We have assisted, in Benin, 1000 patients in purchasing their medicine and found out how severe the drug supply issues are in developing countries. 71% of the prescriptions are off-label-use prescriptions. Only 2,9% of the prescriptions could be purchased at a single pharmacy. 83,2% of prescriptions were purchased partially at different pharmacies. 7,9% were not purchased because the patient procures substitutions at the black market (counterfeit drugs). 6% were purchased abroad. Table 7 summarizes the results of the drugs supply study in Benin.

The high-income countries also face drug supply issues at their way. We analyzed, in Germany, 300 prescriptions all concerning tropical diseases/infections and found out that 95,24% (Table 8) of all pharmacies did not have the sought medicines in stock. An example is a medicine named RIAMET. The pharmacies must order it and deliver it the following day. We have cases where the patients

Table 7. Result of the drugs supply in Benin

Prescriptions	Number of Prescription	Percentage
Off-Label-Use Prescription	710	71%
Label conform prescription	290	29%
Total	1.000	100%
Prescriptions purchased at single pharmacy	29	2,9%
Prescription purchased at many pharmacies	832	83,2%
Prescriptions purchased abroad	60	6%
Prescriptions purchased a black market (Counterfeit)	79	7,9%
Total	1.000	100%

Table 8. Result of certain drugs supply in Germany

Prescription/Pharmacies	Number	Percentage
Prescription purchased with delay	287	95,67%
Prescription purchased immediately	13	04,33%
Total	300	100%
Prescriptions purchased at pharmacies near to the patient place	294	98%
Prescription purchased at pharmacies far to the patient to the place	6	2%
Total	300	100%
Pharmacies, which did not have the drugs in stock	20	95,24%
Pharmacies, which had the drugs in stock	1	4,76%

must urgently use the product and thus cannot wait till to the next day. In these cases, the patients went to the hospital and ask for the product. 2% of the analyzed could not be purchased in the near pharmacy because the pharmacies often do not have a big pack of certain drugs in stock, or the stock is out.

The studies have revealed that the different drug-use regulations applied in several countries worldwide provoke on one hand uncertainty among healthcare professionals and on other hand intended to assure more health safety to patients. Hence, the uncertainty could negatively impact the care delivery due to the legal restrictions. These studies also figure out that most of the practitioner use drugs off-label though without neither inform the patient nor the public healthcare concerning authority.

Most health professionals, pharmacists, health authorities and employees of several pharmaceutical industries consider the Off-Label-Use only as the use of medicine/drugs for an unapproved indication, or in an unapproved age group, unapproved dosage, or unapproved form of administration (Stafford, n.d.). The practicing Over-the-Counter-Drugs (OTCs) purchasing and/or selling can also link to the Off-Label-Use. The discount agreement[1] between German Health insurances and the different pharmaceutical groups are leading to off-label use but are mostly ignored.

SOLUTION APPROACHES

Base on the data analysis we designed and implemented an empirical evidence-based information system for a secure off-label-use and drug prescribing.

To improve the drug supply in developing countries as well as in high-income countries, we also design an E-commerce platform for pharmacies, where the patient can seek for and order pharmaceutical products.

Our proposed evidence-based information system has the potentiality to overcome any uncertainty issue and secure off-label-use and drug prescribing, thus increase patient safety towards medicine adversity.

Drugs Supply Issues

To improve the drug supply particularly in developing countries, we have designed and implemented an adapted E-commerce solution.

Drug Supply Platform

The proposed drug supply platform is a network, a Business-to-Business (B2B) and Business-to-Consumer (B2C) pharmacy marketplace (eCommerce) and a service-oriented Distributed application for the improvement of pharmaceutical care and a communication system or a communication platform (as a computer-controlled co-operation platform) for pharmacies, treating physicians and / or hospitals and patients. The Potential communication axis in the proposed system is based on physician-to-pharmacy, pharmacy-to-pharmacy, Pharmacy-to-wholesaler / supplier as well as pharmacy-to-patient.

The designed drug supply platform consists of two types of E-commerce: (1) B2B (pharmacy-to-pharmacy) and B2C (pharmacy-to-patient and pharmacy-to-physician). Table 9 compares the standard E-commerce with the proposed adapted E-commerce.

ARCHITECTURAL OVERVIEW

This section presents the architectural overview of the proposed drug supply platform.

System Use Cases

Figure 1 presents the use cases of the system. Patients, pharmacies, and physicians could place an order. The patient (or a relative) can purchase medicine for himself using the platform. Since there exist enough illiterates

Table 9. Standard E-Commerce versus updated E-commerce (Drug supply platform for developing countries)

Type of Technologies	Standard E-Commerce	Updated E-Commerce
B2B	Yes, available	Yes, available
B2C	Yes, available	Yes, available
B2G	Yes, available	Not available
C2C	Yes, available	Not available
m-Commerce	Yes, available	Not available
Email	Yes, available	Yes, order can be placed or
SMS	Not standard	Yes, order can be placed through SMS
Telephony	Not standard	Yes, Illiterate can use it to place an order or raise a claim
Fax	Not standard	Yes, Illiterate can use it to place an order or raise a claim
Voice	Not standard	Illiterate can use this way to communicate within the system
Payment	Credit card	Updated payment ways
Delivery	Standard post	Adapted delivery logistics (standard post are not reliable)
Tracking	Standard online tracking system	The supplier informs the customer on demand

Figure 1. Use case of the adapted E-commence solution

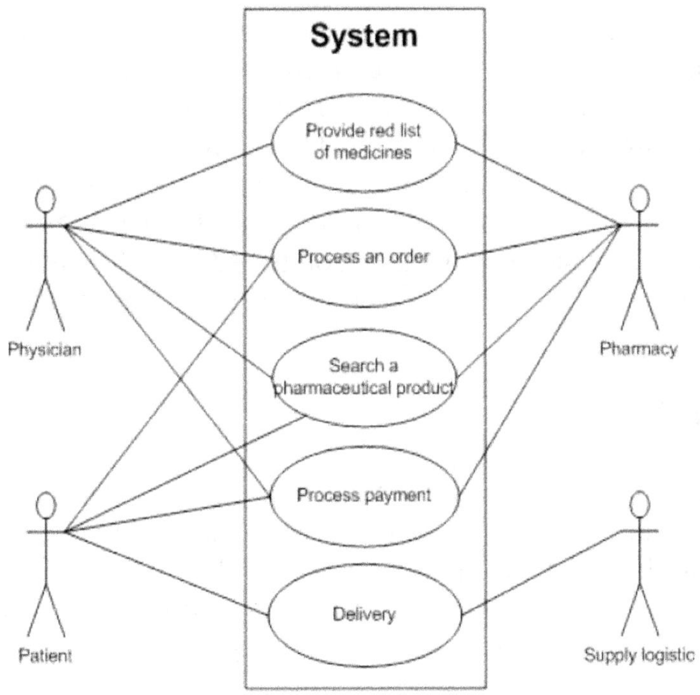

in the developing world, a physician can buy, on behalf of a patient, medicine he prescribes him. A pharmacy near to the patient residence can use the platform to purchase medicine for the patient.

Both pharmacies and physicians would provide an electronic dynamic red list (Available medicine list), The red list should be regularly updated so that only in the entire country available should be mentioned.

The platform features a search subroutine, that can be used by all actors of the system to look for a medicine. A physician can use it to be sure that the product the is prescribing is available at a pharmacy near to the patient residence. Otherwise, the product would be ordered and the pharmacy (supplier) will deliver it at patient home. The patient can track the delivery on the platform. The platform features also a tracking system.

System Component Overview

Figure 2 shows the architectural overview of the drug supply platform. The system consists of three (03) components (i) the user interfaces, (ii) the trade center, and (iii) the backend system (supplier system).

The Trade Center

The trade center, a public service, is the central system component. It is implemented as an application server using a backend database system. The front-end consists of a Web-based interface, an SMS interface, and a call center providing the voice interface and handling SMS messages which do not conform to the template. The basic information is a list of all available pharmaceutical products in the developing world. This list (called red list) is generated as a version and/or variant of the red book. The red list contains a set of information for every product; it must be defined by physicians and pharmacies.

User Interfaces

A set of devices can be used to access the system. The system users could use a traditional mobile phone without internet capability but able to text (send SMS), smartphone, laptop, tablet, and desktop PC with internet access. Any browser can be used to connect to the system and place or track an order. The user can also use a Fax machine to place an order.

Database as Backend

Behind the trade center, several databases are running the stock of each involved pharmacy. This information is replicated to a central database at the trade center, so to prevent latency issues in case of an order. The data replication happens in regular time span so that the local database at the trade center is accurate and updated at any moment. The user can proceed searches only in the trade center database. No user request can reach any pharmacy database. A security mechanism (firewall, etc) separates both trade center and pharmacies database, in order to prevent any attack (SQL Injection, Buffer overflow). Each pharmacy stock database replicates automatically its concerning data into the trade center, but cannot process any request coming from the trade center.

In the case, the pharmacy does not own a database system it can forward the relevant data per email using an XML form.

Deploying cryptographically enforced access control to information in the database at pharmacies ensures the data protection.

Figure 3 shows the firewall-protected supplier's databases. Requests coming from the trade center to the supplier's stock databases will be blocked by the firewall. All order requests use another way to reach the order processing systems at pharmacies side.

Figure 2. Architectural overview of the drug supply platform

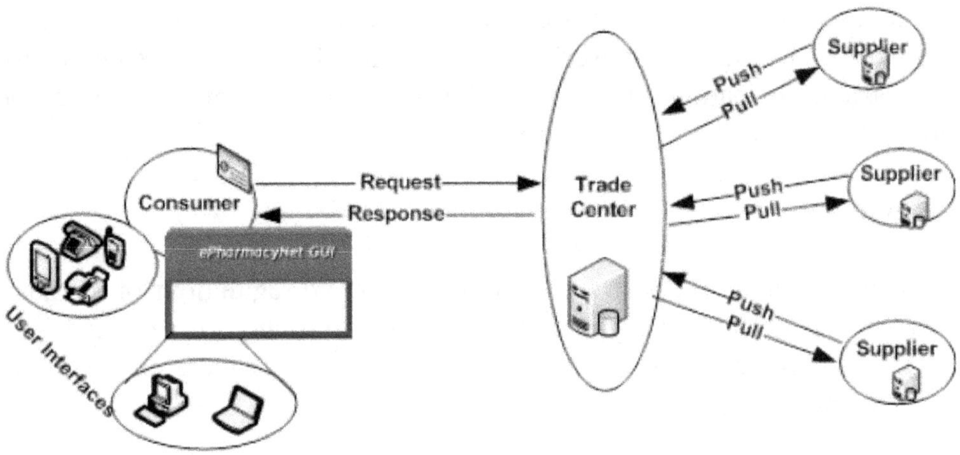

Figure 3. Protecting the supplier stock databases against attack

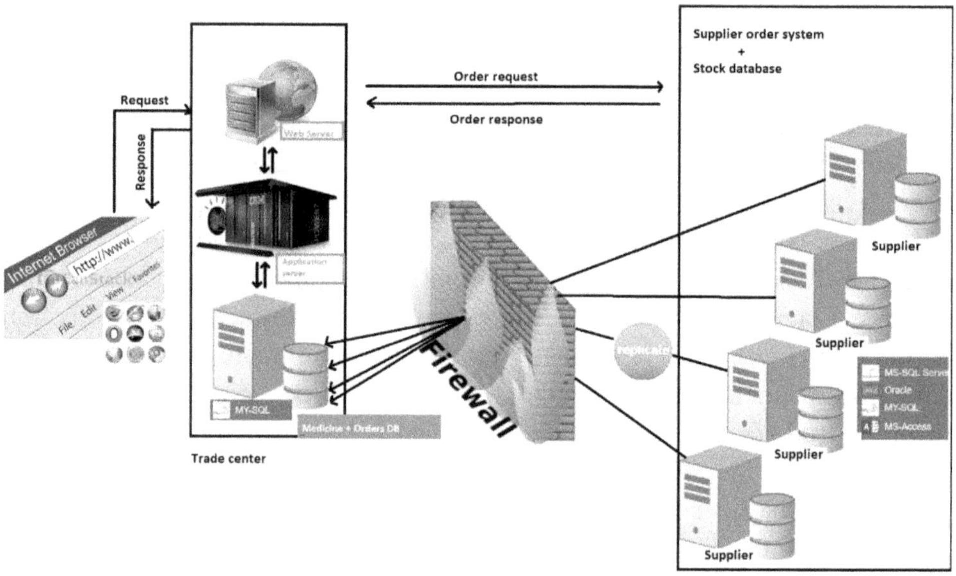

System Functionalities

The system features following functionalities to the system's users.

ePrescription

The ePrescription is the electronic interface for entering searches and orders to the drug supply system. The physician prescribes one or more pharmaceutical products and sends the prescription electronically to the trade center for processing. The patient can also, use the ePrescription interface to order the products by himself.

ePayment

All payment modes need to adhere to the rules and regulations of the bank and financial system. They need to be usable throughout the country – in large cities as well as in rural regions. In Africa today there exist a set of "money transfer-systems:

1. M-Pesa (http://www.vodafone.com/content/index/what/m-pesa.html#)
2. Mobile-money (https://www.mtn.com.gh/personal/mobile-money/about-mobile-money)
3. Flooz (https://www.gsma.com/mobilefordevelopment/wp-content/uploads/2014/02/Snapshot-Etisalat-in-Togo-and-Benin.pdf)
4. Etc.

The payment modes are e-payment (using the internet or telephone to pay a bill), cash on delivery (suited particularly for rural regions) and trust systems.

Pharmacy Support

The system has the potential to provide support and other advantages to the pharmacies. This is an important incentive for them to participate in the system.

First of all, the resulting marketplace improves the revenue for the pharmacies, since they can better sell the products to the patients who require them. The transport costs need not be paid by the pharmacies since for the patients the system already reduces the transportation costs in most cases so that they can pay the remaining costs.

Second, when the trade center supports ordering, delivery, and payment, it decreases the workload for the pharmacies. For example, in an online payment, the trade center verifies the bank data of the customer. There exist today lot of money transfer possibilities in the developing countries such as M-Pesa. These money-transfer-systems are integrated into the ePayment feature so that patients without a bank account can use this possibility to pay for the product they purchase. The trade center can also process the organization and the delivery of the ordered pharmaceutical products. The pharmacy receives the order per email or another communication way and prepares the product. The trade center may also prepare the invoice and process the delivery certificates.

Finally, if a pharmacy uses own ICT equipment for its inventory management, it can further reduce its overhead for participation in the drug supply network by replicating in real time (push mode) its inventory into the central database of the trade center. Another variant of participation is to grant access to the trade center to the supplier's system for querying updates (pull mode).

Teleconsultation and Telediagnosis

The drug supply system enables to provide simple forms of teleconsultation and telediagnosis (telehealthcare). A patient living as far as 10 km from a medical care delivery center, particularly in rural regions, can get a prescription from a physician using his mobile phone to communicate. Alternatively, the physician can directly enter the prescription into the system as an order for the patient, with a confirmation by the patient.

Statistic Data Collection

If the system is widely used, the trade center can provide useful data about the demand and supply of pharmaceutical products in the country. This can be used for automatic statistics processing about certain medicines and optionally its transmission to the health authorities.

Delivery Logistics

The transportation system in the most developing countries is inadequate. The traffic net is in a bad state. In most African developing countries, a new form of transportation is unfolding. As originally in most Asian developing as well as emerging countries, the new transportation consists of using a motorcycle to transport people. This transportation form is revealed efficient with regard to the traffic net, the state of the roads. People can easily travel from point A to point B.

Using a conventional means of transport to deliver pharmaceutical products presents several issues such as late delivery, spoil products, etc. We, therefore, design a smart transport system to secure and quickly deliver the products to the patients.

The requirements for the smart transport are to:

1. Conserve the product temperature during the transport
2. Guarantee that the products would not be exchanged on the way to the patients by counterfeits
3. Monitoring the delivery process
4. Help the deliverer to find the shortest and secure way, avoiding traffic jam
5. Deliver the right product to the person

We design and implement a thermal box to transport pharmaceutical products. The box can itself regulate the interior temperature to keep the products in the good state. As noted above, motorcycles are today the best transport mode in the developing countries. The deliverer carries on his motorcycle the transport box, which regularly communicate with the carrier smartphone (device-to-device communication) in order to inform him about the box interior temperature. RFID technology is identified as included in the Internet of Things Technology (IoT) (Pesonen, Jaakkola, Lamy, Nummila, & Marjonen, 2009) thus can contribute to connecting the different devices in this system into a network. The box also communicates at regular time stamp its geo-position to the cloud, which in turn transmits the data to the monitoring system (machine-to-machine and Internet of things.) The box also features an anti-fraud system that prevents against an exchange of a product against counterfeits. An RFID system reads the data of each product from the box. Each product has its own compartment that can be open only and only if the current position of the box is comparable to the customer provided geo-position through his address. In addition, the patient needs to enter a delivery code he previously gets from the supplier or trade center.

Figure 4a) presents the overview of the logistics for drug supply. Figure 4b) shows how different parts of the system communicate with each other and exchange data. The carrier smartphone communicates with the RFID reader (data logger) using BLE (Bluetooth Low Energy) protocol. At this stage, the communication is device-to-device based. The carrier can regularly check the box interior temperature. The carrier's smartphone receives also data about the transported products. A second RFID tag registers when a product is taken from the box and sends this information to the smartphone, which adds the current geo-position of the box and sends the entire information to the fraud monitoring application/database in the cloud. The trade center would automatically get informed about any fraud tentative and thus react immediately by calling the carrier. This communication uses the machine-to-machine paradigm so that the communication happens without third intervention. RFID can precisely and accurately localize an object indoor (Loeffler & Gerhaeuser, 2013). This ability is used to regularly localize the products in the box.

The carrier is assisted during the travel so to choose the short ways avoiding a traffic jam. A salesman algorithm combined with a crowd sensing (participatory as well as opportunistic) guides the carrier through the city. A cloud-based application initiates the traffic sensing and thus request any smartphone on the potential route to inform the carrier about the traffic.

The smartphone can be requested per SMS if they do not install the client application of the crowd sensing application. The smartphone owners are rewarded by providing the right information. The communication, in this case, is free of charge.

The sensing data are partially processed at the edge so that useless information is removed (fog/edge computing) before sending to the cloud. The data are integrated into the route and new route, if needed, is drawn and send to carrier smartphone in real-time.

RFID for Temperature Measurement

Radio Frequency Identification (RFID) is an effective automatic identification technology for a variety of objects. The most important functionality of RFID is the ability to track the location of the tagged item (Jain & Vijaygopalan, 2010).

Pervasive temperature sensing can improve the cold chain supply operations (Bhattacharyya, Floerkemeier, & Sarma, 2010). The temperature in tropical countries is permanently high, even in the rain season. The transport, of sensible and perishable pharmaceutical products, requires to regularly monitor the ambient temperature to increase the efficiency of the cold chain. RFID temperature sensors can be utilized to monitor the ambient temperature. The RFID technology offers a lot of matter attributes such as standardized communication protocols and low-cost tag (Bhattacharyya et al., 2010).

TempCorder Sense -2,4 GHz, Active RFID Tag – (Figure 5) is an innovative RFID technology capable of measuring with accuracy the cold temperature. According to the vendor, it is:

- Waterproof, dustproof, shockproof, IP68
- Durable, Long battery life
- Wireless temperature sensor
- Accurate thermometers

The RFID Technology is identified to be included into IoT. Thus, as one of the cornerstones of the Internet of Things, RFID can also, like IoT, impact areas such as operational efficiency (cold supply chain efficiency), safety, and security. The pharmaceutical products have to be transported in the best medical condition so to guarantee health safety and security to the customer (the patient). Applying IoT to the drug supply logistics can substantially help to monitor the status of the products (assets) in real-time.

Figure 4. Delivery process and communication during the transportation

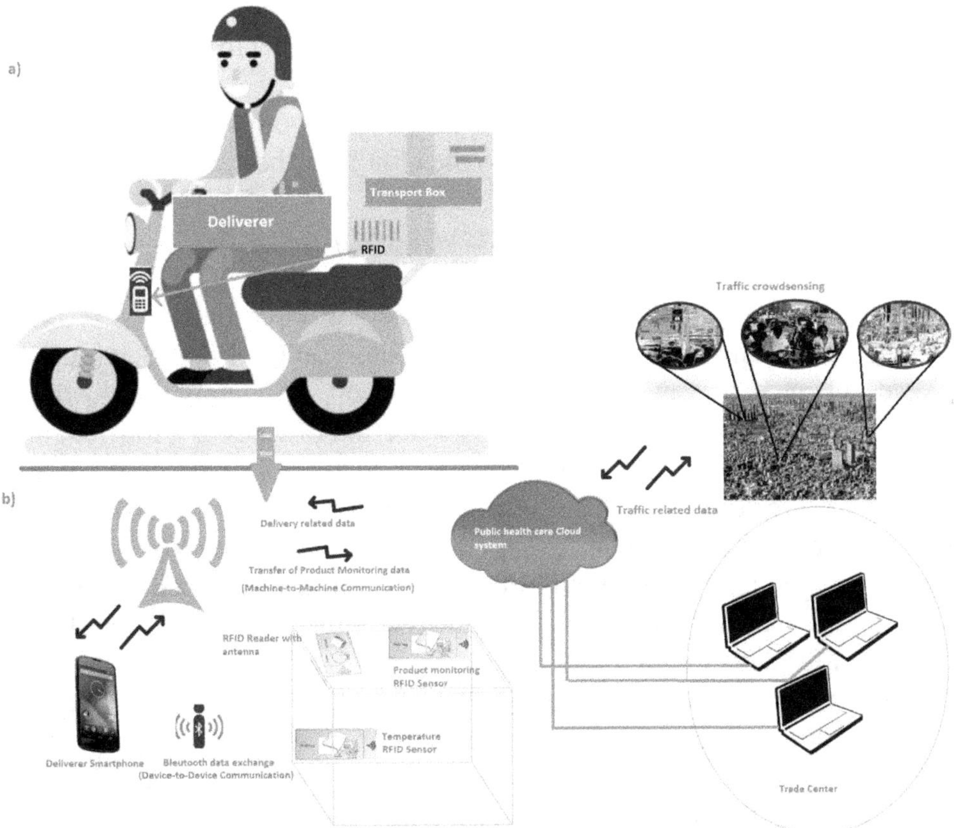

Figure 5. RFID temperature sensor

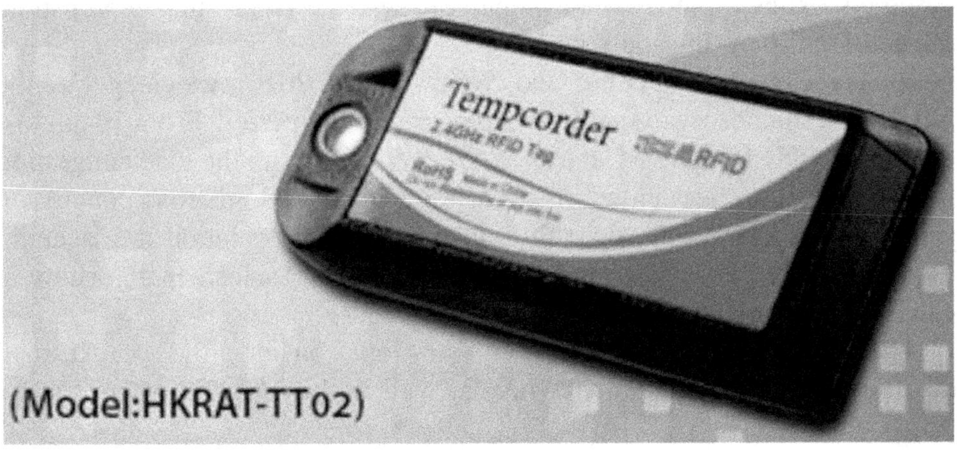

RFID is used to detect the location of assets (Jain & Vijaygopalan, 2010). It is used to itemize the products pharmacy loads into the transport box and configure the appropriate/ideal box temperature in order to efficiently supply the products. The data about each itemized product is sent to the trade center. The data center can, therefore, remote monitor the box temperature through the data the RFID system provides to the cloud via the carrier smartphone.

Avoid the Traffic Jam Using Crowdsensing

Crowdsensing systems are either participatory or opportunistic.

Our concept aims to combine both, participatory and real-time opportunistic crowdsensing and crowdsourcing data to energy-efficiently and low-cost, monitor ad-hoc traffic crowds for early detection of risks of a traffic jam.

A cloud-based algorithm would continuously request participant's mobile phone on a given route to provide information on the traffic. These participants would be requested to activate the client application on their mobile phones. The client application measures the density of the traffic in reporting their GSP coordinates to the cloud. The client could recognize which GSP coordinates are useful for detecting a traffic.

Each traffic has GSP coordinates. Our algorithm monitors every activity within 2 kilometers around the traffic light using all smartphones coordinates in this circle. Thus, we can determine the speed of each vehicle or motorcycle on the given route and thus, detect if a traffic jam is occurring. Similar work is done in (Cárdenas-Benítez et al., 2016) where the authors use the Vehicle-to-Vehicle paradigm to detect traffic congestion. Li Wei et al. propose in (Wei & Dai, 2016) a real-time road congestion detection in estimating vehicle density based on texture analysis and evaluate the system. The results demonstrate the potentiality of this approach.

As Yun Zhu et al. in (Zhu, Gao, Wang, & Liu, 2016), we categorize the traffic, after an observational study, in peak and flat period. From 10 pm to 4 am the next day we have a flat traffic. From 5 am to 9 am the road congestion is high as well as the accident risk. Between 7pm and 9 pm, road congestion can be noted again. Our algorithm takes all this information into account by defining the delivery route. We also use the travel salesman algorithm in calculating the efficient route for a delivery tour.

The planning of the route for a delivery tour considers the context, road congestion at any time and anywhere as well as the road and by-road state.

It takes also into account the season, for example, rain period where most road and way are in the poor state (case of the developing countries). The routing application at the cloud continuously calculates the routes till the carrier delivers the last product.

OFF-LABEL DRUGS USE

System Concept and Design

Knowledge Database

We propose to provide the healthcare professionals with a knowledge-based database (KDB) to help them in prescribing off-label drugs in a secure manner.

A KDB is a system designed for collecting data and data analysis. This system is based on technologies such as data warehousing (data capturing) and data mining[2] (data analysis). Data mining is the analysis of data for relationships that have not previously been discovered (http://searchsqlserver.techtarget.com/definition/data-mining).

The proposed KDB system is consisting of a mechanism for generating pattern lists of off-label-drugs and treatment with high evidence and evidence-based knowledge on Off-Label-Use to help or assist the health professionals

Depending on the legislative situation regarding the off-label-use we propose two data capturing methods by using a web-based user interface: (i) an anonymous (online) off-label-use data capturing and (ii) logged-in (online) off-label-use data capturing with grant access for physicians only.

A Business Intelligence System[3], as backend system of our proposed KDB will take the source of the capturing data in consideration by generating evidence data after automatic analysis of the collected data.

Report Form

To facilitate off-label-use reporting, we proposed a form that we discussed with different interviewees. The improved form after discussing with the interviewees is presented in Table 10. All requested information on the form is mandatory. The form could be anonymized, then the expert's committee

Table 10. Proposed report form

Report on Off-Label-Use Form Nr.:.........
Hospital data: Name .... Address .... P-BOX.. Tel.: ....
Reporter Name .... Tel.: .... Position ....
Treatment provided by Name .... Tel.: .... Professional category. ....
Treatment-Data Date .... Reported Treatment: Diseases/Affection: .... Drug Designation.: .... Relevant active components: .... Result of treatment: ☐ successful ☐ Failed
Patient's State Cured ☐ Palliation/Improvement ☐ Deceased ☐
Course of Treatment Information Regulation for Admission
Application Data Dosage Age group Contraindication (see label) Occurred side effects (see label) Treatment Duration Scope of Application (ex. Psychiatry)
Expected results: .... **The motivation of the use:** .... **Course, Values (Please, compare both data the value bevor and after the use), Result:** ....

needs the personal data of the reporter as well as treating physician's data so that they can be contacted in case complementary information is needed. The form will be provided as workflow chart to guide the reporter. Mandatory data should be inputted at each step before getting allowed to move to the next step.

ARCHITECTURAL OVERVIEW

This section presents the overall architecture of the proposed system. It describes the system use cases, the related functionalities, the activities diagram, and the flowchart of the proposed system.

System Component Overview

Figure 6 illustrates the overall architecture. The system consists of a reporting client running on the mobile phone, desktop PC, and tablet. The reporting application is a web-application. The backend system consists of a medical data server, reporting database (rDB), reviewing database(reDB), and data warehouse management system (DHW) that extracts, transform, and loads data from the rDB and reDB. A business intelligence unit (BIU) uses the data

Figure 6. System architectural overview

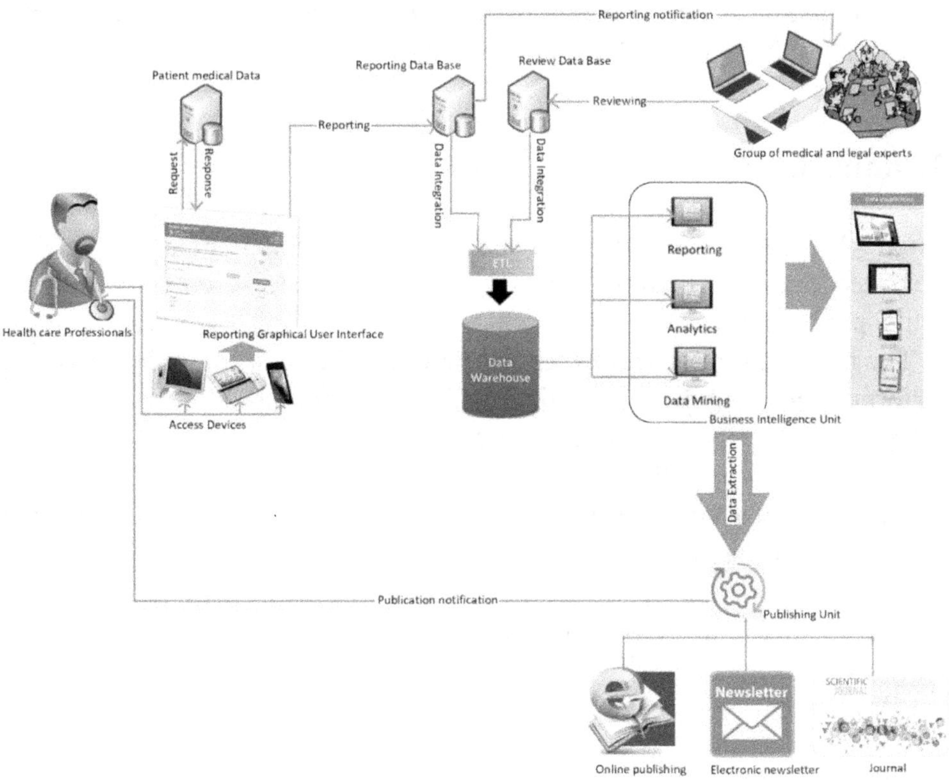

from DWH for data analytics, data mining and reporting. The BIU disposes of an interface for data visualization.

The provides features a publication unit that extracts information from the BIU and generates materials for three (03) kind of publications: (i) online publishing, (ii) newsletters, and (iii) journals

The database could run under MySQL, MSSQL, or Oracle. The client would support all web-browser, such explorer, Firefox, etc. The servers are implemented using Java as a programming language. The client can be implemented using dotNet technology as well as java. The client-server communication can be implemented using dotNet Remoting technology or Java RMI as well as Restful or SOAP web-service.

Flow Chart

Figure 7 illustrates the flowchart of the proposed system. The data acquisition is performed and sent to the next stage where texts are extracted. At the following stage, format/structure check is performed using plausibility rules. The acquired data then stored in the reporting database only if the report is well-formed, otherwise, the report would be corrected before storing into the database.

System Use Cases

Three (03) actors are identified are identified. The system can retrieve requested data/information, perform plausibility check, credential check, online publishing, etc.

The medical doctor and expert's group member can log into the system perform review, submit a reporting, and search for a newsletter,

Figure 8 describes the different use cases backend system, physician, and expert can perform in the system.

The user can access the system only using his credentials. It is important to secure the access to any instruction. The reporting data are also protected against attacks.

These use cases lead us to determine the main system functionalities such as

1. Logging
2. Report
3. Review

Figure 7. Flowchart of the proposed system

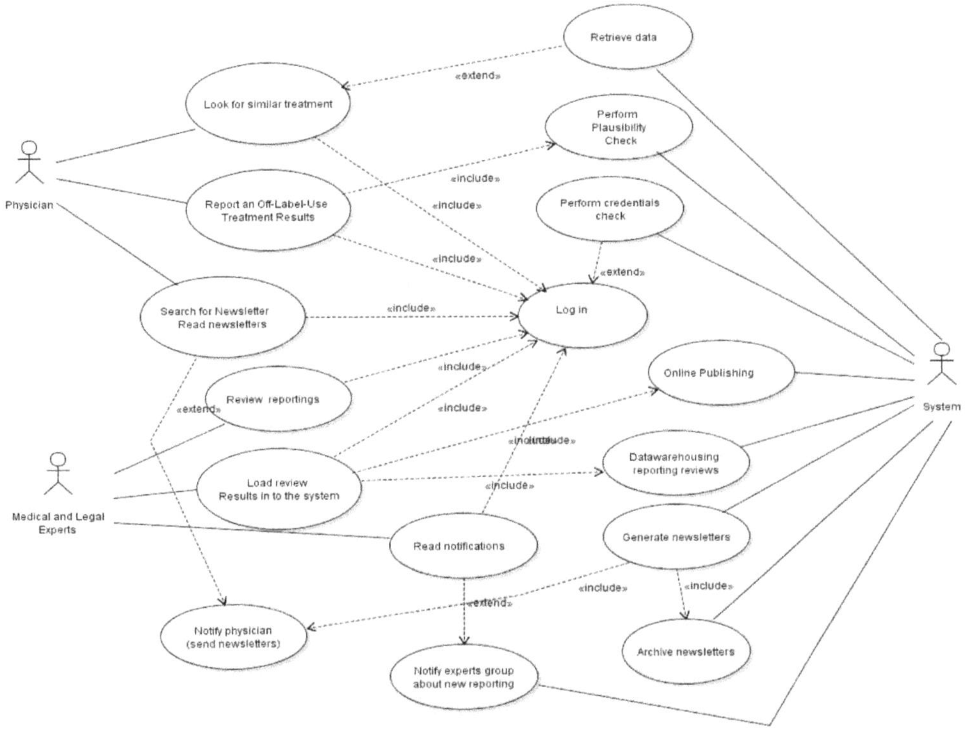

4. Search for information (newsletter, journals, etc.)
5. Notify users
6. Generation publication materials
7. Archive materials

System Components and Functionalities

The KDB will provide the User with following functionalities:

1. **A Module for Treatment Tracking:** This module is a journal where the physician can track how the treatment goes on and documents the methods, the used drug, and indication
2. **A forum for Discussing With Another Health Professionals or Pharmaceutical Companies:** A discussion forum, where the physician can discuss a case or advise another physician, also to report a case or reply to a question

Figure 8. System use cases and actors

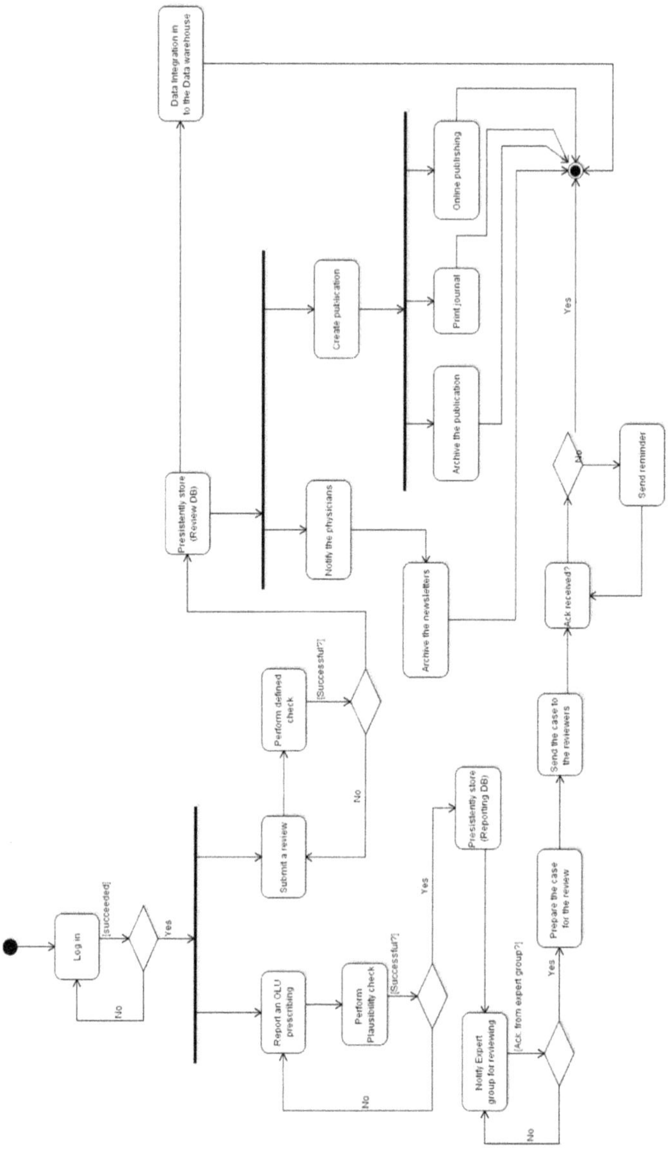

3. **Search Option:** Search for proven and/or succeeded treatment methods, off-label-drug for given diseases, etc.
4. **Reporting Tools:** At end of the treatment, the physician can use this module to report to the central system his experiences and thus described the treatment and the methods also the drugs and indications used. The

system will provide the User with a well-defined form and questions to help the physician to provide all need information.

5. **Approval Tool:** This tool would enable the experts to comment the case, record their proof results. The experts could use this tool to request more empirical evidence from the physician, who recorded the information and other. All registered physicians would be automatically contacted and requested to provide empirical evidence if they have also used the concerning product off-label.

Activity Diagram

Figure 9 illustrates the activity in reporting, reviewing and generating publication materials. Pre- and post-actions each activity.

FURTHER WORKS

Our future work would focus on conducting a long-term evaluation of the proposed system to prove the concept, and collect useful off-label-use data.

Figure 9. Activity diagram of reporting off-label-use

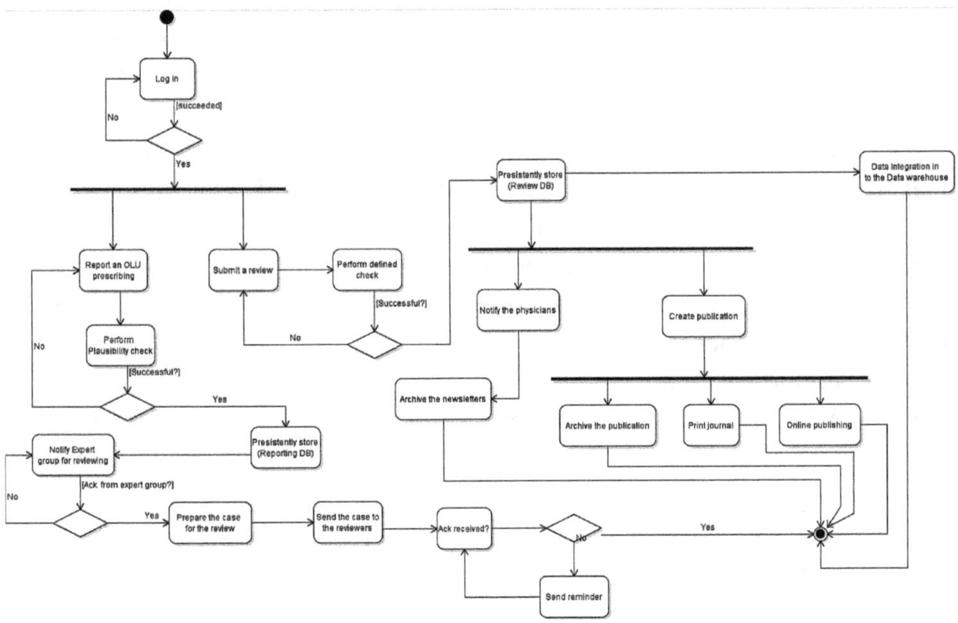

The implementation of the proposed system is in progress and will be presented in the upcoming publication.

CONCLUSION

In a case study, we investigated the problem of the distribution of pharmaceutical products by pharmacies. We found several obstacles for introducing a standard E-commerce system and developed an adapted system. A practical test has shown, that the adapted system has the potential to improve drug supply in the developing countries and help people in western countries to quickly find and purchase scarce medicines.

A survey showed that all Sub-Saharan African countries (except for South Africa) suffer from similar problems and have a similar situation according to ICT introduction. The same holds for rural regions of North African countries. Hence, it can be expected that the designed, implemented, and successfully tested drug distribution approach can be transferred successfully to those countries. Additionally, the system can also be used in western countries.

The legislative and administrative hurdles may hinder to assure safe off-label-use since more proven evidence is needed before authorizing drugs in unapproved indication.

Beyond the drug supply issues, we investigate the off-label-use practices in developed as well developing countries. We point out that off-label-use in the developing countries is due to poor drug supply and lack of essential drugs in these countries. In developed countries, off-label-use is more practiced in the pediatric and geriatric medicine.

To extend the indication of an already authorized medicinal product, a pharmaceutical manufacturer must provide new clinical trials of phase II and III. However pharmaceutical manufacturers would not spend the amount of sum to extend some of their drug's indication or to provide evidence for any off-label-use of those drugs that are already authorized for sale. Therefore, only the practitioner can provide some evidence for drugs to be used for unapproved indications.

Priv. Doz. Dr. med. H.E. Langer reported on 04.02.2002, Paul-Ehrlich-Institute has reported about 29 death cases registered till to 31st of December 2001 in Germany due to the use of Remicade (Infliximab). The institute has further reported that 10 death cases among the 29 death cases occurred because of the use of the concerning drug for unapproved indications (Steiner, 2007). Since most off-label-use treatments are not documented it is difficult to show how off-label-use drugs can also cause health damage to the patient. The health bodies should find solutions and ways to protect the patient on one hand and on other hand enable the patient to be treated in the case where off-label-use drugs are the last possibility to provide a possible successful treatment. Therefore. regulations are needed to help the patient, protect him by preventing an illegal Clinical trial. We can then conclude the different legislative, administrative guidelines hurdles and reimbursement politics of the health insurance companies hinder on one hand to provide enough evidence for off-label-use drugs and on other hand increase the uncertainty among the practitioners, but increase the patient protection against possible health damages or death by using unproven off-label-use drugs.

Regarding the facts presented above, we design a system based on empirical evidence to make off-label-use of the pharmaceutical product more secure and safe for the patient. Our concept consists of using knowledge database and business intelligence system as technical support of all system actors. The central point of the system is the expert's group, which examines the provided information and approve or disapprove the use.

The proposed system presents the advantage to improve information dissemination among the community and increase the certainty among the healthcare professionals.

REFERENCES

Bhattacharyya, R., Floerkemeier, C., & Sarma, S. (2010). *{RFID} tag antenna based temperature sensing*. Academic Press. 10.1109/RFID.2010.5467239

Cárdenas-Benítez, N., Aquino-Santos, R., Magaña-Espinoza, P., Aguilar-Velazco, J., Edwards-Block, A., & Cass, A. M. (2016). Traffic congestion detection system through connected vehicles and big data. *Sensors (Switzerland), 16*(5), 599. doi:10.339016050599 PMID:27136548

De Decker, R., Gordon-Graham, E., & Seller, N. L. J. (2009). Surprises of off-label drug use: Where had all the Prostin gone? *South African Medical Journal*, (99): 432–434. PMID:19736841

Edoh, T. O. (2010). *ICT-Systeme zur Verbesserung der Gesundheitsversorg ung in den Gesundheitssystemen der afrikanischen Entwicklungsl änder. Fallstudien: Benin*. Universität der Bundeswehr. Retrieved from https://athene-forschung.unibw.de/doc/88986/88986.pdf

Edoh, T. O., & Teege, G. (2011). Using information technology for an improved pharmaceutical care delivery in developing countries. Study case: Benin. *Journal of Medical Systems, 35*(5), 1123–1134. doi:10.100710916-011-9717-y PMID:21519942

Fukada, Kohler, Boon, Austin, & Krahn. (n.d.). Prescribing gabapentin off label : Perspectives from psychiatry, pain and neurology specialists. *Can Pharm, 145*(6), 280–284.

Goldbeck, Plener, & Resch. (n.d.). *Psychiatrie und Psychotherapie des Kindes- und Jugendalters*. Springer-Verlag Berlin. 10.1007/978-3-642-19846-5_1

J., B. (2003). Off label use — label off use? *Ann Oncol*, (14), 1–5.

Jain, P. C., & Vijaygopalan, K. P. (2010). RFID and Wireless Sensor Networks. *Proceedings of ASCNT--2010, CDAC, Noida, India*, 1–11.

Jansen, R.-M. (2009). The off-label use of medication in South Africa – what about some information for medical practitioners? *South African Medical Journal, 99*(438), 438–439. PMID:19736843

Jansen, R.-M. (2011). *Dissemination of information on the off-label (unapproved) use of medication: a comparative analysis*. Academic Press.

Krzyzaniak. (2016). *Review of drug utilization patterns in NICUs worldwide*. Academic Press. 10.1111/jcpt.12440

KVBW. (2012). *Verordnungsforum 24*. Retrieved April 9, 2017, from http://www.kvbawue.de/index.php?id=870&no_cache=1&user_kvbwcontenttabelle_pi2%5Bid_detail%5D=3203&user_kvbwcontenttabelle_pi2%5Bpid%5D=300

Loeffler, A., & Gerhaeuser, H. (2013). Localizing with Passive UHF RFID Tags Using Wideband Signals. *Radio Frequency Identification from Systems to Applications*, 85–110. 10.1109/COMCAS.2011.6105824

Off-label drug use. (2009). *South African Medical Journal, 99*(6), 411.

Pesonen, N., Jaakkola, K., Lamy, J., Nummila, K., & Marjonen, J. (2009, February). Smart RFID Tags. *Development and Implementation of RFID Technology*, 159–178. 10.5772/6523

Research, A. D. (n.d.). *Investigators use EHR data to study off-label use of asthma medications*. AAP News.

Stafford, R. S. (n.d.). Regulating Off-Label Drug Use - Rethinking the Role of the FDA. *N Engl J Med*, *358*(14), 1427–1429. 10.1056/NEJMp0802107

Steiner, G. (2007). Retrieved April 9, 2017, from https://www.bundesverfassungsgericht.de/entscheidungen/rk20070206_1bvr310106.html

Thomas, D. A. (2014). *The use of unlicensed and off label drugs in Tygerberg - Hospital neonatal intensive care unit*. Stellenbosch University.

Wei, L., & Dai, H.-Y. (2016). Real-time Road Congestion Detection Based on Image Texture Analysis. *Procedia Engineering*, *137*, 196–201. doi:10.1016/j.proeng.2016.01.250

Zhu, Y., Gao, N., Wang, J., & Liu, C. (2016). Study on Traffic Flow Patterns Identification of Single Intersection Intelligent Signal Control. *Procedia Engineering*, *137*, 452–460. doi:10.1016/j.proeng.2016.01.280

ENDNOTES

1 Discount Agreement: German healthcare legislatives prescribe discounts on the drugs' price. Every health insurance company should negotiate with pharmaceutical companies for off-patent and/or not patented medicines discounts. Pharmacies must then exclusively sell to the patient drugs from the manufacturer's drug with which the fund has entered a contract. Since July 2014 about 53 percent of all drugs sold with the same agent are covered by health insurance's discount agreement. The benefit to the insured: insurance companies can exclusively provide their insured with molecules concerned without supplement costs.

2 A process used by companies to turn raw data into useful information. By using software to look for patterns in large batches of data, businesses can learn more about their customers and develop more effective marketing strategies as well as increase sales and decrease costs. Data mining depends on effective data collection and warehousing as well as computer processing (http://www.investopedia.com/terms/d/datamining.asp).

3 According to CIO, business intelligence as a discipline is made up of several related activities, including data mining, online analytical processing, querying and reporting. Companies use business intelligence to improve decision making, cut costs and identify new business opportunities.

Business intelligence is more than just corporate reporting and more than a set of tools to coax data out of enterprise systems. Chief information officers use business intelligence to identify inefficient business processes that are ripe for re-engineering (http://www.ask.com/business-finance/data-mining-vs-business-intelligence-278d8f619f678338).

Chapter 4
Challenges Facing Adverse Drug Reactions Reporting and Counterfeit Drugs Monitoring

ABSTRACT

This chapter investigates in a case study the limitations of adverse drug reactions reporting (ADRr) and the challenges facing counterfeit drugs monitoring in the African developing countries with a focus on the Republic of Benin and proposes solutions to improve the adverse drug reporting method and infrastructures as well as the counterfeit drugs monitoring. The study aims at implementing an ADRr system using the m-health technology to overcome the limitations and ease the use of the "yellow card" in the developing world. Furthermore, a real-time notification system is provided to promptly disseminate among the populations any registered and proved ADR.

INTRODUCTION

Pharmacovigilance History

WHO defines Pharmacovigilance (PV) as the science and activities relating to the detection, evaluation, understanding, and prevention of drug adverse reactions or other drug-related problem (WHO, n.d.). The pharmacovigilance is consisted of recording and evaluating side or adverse effects resulting from the use of drugs. Its roles are to (i) report adverse drugs reactions by healthcare

DOI: 10.4018/978-1-5225-5528-5.ch004

professionals, companies dealing with drugs, and collect information by the public pharmacovigilance organization, (ii) register, evaluate, and use the collected information, (iii) monitor drug safety.

Although, it is reported in the Hippocrates: "*primum non nocere*" that in the ancient time, the doctors who prescribed a medicine (opium, strychnine ...), also monitored the individual tolerance. The pharmacovigilance is, however, a recent science, unlike the medicine. The pharmacovigilance began in the USA in later 1938 after President Franklin Roosevelt signing the ''Federal Food, Drug and Cosmetics Act''. This law foresees the necessity and the obligation for pharmaceutical companies to report to the FDA concerning the safety of all medicinal drugs. (Caron, Rochoy, Gaboriau, & Gautier, 2016). European countries like France start their pharmacovigilance in earlier 1950. The pharmacovigilance was subsequently widely implemented in all high-income countries and only recently developing countries (Sommet, Bagheri, & Montastruc, 2007).

The main event leading to the adoption and implementation of the pharmacovigilance as known nowadays are among others:

1. In 1937 the sulphanilamide elixir causing 105 deaths as a result of poisoning due to a lack of formulation enabled the improvement of pharmaceutical regulation. (Akst, 2013; FDA, n.d.)
2. In 1961 thalidomide causing phocomelia in infants whose mothers took the drug. This event allowed WHO to create an international drug surveillance program (the birth of the first national pharmacovigilance systems).
3. In 1969, subacute retrobulbar optic neuritis with clioquinol in Asia revealed an ethnic susceptibility to drugs and their adverse effects.

The Program for International Drug Monitoring (PIDM), which, in 1960, was consisted of ten (10) developed countries and expanded over the years, was launched in 1992 in Africa. Morocco and South Africa have joined the PIDM as the first two African countries. In 2006 the majority of African countries joined the PIDM. In 2015, 35 of 54 African countries are already members of the PIDM (Ampadu et al., 2016). Among the African countries joined the PIDM, 24 countries have the status of full members and 9 are associate members in 2010. The Republic of Benin is till 2010 an associate member(Isah, Pal, Olsson, Dodoo, & Bencheikh, 2012) and becomes a full member from 2011 PIDM (Ampadu et al., 2016).

Adverse Drug Reactions Reporting in Developing Countries: State-of-the-Art

The tragedies mentioned above and other disasters, for example, oral contraception (1970), Practolol (1975), AINS (1980) have shown the extreme importance of monitoring adverse drug reaction and thus the need for implementing monitoring and reporting systems.

The main concern of pharmacovigilance remains to collect unknown adverse drug reactions and report them to WHO.

The pharmacovigilance in Africa is still considered to be low due to their low reporting quota into the UMC database (Isah et al., 2012). By 2015 the rate of reporting sent by African countries represents 0.88% of the total reporting received (Ampadu et al., 2016).

... While the total number of adverse event reports has increased steadily over the past several decades, reporting of adverse drug reactions and suspected adverse drug reactions have always been low...(Dal Pan, 2014)

... Although the number of ICSRs from Africa has increased substantially, ICSRs from Africa still make up < 1% of the global total in VigiBase... (Ampadu et al., 2016).

Many studies carried out in the developing world, particularly in African developing countries reveal the poor ADRr from these countries and the challenges facing the events or signals collection regarding certain affections. For example, pharmacovigilance of antimalaria treatment is facing several challenges in collecting the adverse drugs signals. In (Talisuna, Staedke, & D'Alessandro, 2006) the authors describe a set of challenges facing the pharmacovigilance of antimalaria treatment. The described challenges, such as difficulty to distinguish adverse drug events from malaria symptoms, could lead to poor ADRr in the endemic countries. Andrea Kuemmerle et al. found out that only 51 out of 21,312 submitted number of individual case safety reports (ICSRs) of antimalarials come from sub-Saharan countries (Kuemmerle et al., 2011).

In 2009 Ezeoke, Ogochukwu M. et al. conducted in Nigeria and Benin a study (Ezeoke, Ezeoke, & Chukwujindu, 2016) on the evolution of the pharmacovigilance in western Africa and point out the causes of the poor ADR in these countries. They found out that the healthcare professionals who fill the "Yellow Card" (Figure 1), intended to be used to collect ADR, found the yellow card to be too complex to complete. Furthermore, few physicians had been trained to complete the ADR reporting procedure. Some physicians assert that reporting is not part of their professional duties. In 2013, a survey (Hardeep, Bajaj, & Kumar, 2013)conducted in India also reveals that the physicians are undertrained regarding the ADR reporting. The healthcare personnel find the reporting process tedious and lack time to perform the reporting. The survey concludes as follow:

... There is a need for a regular training and the re-enforcement for the ADR reporting among the healthcare personnel. The perception of the reporting process is tedious, the lack of time, a poor knowledge of the reporting mechanism and inadequate expertise seemed to be the main reasons for not reporting the ADRs.

Figure 1. Sample of the yellow card (Nigeria)

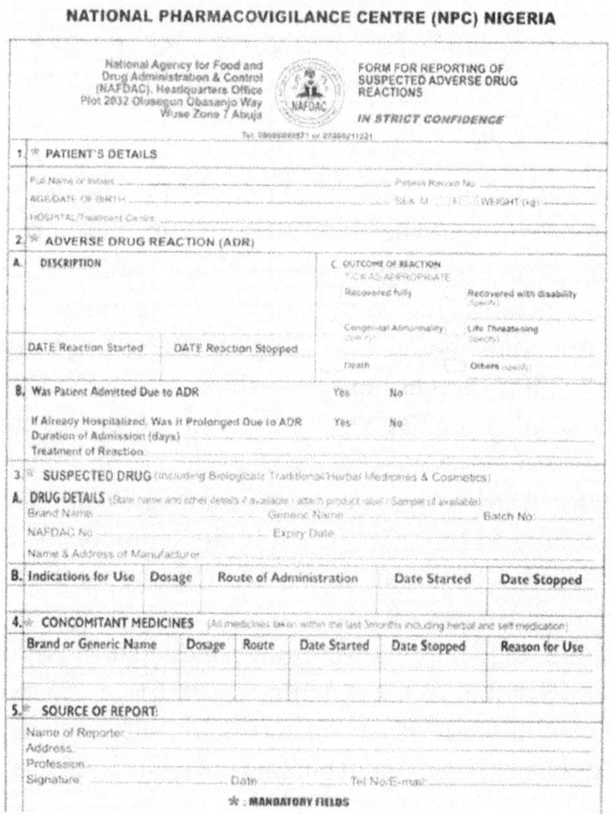
NATIONAL PHARMACOVIGILANCE CENTRE (NPC) NIGERIA

National Agency for Food and Drug Administration & Control (NAFDAC), Headquarters Office Plot 2032 Olusegun Obasanjo Way Wuse Zone 7 Abuja

FORM FOR REPORTING OF SUSPECTED ADVERSE DRUG REACTIONS

IN STRICT CONFIDENCE

1. * PATIENT'S DETAILS

Full Name or Initials ... Patient Record No ...

AGE/DATE OF BIRTH ... SEX M F WEIGHT (kg) ...

HOSPITAL/Treatment Centre ...

2. * ADVERSE DRUG REACTION (ADR)

A. DESCRIPTION

DATE Reaction Started | DATE Reaction Stopped

C. OUTCOME OF REACTION

TICK AS APPROPRIATE

Recovered fully | Recovered with disability (Specify)

Congenital Abnormality (Specify) | Life Threatening (Specify)

Death | Others (specify)

B. Was Patient Admitted Due to ADR Yes No

If Already Hospitalized, Was it Prolonged Due to ADR Yes No

Duration of Admission (days) ...

Treatment of Reaction ...

3. * SUSPECTED DRUG (including Biologicals Traditional/Herbal Medicines & Cosmetics)

A. DRUG DETAILS (State name and other details if available / attach product label / Sample (if available))

Brand Name ... Generic Name ... Batch No ...

NAFDAC No ... Expiry Date ...

Name & Address of Manufacturer ...

B. Indications for Use	Dosage	Route of Administration	Date Started	Date Stopped

4. * CONCOMITANT MEDICINES (All medicines taken within the last 3months including herbal and self medication)

Brand or Generic Name	Dosage	Route	Date Started	Date Stopped	Reason for Use

5. * SOURCE OF REPORT:

Name of Reporter ...

Address ...

Profession ...

Signature ... Date ... Tel No/E-mail ...

* : MANDATORY FIELDS

In 2014, a study (Allabi & Nwokike, 2014) has assessed the pharmacovigilance system in the Republic of Benin and thus pointed out significant results. This study is the first and complete ever conducted to assess the pharmacovigilance system in Benin. One of the significant results is that

... no Physicians or pharmacists (0.0%) had ever reported ADRs to pharmacovigilance service...

The lack of the yellow card is the principal point why no reporting has never been submitted. Further, the healthcare personnel and pharmacists are not aware of the existence of the pharmacovigilance system and additionally lack of knowledge on how to find the reporting form. The study in 2014 paints an exhaustive and comprehensive picture of the pharmacovigilance system in Benin This study

The main objective of this present study is to investigate the limitations of the ADRr and figure out how to improve the process to increase the ADRr rate. As many studies reveal the use of the yellow card is tedious for the healthcare personnel. The lack of time to perform the reporting is also a challenge to overcome. A computerized system could help to ease the reporting procedure. In (Allabi & Nwokike, 2014) the results of the questionnaire are summarized in a table (Table 1). We can notice that more 96% of interviewed physicians have been once reported by patients on ADR. However, the physicians do not forward the report to the national pharmacovigilance center because of the lack of the yellow card at their office. Therefore, a simplified reporting system supported by the mobile distributed application can be provided to the population so that people can report by themselves the ADR. Additionally, a training module on pharmacovigilance would also be provided so that the users get trained on how to report the ADR.

RESEARCH METHODS AND MATERIALS

Materials and Samples Selection

Literature Sampling

The Republic of Benin represents the study subject of this case study. We select a set of 35 materials (published papers) from different publication libraries: PubMed, Scopus, Google-scholar using the snowball process as defined in Chapter 4/STUDY METHODS AND DATA. 15 papers deal with the pharmacovigilance in Africa, 10 papers handle the state-of-the-art, the history and the reporting of pharmacovigilance in low- and middle-income countries. The other 10 papers deal with the pharmacovigilance in high-income countries, compare the pharmacovigilance procedure in the high-income countries with that is running in low- and middle-income countries. The challenges facing the pharmacovigilance of antimalaria treatment and other affections are also described in the selected papers. Among the selected papers,

- 2 papers deal with the pharmacovigilance procedure in Benin, 2 papers for Nigeria, 1 for Ivory Coast (Abidjan)
- 2 papers present implemented spontaneous reporting systems for example "*A computerized system for signal detection in spontaneous reporting system of Shanghai China*"

Testing: Cohort Sampling

We qualitatively and quantitatively collected in 2016 (for 6 months – March to September) data related the pharmacovigilance procedure in the Republic of Benin, we have interviewed physicians and patients (Table 1).

We built in afterward a cohort for test purpose. The main objective of the test is to investigate whether the proposed system and infrastructure would contribute to overcoming the challenges facing the ADRr in Benin. The results of this test can be generalized to other sub-Saharan African countries.

Table 1. Participants structure

Hospitals/Clinics-Level	# Number	Participants Category	Number of Participants
University Hospital	1	General Physician	13
		Pediatric	2
		Emergency care	5
		In-Patient	10
Private Clinics	1	General Physician	3
		In-Patient	2
Medical practice	1	General Physician	5
		In-Patient	4

- **Qualitative Research Approach:** To collect qualitative data we use the qualitative research approach and accordingly sample the cohort (Table 2/Table 3) consisting of diverse categories of persons: (i) Healthcare professionals (HCP), (ii) Pharmacists, (iii) the population/patients. In this dummy test, we like to know if the involved pharmacists and HCP find the necessary time to complete the reporting, and how they find the procedure since they complain that it is complex to complete yellow-card, however. We identified patients following a medical treatment. The goal of the test involving the patient is to know: (i) if the patients could make difference between diseases symptoms and adverse drugs reaction, (ii) if are they able to correctly complete the forms, and (iii) what is the quality of the information they provide. The patients are divided into three categories: (i) illiterates, (ii) semi-illiterates, and (iii) high educated.
- **Quantitative Research Approach:** In this study, we like to know how many people are interested in using the system to report ADR. For this purpose, we inform the healthcare professionals and pharmacists association about the online variant and advertise in the different social network such as Facebook, LinkedIn, in some schools and universities so that many persons get informed on the system. We also use the snowball approach to reach many people.

Table 2. Structure of the care professional's cohort

Category	Number	Are Trained on Pharmacovigilance (%)	
		Yes	No
Pharmacists	12	16,67%	83,33%
Health care Personnel	28	32,14%	67,86%

Table 3. Structure of the patient cohort

Category	Number	Are Trained on Pharmacovigilance (%)		Diseases
		Yes	No	
Illiterates	9	0%	100%	Malaria Injuries
Semi-illiterates	4	0%	100%	Malaria Heart diseases Lung diseases
High-educated	3	0%	100%	Severe malaria Gastro-enteric

Data Collection

Assessment and Interview on Pharmacovigilance in Benin

We used a semi-structured questionnaire to get insight into the ADRr process in the country (Benin) and investigate the knowledge of the healthcare personnel. The main reason for using the semi-structured interview in this case study is that a semi-structured questionnaire is that to the set questions we used we expect that the qualitative responses from participants, which may vary despite that everyone gets asked the same questions.

The qualitative data analysis conducted the authors in (Allabi & Nwokike, 2014), pointed out the causes of the poor ADRr in the country. The causes are according to the results of the study are that the yellow card is neither available at the hospital nor at the pharmacies. Furthermore, most of the healthcare personnel are not aware of the existence of the pharmacovigilance center in the country. The training on pharmacovigilance reporting remains a challenge facing the system.

We, therefore, use the finding from the 2014 study together with the data we collected in 2016 to design and implement a prototype of the proposed system.

Resulting Application for Reporting Improvement

NetBeans was used as IDE and Java 1.7 was the programming language we used to implement the reporting system. MySQL was used to implement the database management system. The application system consists of web interfaces (running on any web-browser) and a desktop client which can communicate with the server-side application over a Remote Method Invocation (RMI). It is also possible to use web services to access to the remote functions. This implemented system considers the results of the data analysis, thus the challenges facing the ADRr in Benin.

A training unit is provided to enable the users (healthcare professionals, pharmacists, population) to receive a training on pharmacovigilance reporting procedure and to spontaneous report any ADR. We provided a mobile version of the application which can run on the mobile phone. Smartphones are more used in Benin. More than 95% of the population has a mobile phone, but only a few people own a computer (Edoh, 2010). Each citizen, healthcare personnel have 4 possibilities to access to system and report an ADR (Figure

Figure 2. Data acquisition and reporting generating

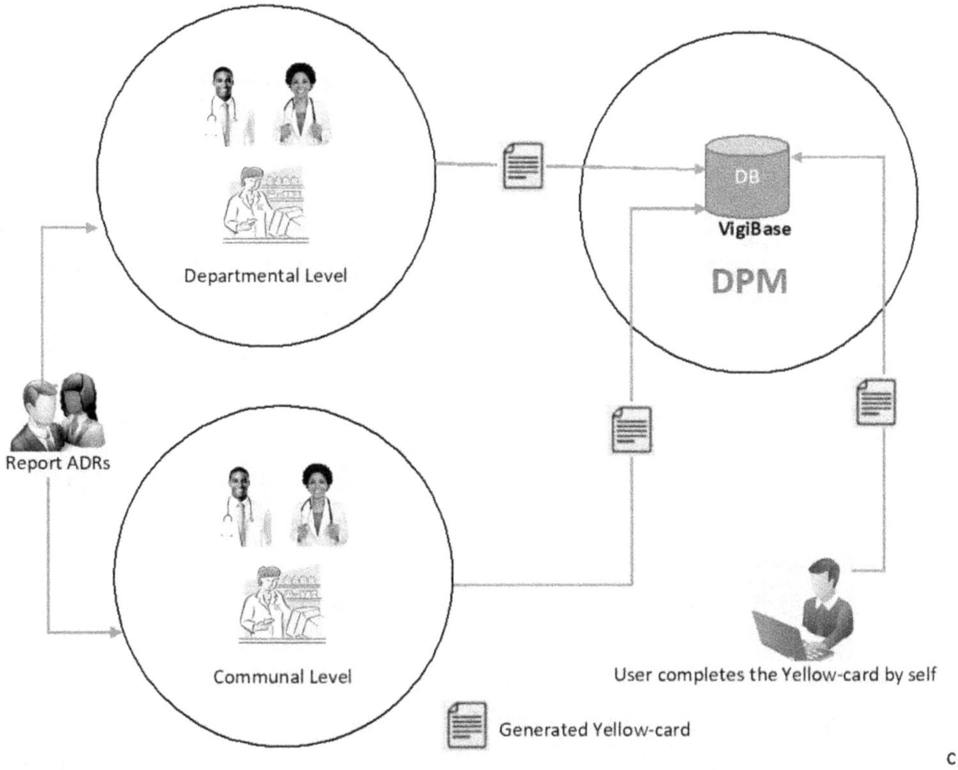

2): (i) use a browser to connect to the system anytime, anywhere, (ii) use the desktop variant, (iii) use the SMS to report the ADR, (iv) use the telephony to connect to the system and report the ADR. The reported ADRs are either directly forwarded and automatically insert into the VigiBase at the DPM or would manually be added to reporting Database.

Figure 3 illustrates the flowchart of the proposed system. Data are collected and processed following a defined workflow: (1) the user completes the reporting form. (2) The acquired data are pre-processed where the inputs are verified against the yellow card to figure out any missing information. (3) If the data pass the step 2, then the generic name of the medicine will be verified. If the name used is not valid so the system refers to the generic name database (gnDB) to retrieve the valid name and complete the intern form. Otherwise, the report is sent to the closest health center, where the report would be manually re-processed. (4) At this stage, an electronic yellow card is generated and automatically sent to the DPM to be inserted into the VigiBase.

Figure 3. The flowchart of the proposed reporting system

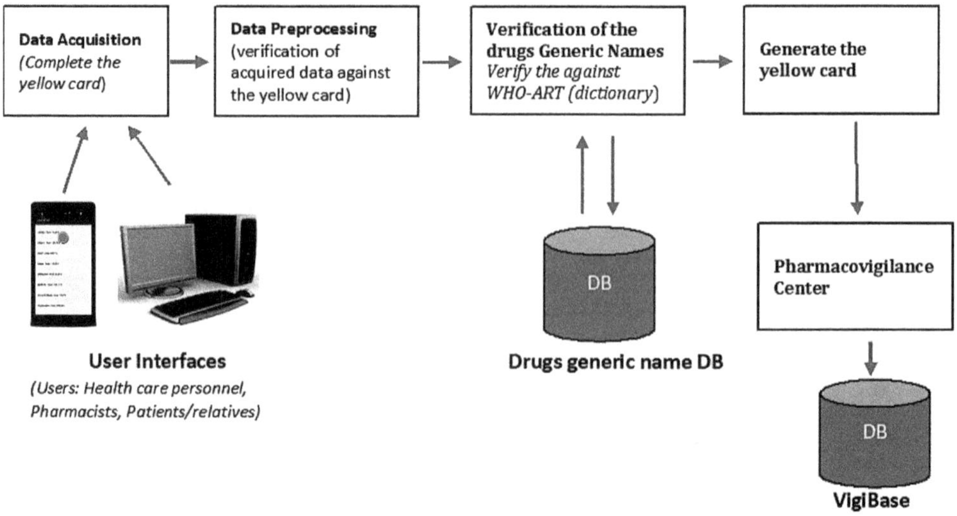

Collected Data Using the Proposed System

The proposed system enables to collect important data. The collected data through the test allow us to find out the limitations of the proposed system and the feasibility and the flexibility of the system. The following data are collected and processed:

- Drug information (name and generic name, does the system always detect and correct invalid generic name?)
- Are the ADRs (to what extent are the ADRr correct?)
- Locality/residence of the respondents (rural or urban)
- Professional status (Worker, HCP, pharmacist, farmers, jobless)
- Education Level
- Level of difficulty in completing the forms
- Consuming time
- User observations
- Usability and operability
- Impact of the training unit on the quality of the ADRrs

Study Limitations

We conducted a literature research at the first step to identify the open questions and to verify if the study main question is still up to date or already solved. The question was to know why the healthcare professionals in Benin are not aware of the pharmacovigilance system available in the country and how can this get situation get improved so that each healthcare professional will be aware of the system, get trained, and easily get access to the system and spontaneous report ADR.

We find many studies on the topics, however, only one study (Allabi & Nwokike, 2014) has completely assessed the pharmacovigilance system in Benin and presented the finding in detail. Another study (Ezeoke et al., 2016) in 2016 has presented a brief outline on topic.

We found no study that is dealing with how to increase the access to the pharmacovigilance system and prevent from tedious reporting. We, therefore, conducted a survey to get our research questions answered.

DATA ANALYSIS

Quantitative Data Analysis

We define a set of research hypotheses, which we verify within this analysis approach. The hypotheses are:

H1: Adults (40 to 59 Years old) would adhere more to the system than young people
H2: High educated people would be more interested in the system than illiterates
H3: Women would use the system more than men
H4: Young doctors and pharmacists would use the system more than elder peers
H5: The education level and the training on pharmacovigilance would impact the quality of the ADRr

Qualitative Data Analysis

We use Microsoft Excel to analyze the data collected through the test. We follow the 4 steps of the qualitative data analysis approach in:

- Organizing the data
- Identifying the framework
- Sorting the data into the framework, and
- Using the framework for descriptive analysis

The main objective of this analysis is to detect why and how many persons have difficulty in completing the forms. Further, we like to know who (education level, professional status) mostly face difficulty, and what was the impact of the training on the quality of the ADRr. Therefore, we group the ADRr in two (02): No-Health Care Workforce and Health Care Workforce. The first consists of patient, common citizen, while the one consists of doctors, pharmacists, nurses, etc.

Both groups are in turn divided into sub-groups with respect to the education level for the first group and in a category such as a nurse, a doctor for the second group.

RESULTS

Recommendations

The interviews results reveal that there is a need to improve the effectiveness and safety of drugs use, to have a better knowledge of the adverse drugs in certain situations and to warn health personnel of any risk for health.

The few literature (Allabi & Nwokike, 2014; Choi, Jude Nwokike, & Lee, 2011; Ezeoke et al., 2016) available, which has dealt with the pharmacovigilance in Benin has shown that:

- A pharmacovigilance (PV) center with a clear mandate, structure, roles, and responsibilities exists in Benin

- No National PV guideline exists
- No National safety advisory committee exists
- No Mechanism for coordinating PV activities across all stakeholders exists
- Database exists, containing partial sources of information for Coordination and collation of PV data from all sources in the country
- Few Spontaneous reporting on ADRs
- No Spontaneous reporting on product quality
- No Spontaneous reporting on medication error
- No Spontaneous reporting on treatment failure
- No existing medicines safety newsletters or bulletins published
- No Mitigation plan for high-risk medicines in place
- No locally relevant safety issues identified and acted on from outside sources
- No public education activities on ADRs and medicine safety
- No safety alerts distributed
- No regulatory actions were taken

We, therefore, propose to create a local pharmacovigilance center at each health center (about 500 at communal and rural level and 12 at departmental level), which will communicate with the departmental pharmacovigilance centers or directly with national pharmacovigilance center, which in turn will ultimately be linked to the national pharmacovigilance center, Direction des Pharmacies et Médicaments (DPM). Figure 4 Illustrates the structure of the proposed pharmacovigilance.

This recommendation can be generalized to other sub-Saharan African countries since their structures and infrastructures, as well as the challenges facing, are similar.

Additionally, we propose to grant to the population access to the yellow card in a light way so that the citizens can report online any ADR to the local pharmacovigilance center.

An electronic yellow card available anytime anywhere would ease the reporting and thus overcome the time issues the physician have reported to be facing.

Figure 4. Proposed structure of the pharmacovigilance

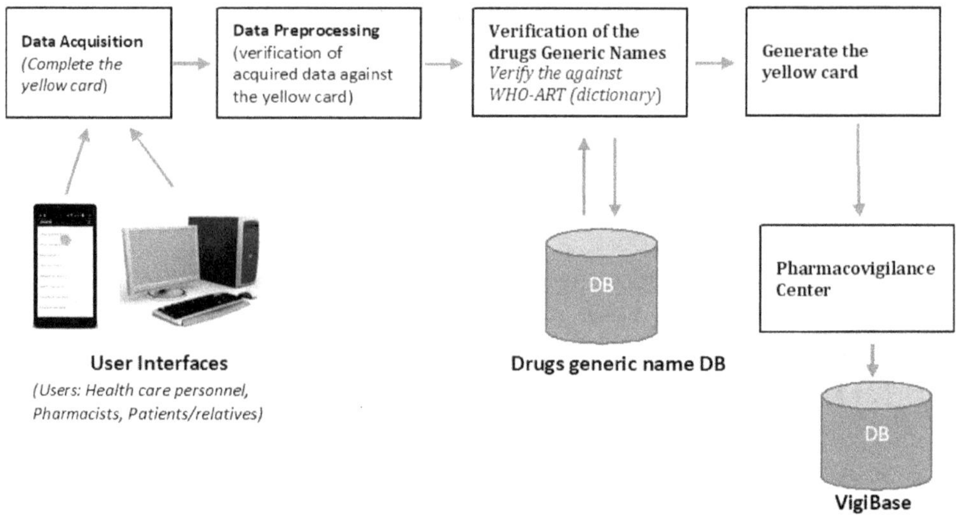

Test Results

Impact of Education level

The goal was to investigate the impacts of the education level (education level, professional status) and training on the quality of the ADRr

Table 4 summarizes the behavior of healthcare professionals toward our system and its usability. Figure 5 illustrates the results. It indicates that nurses lack time to report ADR. This is since they are assigned to many tasks. Our interview reveals that they also less confident in reporting the ADR then they have no training on pharmacovigilance. Thus, it matters to train all healthcare professionals on pharmacovigilance, so that they get confident to report ADRs.

To get better insight, we analyze the collected data in the light of the age range of the participants. Table 5 indicates that elder participants show more resistance towards the system. We interview them and find out that most of the elder have few ICT-knowledge and have more difficulty to use electronic systems. The young participants were more comfortable using the system. Figure 6 compares the results obtained in each age-group with each other.

Table 6 presents the results obtained from patient group. Illiterate produce worst reporting. This result shows that the system needs to be extended with functionalities, which may help illiterates to easily access the system, that means the reporting should be in the local tongue so that this group of patients

Table 4. Overall results of the test (group: healthcare workforce)

Category	Number	Challenges					
		Lack Time		Find the Form Complex		Are Trained on Pharmacovigilance	
		Yes	No	Yes	No	Yes	No
Pharmacists	12	2	10	1	11	3	9
Medical doctors	19	5	14	6	13	1	18
Nurses	9	9	0	8	1	0	9

Figure 5. Overall test's results on usage of electronic ADRr

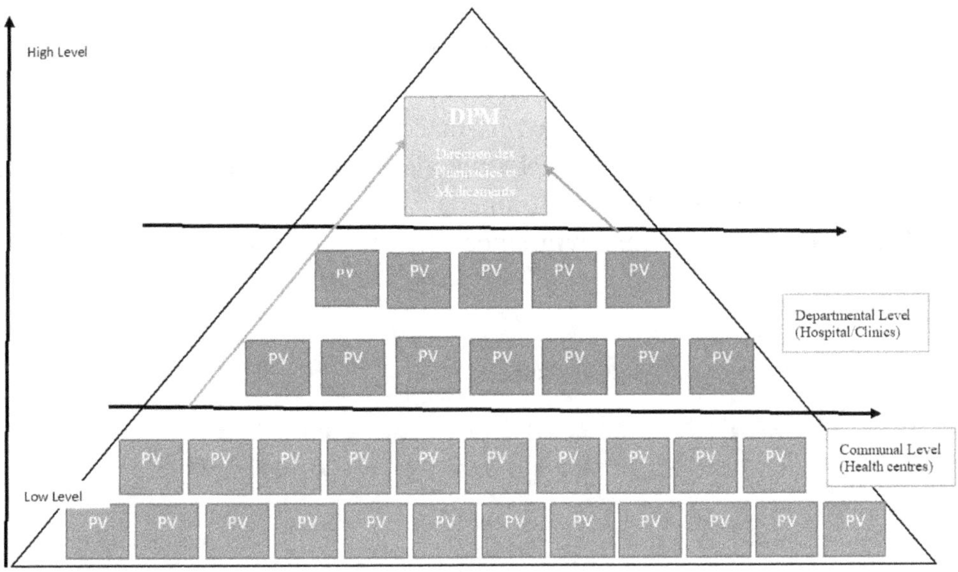

Table 5. Results regarding the age ranges

Category	Find the Form Complex		Are Trained on Pharmacovigilance		Age Ranges
	Yes	No	Yes	No	
Pharmacists	1	0	1	2	≥ 50
	0	1	2	7	≤ 49
Medical doctors	6	1	1	0	≥ 50
	0	12	0	18	≤ 49
Nurses	6	0	0	5	≥ 50
	2	1	0	4	≤ 49

can understand the questions and correct answer. The system should able to translate the questions. These results further indicate that the education level is an important factor that strongly impacts the quality of the ADR reporting. The training on pharmacovigilance also impacts the quality, but its impact is minor towards the age factor. Figure 7 compared the results produced by each group of patients with each other.

Difficulty in Completing the Forms

One of the objectives of the study and relating tests was to find out why and how many persons have difficulty in completing the forms.

We compare the difficulty of completing our simplified reporting form with that of completing the actual paper-based form. The test reveals that the paper-based form lacks an explanation of each point, which can be completed only if the user was trained on the pharmacovigilance. Our proposed system provides the user during the completing phase necessary information so that he can complete without getting trained.

The training on pharmacovigilance, therefore, reduces the difficulty of completing.

Figure 6. Test's results per age ranges

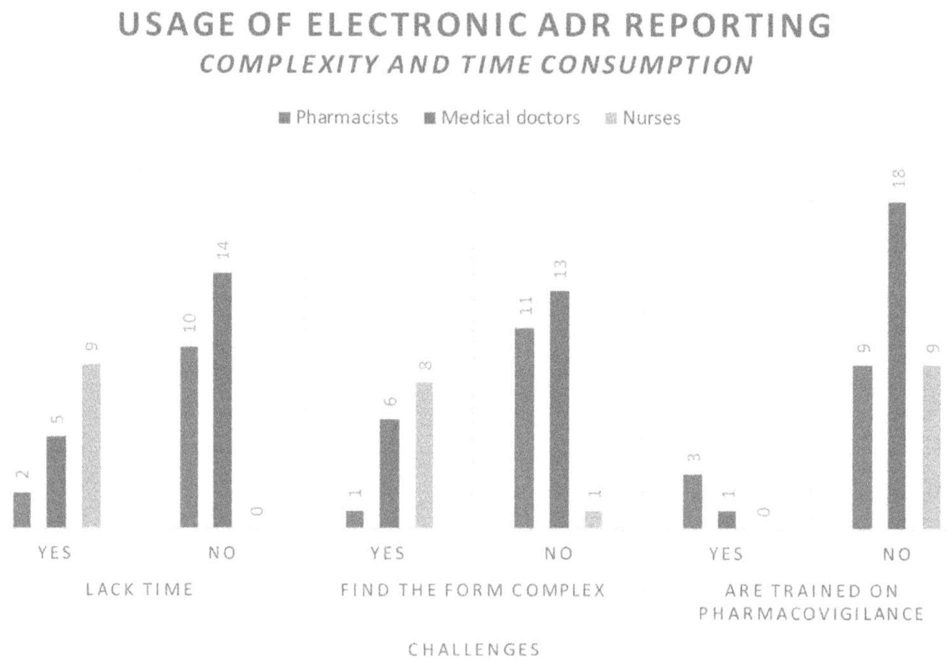

Table 6. Results of the test (group: patient)

Category	Number	Quality of Collected Information (%)		Is It Difficult to Complete the Form? (%)		Can Make Difference Between ADR and Symptoms	
		Good	Bad	Yes	No	Yes	No
Illiterates	9	0%	100%	100%	0%	0%	100%
Semi-illiterates	4	25%	75%	75%	25%	50%	50%
High-educated	3	100%	0%	0%	100%	75%	25%

Figure 7. Quality of reported data by patient

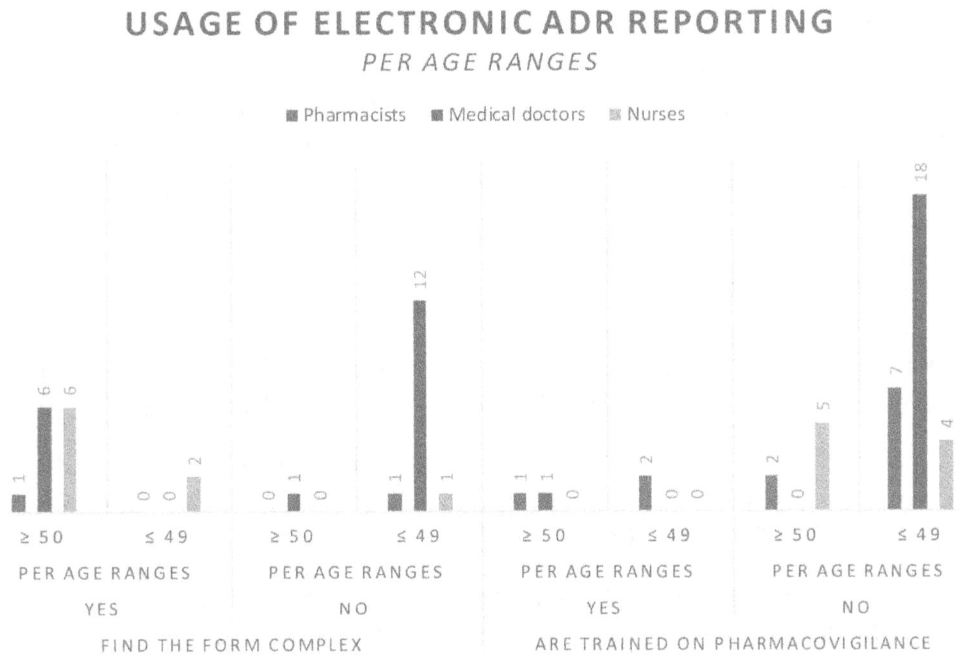

CONCLUSION

This study presents a matter factor in improving the healthcare in developing countries. An improved pharmacovigilance system can save a life. Involving patients in this process can increase their empowerment and awareness of the ADR and thus educate them. Health literacy is today an important research field. Several research works have been conducted on the topic.

ADR is a worldwide phenomenon. This study demonstrates the need to involve the world population in the reporting operation, train the population on this topic.

As it is shown in (Edoh, 2010) counterfeit drugs, illegal drug testing are challenges facing most public health care systems in the developing countries. It is worth to notice that these drugs are mostly not labeled; thus, the adverse effects are unknown. The population is not educated to report such adverse, Additionally, the concerned people are mostly illiterate.

This chapter has discussed what the pharmacovigilance is and the challenges the global health care system are facing. The origin of the topic is presented. This study has shown that the public health care systems in the low- and middle as well as high-income are facing the pharmacovigilance and ADR issues at different levels, Therefore, the presents adequate solution approaches to meet the different challenges.

Recommendations are made with focus on the developing countries, then this chapter has dealt with a case study in order to point the pharmacovigilance issues facing the global health care.

REFERENCES

Akst, J. (2013). *The Elixir Tragedy, 1937*. Retrieved from http://www.the-scientist.com/?articles.view/articleNo/35714/title/The-Elixir-Tragedy--1937/

Allabi, A. C., & Nwokike, J. (2014). A Situational Analysis of Pharmacovigilance System in Republic of Benin. *Journal of Pharmacovigilance*, *2*(4), 4–11. doi:10.4172/2329-6887.1000136

Ampadu, H. H., Hoekman, J., de Bruin, M. L., Pal, S. N., Olsson, S., Sartori, D., ... Dodoo, A. N. O. (2016). Adverse Drug Reaction Reporting in Africa and a Comparison of Individual Case Safety Report Characteristics Between Africa and the Rest of the World: Analyses of Spontaneous Reports in VigiBase®. *Drug Safety*, *39*(4), 335–345. doi:10.100740264-015-0387-4 PMID:26754924

Caron, J., Rochoy, M., Gaboriau, L., & Gautier, S. (2016). The history of pharmacovigilance. *Therapie, 71*(2), 129–134. 10.1016/j.therap.2015.12.007

Choi, H. L., Nwokike, J., & Lee, D. (2011). *Strengthening Pharmaceutical Systems (SPS) Program. 2011. Safety of Medicines in Sub-Saharan Africa: Assessment of Pharmacovigilance Systems and their Performance.* US Agency for International Development. Retrieved from http://projects.msh.org/projects/sps/SPS-Documents/upload/SPS-FDA-PV-Report-March-2012.pdf

Dal Pan, G. J. (2014). Ongoing challenges in pharmacovigilance. *Drug Safety, 37*(1), 1–8. doi:10.100740264-013-0123-x PMID:24264884

Edoh, T. O. (2010). *ICT-Systeme zur Verbesserung der Gesundheitsversorg ung in den Gesundheitssystemen der afrikanischen Entwicklungsl änder. Fallstudien: Benin.* Universität der Bundeswehr. Retrieved from https://athene-forschung.unibw.de/doc/88986/88986.pdf

Ezeoke, O. M., Ezeoke, E. U., & Chukwujindu, J. (2016). The Evolution of Pharmacovigilance in Western Africa Current Practice of Pharmacovigilan ce. *Research, Innovation and Scholarship Expo.* 10.4314/gm

FDA. (n.d.). *Taste of Raspberries, Taste of Death The 1937 Elixir Sulfanilamide Incident, 2010.* Retrieved from https://www.fda.gov/aboutfda/whatwedo/history/productregulation/sulfanilamidedisaster/

Hardeep, Bajaj, J. K., & Kumar, R. (2013). A Survey on the Knowledge, Attitude and the Practice of Pharmacovigilance Among the Health Care Professionals in a Teaching Hospital in Northern India. *Journal of Clinical and Diagnostic Research, 7*(1), 97–99. doi:10.7860/JCDR/2012/4883.2680 PMID:23449824

Isah, A. O., Pal, S. N., Olsson, S., Dodoo, A., & Bencheikh, R. S. (2012). Specific features of medicines safety and pharmacovigilance in Africa. *Therapeutic Advances in Drug Safety, 3*(1), 25–34. doi:10.1177/2042098611425695 PMID:25083223

Kuemmerle, A., Dodoo, A. N. O., Olsson, S., Van Erps, J., Burri, C., & Lalvani, P. S. (2011). Assessment of global reporting of adverse drug reactions for anti-malarials, including artemisinin- based combination therapy, to the WHO Programme for International Drug Monitoring. *Malaria Journal, 10*(1), 57. doi:10.1186/1475-2875-10-57 PMID:21388536

Sommet, A., Bagheri, H., & Montastruc, J. L. (2007). *De la pharmacovigilance à la gestion des risques – From pharmacovigilance to risk management plans.* Academic Press.

Talisuna, A. O., Staedke, S. G., & D'Alessandro, U. (2006). Pharmacovigilance of antimalarial treatment in Africa: Is it possible? *Malaria Journal*, *5*(1), 50. doi:10.1186/1475-2875-5-50 PMID:16780575

WHO. (n.d.). Retrieved from http://www.who.int/medicines/areas/quality_safety/safety_efficacy/pharmvigi/en/

Section 3

Diseases Monitoring and Prevention

Chapter 5
Novel Approach to Anticipate Emerging Infectious Diseases Spreading and Epidemics

ABSTRACT

In recent years, especially in 2014, Africa, as well as the whole world, has faced an Ebola epidemic. The facts have demonstrated the weakness of the global crisis management and limitation of existing diseases prediction, prevention, monitoring, and surveillance systems and policies. From 2015 until today, many studies have been carried out and systems have been implemented to improve the global infectious diseases monitoring. Most proposed monitoring systems consist of using wearable sensors for the remote sensing vital parameter in an individual. These monitoring systems are, however, limited. This chapter proposes a novel infection monitoring and prevention system using a hybrid crowdsensing paradigm to overcome the limitation of existing systems. The proposed system uses large-distance optical sensors (e.g., fiber Bragg grating sensors) for sensing bio-signals in individuals within (ad-hoc) crowds to anticipate any risks of emerging infectious diseases spreading or epidemics.

DOI: 10.4018/978-1-5225-5528-5.ch005

INTRODUCTION

Infectious diseases can quickly spread to a crowd at a market or supermarket, festivities, dancing clubs, schools, universities, etc. Therefore, it matters to monitor any (ad-hoc) crowds, especially in regions and eventual in season at high-risk for infectious diseases.

The tendency today in diseases surveillance consists of collecting epidemiological data on emerging infectious diseases through social media, wearable sensors systems, or mobile applications and carrying out the analysis by examining the collected epidemiological data. Screening for diseases is one of the oldest traditional diseases surveillance methods. It consists of asking and medically examine a patient or an asymptomatic individual in order to early detect diseases. This method presents certain limitations in early detecting the pathology. In much of cases, diseases are quite late detected and can only be treated than prevented, people do not adhere enough to the screening programs. Additionally, the results of screening for diseases can be wrong or biased.

In the age of information and communication technology, many social web-platforms are used to collect epidemiological data to predict and prevent (infectious emerging) diseases and health conditions. For example, Foodborne Chicago[1] and Flu Near You[2] are social media application used to collect diseases and health condition related data (Christaki, 2015). Though, collecting data through social media applications is limited in its "participatory" and/or voluntary aspect. Furthermore, they present a geographical surveillance gap due to limitations in communication infrastructures in low- and middle-income countries. To overcome this limitation, mobile phone application is using to collect epidemiological data on infectious diseases, since the mobile phone is widely distributed in these areas (Christaki, 2015). In (Brownstein, Freifeld, Reis, & Mandl, 2008) have discussed the limitations of the internet based diseases surveillance using the example of the Health Map system. The authors summarize the limitations of the HealthMap as follow:

... While Internet-based online media sources are becoming a critical tool for global infectious disease surveillance, important challenges still need to be addressed. Since regions with the least advanced communication infrastructure also tend to carry the greatest infectious disease burden and risk, system development must be aimed at closing the gaps in these critical areas...

Influenza is endemic in Europe. Several Influenza monitoring and surveillance systems exist at national level. The authors in (Paolotti et al., 2014) have discussed the limitations of existing Influenza monitoring and surveillance systems and propose an innovative web 2.0 based monitoring system that is an improvement compared to the existing system. However, the authors conclude that *"Internet surveillance of healthcare usage can be used to complement traditional surveillance"*. This conclusion reveals another limitation of internet-based diseases surveillance.

In (Steinhubl, Marriott, & Wegerich, 2015), the authors present a system consisted of wearable sensors to remote sensing vital parameter in the patient. The system can detect any change in patient's status quickly than conventional monitoring. The tests conducted are conclusive. However, this system can only monitor a unique individual, thus, it is limited in monitoring a crowd.

The few, but representative, Internet-based monitoring systems presented above have demonstrated the limitations of such systems, which are not applicable everywhere. Most of them are more focused on diseases monitoring than surveillance. Monitoring is when an individual is suffering from an affection and healthcare professionals are sensing changes occurring in his medical status. Diseases surveillance is when a population at given areas are screening to detect any abnormal indices pointing to any infection.

Collecting epidemiological data through internet based, social media, or wearable sensors applications requires that the user should have access to the internet, be literate (can read and write) and is willing to provide the requested information. Further, it possible that the provided information can be biased or fanciful. To our best knowledge, there exists no study that analyzes the accuracy and scientific soundness of data containing in such diseases surveillance and monitoring systems.

Preventing risks of emerging infectious diseases spreading and epidemics, pervasive screening asymptomatic individuals for diseases, and remote diseases monitoring, in regions at high-risk present more than ever challenges. The case of Ebola epidemics in Africa in recent years has, however, demonstrated the limitation of existing diseases surveillance systems. These surveillance systems are mostly enabled to visualize extracted data (events or stories) in form of map (Haddawy et al., 2015), for the HealthMap system (Brownstein et al., 2008).

Crowdsensing offers interesting opportunities in providing real-time and detailed information for example in a crisis situation (Haddawy et al., 2015). The authors in (Haddawy et al., 2015) have presented approaches used to bring people to actively report diseases. These Approaches are, under other, analysis of search queries, web-blogging activities, and web-platforms. Compared with the internet-based approach described above, the crowdsensing approaches presented in (Haddawy et al., 2015) are also limited, then they request the user to actively participate in the data collection. So, if the users do not trust the system, they would not provide their data. In (Gong, Fang, & Guo, 2016), the authors propose to guarantee their data privacy so the users are motivated to trust their data to the system.

Using a hybrid crowdsensing (opportunistic and participatory) system to autonomously collect early diseases related data can help to overcome the limitations presented above. Sensors can collect accurate data without human involvement. The data accuracy depends then on the quality of the sensors: (i) accuracy and (ii) sensibility.

To overcome the limitations, we propose an innovative crowd-sensing framework for the Internet of Health Things (IoHT) for diseases surveillance. The proposed IoHT system features a Hybrid Crowdsensing functionality that consists, on one hand, of using sensor for long-range (up to 50 km) and biomedical measurements to collect medical data such as temperature and detect signs of infectious disease such as fever (for ex. in case of Ebola); on other hand of using participant's smart devices to identify and isolate the sick person.

The main intention is to provide a balloon with long-range sensors and IR-cameras for monitoring and measuring: (i) Blood temperature, (ii) Continuous Respiratory air temperature, and (iii) Humidified oxygen heater temperature. Unlike traditional temperature sensors, fiber sensors for long-range can measure biomedical data at long-distance (up to 50 km: Ex. Fiber Bragg Grating Sensor).

Methods of Epidemiological Data Collection

The trend today in diseases surveillance is consisting of epidemiological data collection about emerging infectious diseases using social media, wearable sensors systems, or mobile applications and data analysis.

Screening for diseases is one of the oldest traditional diseases surveillance methods. It consists of asking and medically examining a patient or an asymptomatic individual to early detect diseases. This method presents certain limitations in the case of early detection of pathology. In many cases, diseases are detected quite late and can only be treated than prevented, as people do not adhere enough to the screening programs. Additionally, the results of screening for diseases can be wrong or biased.

In the age of information and communication technology (ICT), many social web-platforms are used to collect epidemiological data in order to predict and prevent (emerging infectious) diseases. For example, Foodborne Chicago3 and Flu Near You4 are social media application used to collect diseases and health conditions related data (Christaki, 2015). Collecting data through social media applications, however, is limited in its "participatory" and/or voluntary aspect. Furthermore, they present a geographical surveillance gap due to limitations in communication infrastructures in low- and middle-income countries. To overcome this limitation, mobile phone application is using web-based surveillance tools and epidemic intelligence methods to collect epidemiological data on infectious diseases, since the mobile phone is widely distributed in these areas (Christaki, 2015). In (Brownstein et al., 2008), the authors have discussed the limitations of the internet based diseases surveillance using the example of the Health Map System. The authors summarized the limitations of the HealthMap as follow:

...While Internet-based online media sources are becoming a critical tool for global infectious disease surveillance, important challenges still need to be addressed. Since regions with the least advanced communication infrastructure also tend to carry the greatest infectious disease burden and risk, system development must be aimed at closing the gaps in these critical areas...

Crowdsensing

Crowdsensing presents various advantages in collecting epidemiological data and can contribute to overcome the limitations described earlier.

An innovative crowd-sensing framework is proposed for the Internet of Health Things (IoHT) for the diseases monitoring. The proposed IoHT system features a Hybrid Crowdsensing functionality that consists, on the one hand, of using non-contact sensors for long-distance (up to 50 km) and biomedical measurements to collect medical data such as body temperature and detect signs of infectious disease such as fever (for example in the case of Ebola); on the other hand of using participant's smart devices to identify and isolate the sick person.

The main intention is to provide a balloon with long-range sensors and IR-cameras for monitoring and measuring: (i) blood temperature, (ii) continuous respiratory air temperature, and (iii) humidified oxygen heater temperature.

Precisely for the unique reason that smartphone embedded sensors are limited in collecting accurate data, non-contact fiber optic sensors would be used for the data collection. Unlike traditional temperature sensors, non-contact fiber sensors for long-distance can measure biomedical data at long-distance (up to 50 km: Example Fiber Bragg Grating Sensor).

RESEARCH OBJECTIVES

This ongoing research work would focus on ad-hoc outdoor crowd surveillance in regions and seasons/periods at high-risk of infectious diseases and autonomously detecting in a crowd ill subjects using a novel hybrid crowdsensing paradigm.

Overcome the Limitations of Smartphone Embedded Sensors

The proposed novel hybrid crowdsensing aims to use smartphone extended with optical fiber sensors for opportunistic crowdsensing thus, overcome the limitation of embedded sensors.

Close the Geographical Gap

The work would mainly focus on closing geographical surveillance gap due to limited communication infrastructures in certain areas, such as developing countries. Data acquisition would be performed by a central unit, a flying balloon. Care units would then get needed data from the central database using mobile phones. The mobile phone is widely distributed in developing countries and mobile communication is relatively good.

Reduce the Human Active Involvement in Data Gathering

This work aims at reducing the participatory part of the data collection to a minimum. Data manually provided by system user could be biased, incomplete, are fanciful. So, the implemented system would autonomously collect all epidemiological data and carry out the analysis. Users are only actively involved non-epidemiological data collection.

CONCEPT OF HYBRID CROWDSENSING SYSTEM

This section presents the concept of the proposed novel hybrid crowdsensing approach and the major limitations that the proposed infrastructure presents and how to overcome the limitation.

Our concept aims to combine both, participatory and real-time opportunistic crowdsensing and crowdsourcing data to energy-efficiently and low-cost, monitor ad-hoc outdoors crowds for early detection of risks of diseases spread. Traditional opportunistic crowdsensing and crowdsourcing data is energy-efficient but has poor real-time performance (J. Liu, Shen, & Zhang, 2016). Figure 1 presents the general mobile crowd sensing (MCS) framework, where participants open call, sense and collect data, aggregate analytics and send collected and transformed data to the data center. The MCS strategy consists of participatory, opportunistic and context-aware crowdsensing. Context-aware data sensing is triggered by pre-defined context (J. Liu et al., 2016) (Chatzimilioudis, Konstantinidis, Laoudias, & Zeinalipour-yazti, 2012).

We propose a smart health system that collects data, communicates with other smart devices and people (e.g. emergency teams) to monitor outdoor (ad-hoc) crowd to prevent diseases spread. The proposed smart health system will integrate the physical and digital world (IoT/IoHT), where they interact with each other using object with network connectivity.

Our Smart Health System, an Internet of Health Things, combines two paradigms: (i) crowdsensing and (i) Internet of Things. IoT is defined as a paradigm in which computing, and networking are embedded in objects, (Pena-Lopez et al.) equipped with embedded sensors, which could be used to collect (crowdsourcing) data.

In the scope of this project, we foresee to use balloons and drones provided with fiber optic sensors and infrared cameras. The balloons and/or drones equipped with infrared cameras (IRC) and sensors will permanent overfly cities and seek for (ad-hoc) crowd in order to collect crowdsourcing data such as temperature. Our system application would able to detect outdoor overcrowding (congestion) and thus contextually start collecting crowdsourcing data, which would be transformed into useful information. Fiber-optic sensing is an excellent solution to overcome the limitations of smartphones embedded sensors.(National Instruments, 2016). Furthermore, a pedestrian detection method in infrared images would be implemented for automatic crowd detection using the images produced by the IRC that is fixed on the balloon. A shape-based pedestrian detection method is presented in

(S. Liu, Luo, & Yang, 2007) and a real-time pedestrian detection system that works on low-quality infrared videos is implemented in (Nanda & Davis, n.d.).

In the case of detecting a risk of diseases spread within a crowd, the system will autonomously detect smartphones available in the crowd and will request them to opportunistically collect crowdsourcing data to isolate the sick person. Participants would be requested per SMS to actively be involved in the crowdsourcing data collection. The balloon will communicate the geo-position of the detected person to a closer drone, which will follow the person in his displacement. The person's (smart) phone will then requested to provide in real-time its geo-position so that emergency service can easily find the person. In case no smartphone is available to determine the geo-position, the drone would monitor the person per video and additionally requested any detected smartphone near to the detected person to provide the geo-position. Similar work was implemented in SmartTrace project.(Chatzimilioudis et al., 2012)

It is required that smartphones would be provided with an application, that would run in the backend and enable to purposely use the device without the explicit action of the owner.

CHALLENGES AND SOLUTION APPROACHES

This subsection discusses the limitations of using smartphones embedded sensors for sensing data and challenges facing participatory crowdsensing. It further proposes solution approaches to meet the challenges

Smartphone Embedded Sensors

Limitations

Crowdsensing paradigms (participatory and opportunistic) are intended to help to collect crowdsourced data and forward them to a central unit for processing. Participants can be requested to collect bio-signals such as body temperature to detect fever, continuously monitor individual respiration, etc.

Sensing and processing in- and outdoor temperature using a smartphone or tablet is theoretically an ideal method. Unfortunately, applications running on a smartphone for sensing temperature do not deliver accurate values since smartphones are not intended to be used as a thermometer. An accurate temperature measurement with a smartphone or tablet embedded sensors is therefore not possible without extension. These limitations are due to the electrical sensors smartphones actually feature (Van Hoe et al., 2012). Electrical sensors have inherent limitations such as transmission loss and susceptibility to electromagnetic interference (noise) that make their usage challenging or impractical in many applications. (National Instruments, 2016) An application running on the smartphone can only read temperature values provided by an integrated sensor. However, the device and/or battery temperature can bias the measurement.

In (Kos, Tomazic, & Umek, 2016), Kos Anton et al. have evaluated the accuracy of the smartphone sensors and figure out biases between measurement from smartphone models. They conclude following:

... that the parameters of measured smart-phone sensors vary considerably between different smartphone models and some of the parameters also within the same model...

There are smartwatches that can sense bio-signals such as ECG, PPG, temperature. These smart devices can though be used for crowdsensing, where participants could collect their own data as input for crowdsourcing systems or the devices could automatically collect the data and perform computations for opportunistic systems. However, these devices present limitation regarding the accuracy of the sensitivity or specificity of the sensor (Carpenter & Frontera, 2016). Rahul Majethia et al. have evaluated in (Majethia et al., 2015) the sensitivity and accuracy of the onboard ambient temperature sensor under various circumstances and measure its performance against standardized weather monitoring equipment. They had outlined four (04) key challenges to get domain specific accuracy in using smartphone sensors. They use Acru-rite temperature sensor (indicated to be accurate to 0.50 C within its operating temperature range, i. e. -20°C to 60°C) to evaluate if the sensor in a smartphone can provide accurate data as delivering by weather-sensing equipment. The results of their work figure out that temperature measurement using the smartphone sensors can cause biased data due to several device-dependent and context-dependent factors.

Therefore, using smartphone sensors for collecting body temperature presents some limitations, since smartphone sensors are limited in measuring accurate in- and outdoor temperature as well as body temperature (Kos et al., 2016).

To overcome the limitation of sensing with smartphone embedded sensors, Fraden Corporation invents an instant, the non-contact medical infrared thermometer for augmenting any smartphone temperature sensing capability. Accurate temperature measurement is only possible using an external sensor.

Regarding the above mentioned key challenges and limitations of using smartphone sensors in measuring the body temperature of individuals within a crowd, a question then arises, *how to meet these challenges and collect accurate medical crowdsourced data to detect emerging infectious diseases?*

Fiber Bragg Grating Sensors (FBG) as Solution Approach

FBG sensors are the most used Fiber-optic sensors. They can measure strain and temperature (see Figure 1) and present the advantage to overcome the limitations of electrical sensors by using light rather than electricity and standard optical fiber in place of the copper wire (National Instruments, 2016). FBG signals are not distance-dependent and can precisely be collected from at least 50 km transmission distance.(Soto, Bolognini, Pasquale, & Thévenaz, 2010).

We propose to use Fiber Bragg Grating sensors for context-aware crowdsourcing data collection. FBG sensors are suitable for strain measurement from a large distance too, so this capability would help to exactly determine the nature of the sensing objects and thus to prevent false alarm within the system.

Participatory Crowdsensing

Limitations

Nobody would voluntarily accept to deliver his medical data to diseases monitoring systems if they do not have the guarantee of data privacy (Gong et al., 2016). However, participants' devices cannot be used as sensing device from which data will be collected, since: (i) participants must be enrolled before starting collecting needed data, though (ad-hoc) crowd participants are not known in advance, (ii) it will be difficult to find and/or to enroll participants who would accept to sense own medical data and send it to health monitoring system. In (Chessa, Corradi, Foschini, & Girolami, 2016) Chessa Stefano et al point out the biggest challenge of real long-running participatory mobile crowd sensing in the theme of the capacity to keep existing volunteers involved

Figure 1. Fiber Bragg Grating technology
Source: http://www.scaime.com/en/335/article/la-technologie-advoptics.html.

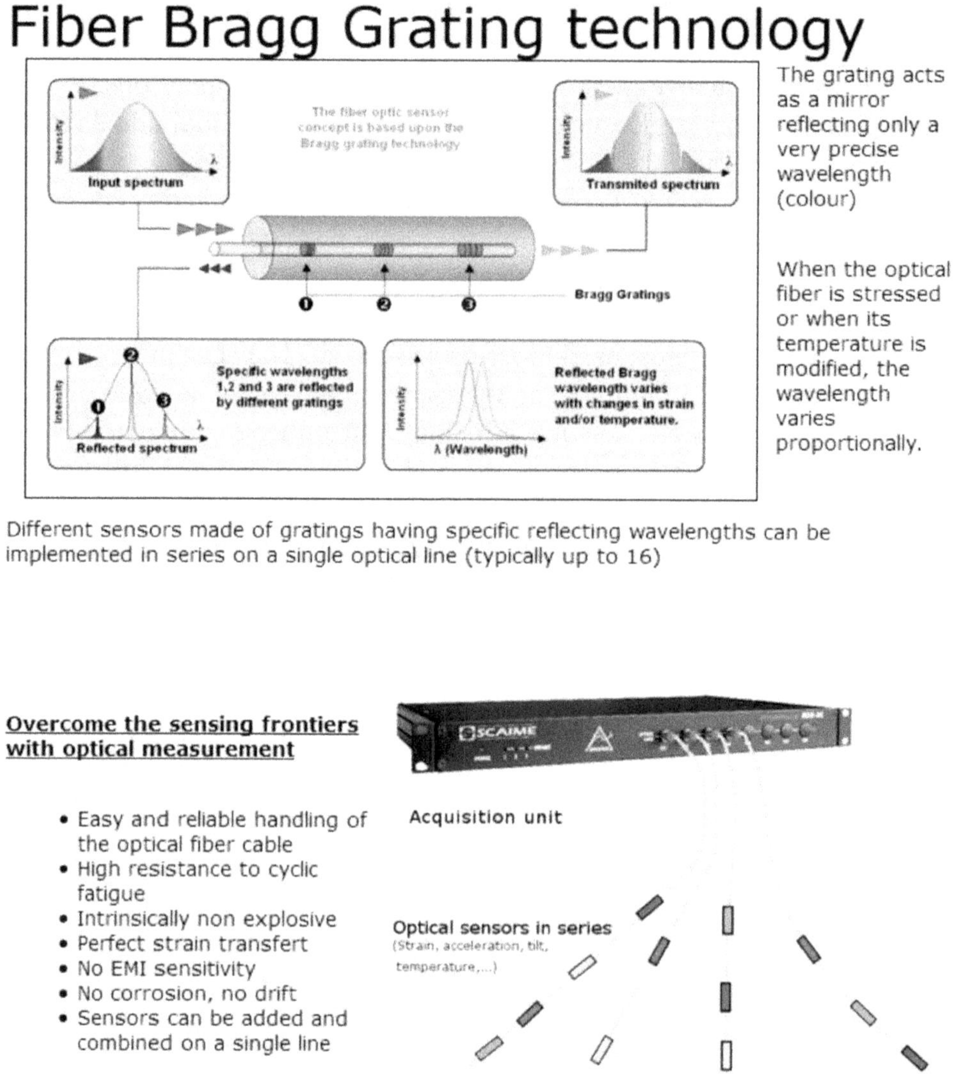

in the sensing communities. A diseases surveillance system that only relies on participatory crowdsensing paradigm could face challenges described above. The key challenges are to hire volunteers before the crowd is built, keep the volunteer's community as long as the crowd is existing. Beyond this challenge, can participants use their smartphones to contactless measure the body temperature of their crowd neighbor? This is only possible if their smart devices feature non-contact temperature sensors and are authorized to sense the medical data or get the neighbor consent to do this, then nobody within a crowd would accept that another participant measures his temperature, even contactless. No smartphone is today capable of contactless tracking body temperature.

Hybrid Crowdsensing as Solution Approach

Monitoring ad-hoc crowd using opportunistic crowd-sensing paradigm requires that participant's devices may be used to passively collect and process crowdsourced data, or (wireless) sensor networks are available and can collect crowdsourced data. In contrast to participatory sensing, opportunistic sensing does not require human involvement. An application may run on a device and collect data. Huadong et al. define, in (Ma, Zhao, & Yuan, 2015), participatory sensing as conscious and opportunistic sensing as fully unconscious. Combining both, unconscious and conscious sensing paradigm, would compensate the limitations of one or other.

System Overview and Components

Our proposed IoHT would be consisted of (i) crowdsensing units using hybrid crowdsensing paradigms, (ii) video surveillance units [using controllable drones], (iii) a cloud, and (iv) emergency centers, that coordinates the entire diseases monitoring.

Figure 2 shows the framework of the proposed data sensing system.

Set of Balloons, Which Permanent Overfly Cities

Balloons are featured with smartphones acting as a gateway, FBG sensors, IR cameras, During the fly IR camera produces images, which the system uses to detect crowd, congestion. The FBG sensors then start collecting data from the detected crowd. The control unit on board of the balloon can request any smartphone, near the scene and connected to the internet, to sense and collect data,

Figure 2. Proposed crowdsensing framework

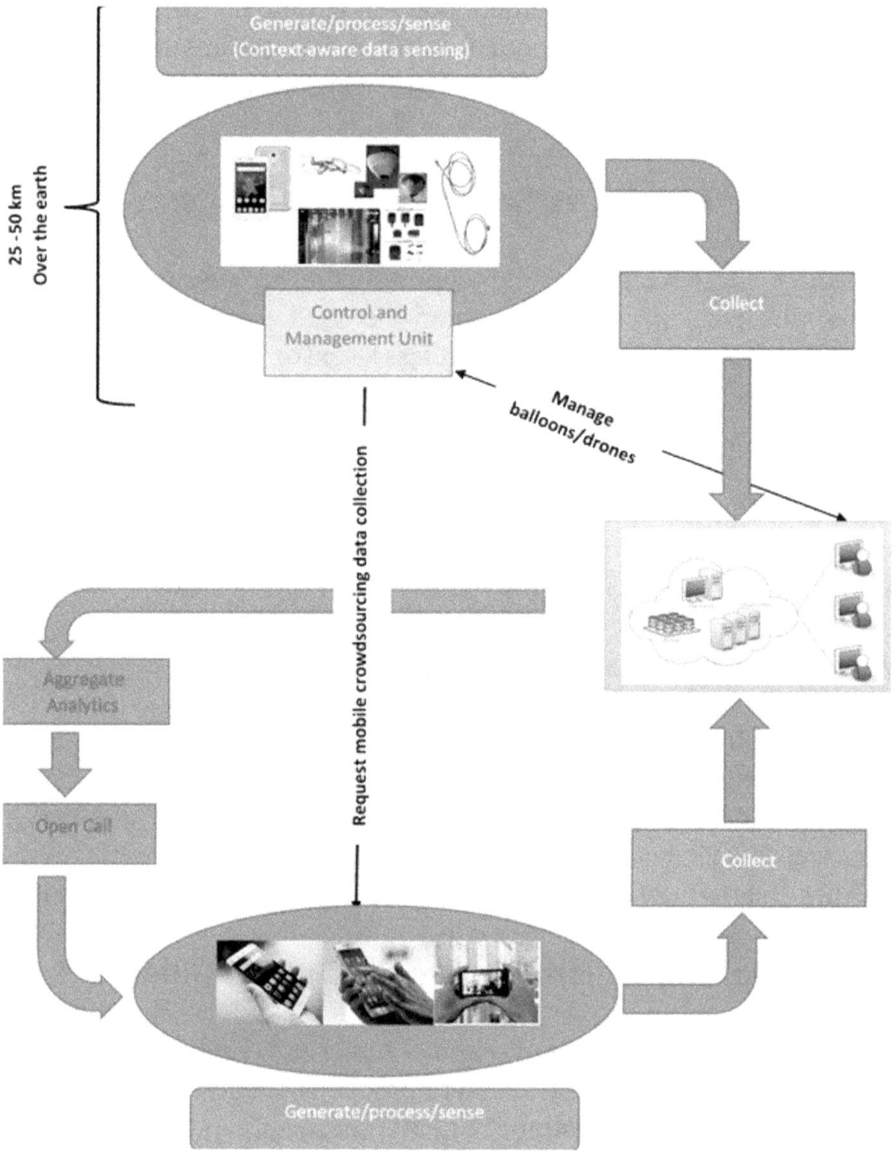

Using a Smartphone as Gateway

Marko Pesko et al. investigated in (Pesko et al., 2014) how a smartphone can be used as a gateway, a bridge between sensors network and the remote server. They prove their concept of connecting Samsung i8910 phone and a

VESNA sensor node via Bluetooth. G. Aloi et al. also show in (Aloi et al., 2017) that smartphone can be used to serve as a gateway in an IoT network. Furthermore, they use this solution approach to overcome the interoperability issues between different IoT-Devices.

We, therefore, propose to use a smartphone as a gateway to connect our sensors network with the cloud.

We would choose appropriate architecture to overcome the high energy consumption issues as the authors have been faced and reported in (Aloi et al., 2017). The results of the tests and evaluation conducted in (Morón, Luque, & Casilari, 2014) reveal that the selected Bluetooth profile, the use of GPS device or the data buffering impact the battery lifetime. The energy and battery lifetime would be investigated, and solutions would be implemented to reduce energy consumption and increase battery lifetime.

Cloud-Based Applications and Infrastructures

The cloud will host the necessary applications such as machine learning application, analytics, prediction, geo-localization, etc., it could be hybrid or public. OpenSource systems could be used to implement low-cost hybrid cloud.

Data Center

The data center can be in a public cloud since all collected data are anonym

Ad-Hoc (Mobile) Crowdsensing

An application for the purpose will be implemented and deployed on all smartphone in the entire country. Participants would start the application once they are requested per SMS to participate (actively or passively). The only user who is closer to the scene would be requested. Since each mobile is connected to the closer relay station, it will easy to identify the appropriate devices and send to them a request. They would be rewarded for this service-

Emergency Center

This center would decide and coordinate any emergency action. It can send ambulances, doctors to the crowd scene for medical means.

Energy Consumption and Supply

We proposed to use photovoltaic and/or solar energy on the balloons as an energy supplier.

Our intention is to use an external battery to operate the entire system including the smartphone. Figure 3 shows our concept of energy supply.

Figure 3. Energy supply system

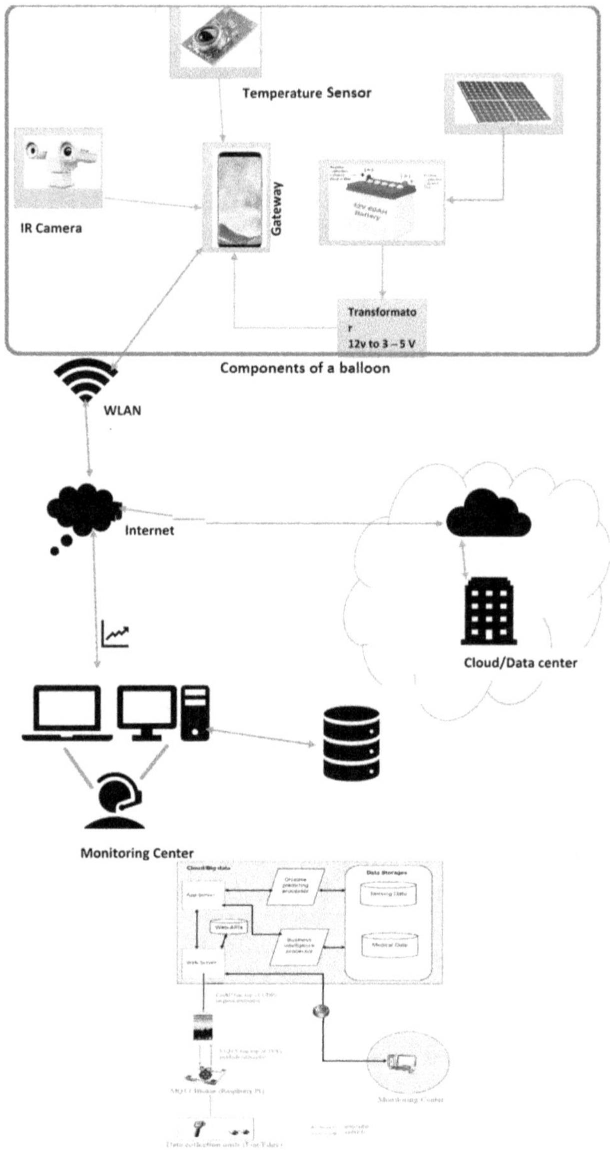

Architecture Approach

As described above, our concept foresees to use a smartphone as a gateway at the data hub. Collected raw data would be short-term processed at the edge (for short-term analytics). This will, therefore, reduce the amount of data to be sent to the cloud for long-term analytics. We will, therefore, implement an edge or fog computing. Fog is more scalable, though it presents some weakness as security issues (IP address spoofing, man-in-the-middle), privacy, trust and authentication concerns. These points would especially be considered during the implementation.

Additionally, edge/fog computing, cloud computing has to be considered. However, cloud computing can support IoT, though soon a huge amount of device and incredibly latency sensitive transactions are added to the system, the cloud could fall apart by computing all these collected data. A Fog/edge computing can help to overcome this issue.

Figure 4. The System functional architecture

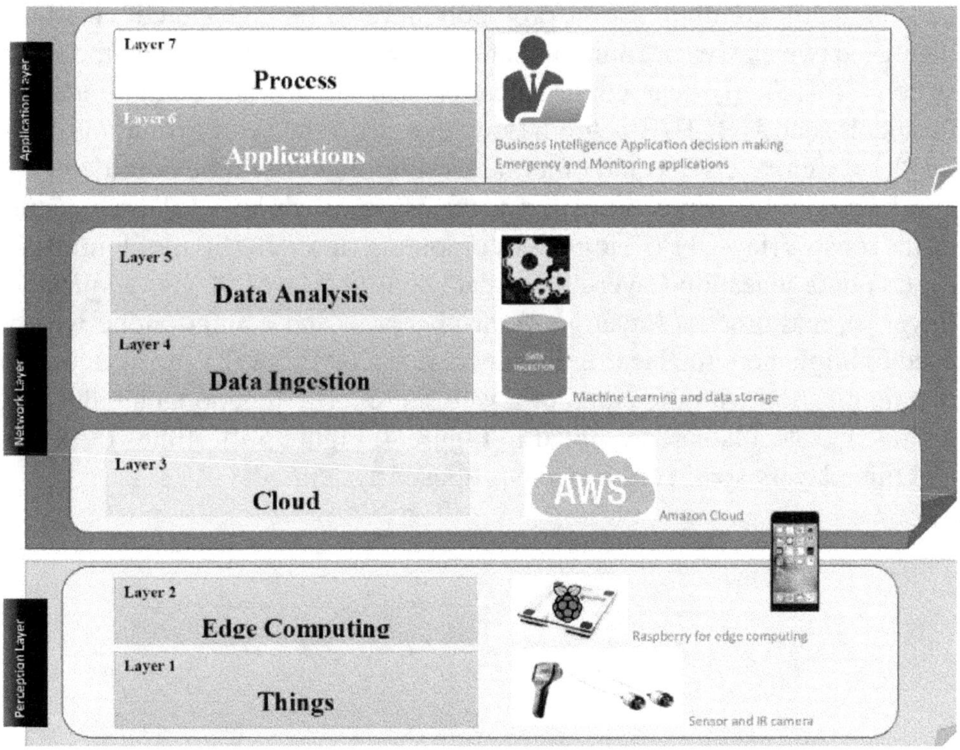

Figure 5. The seven and three layers of the system architecture

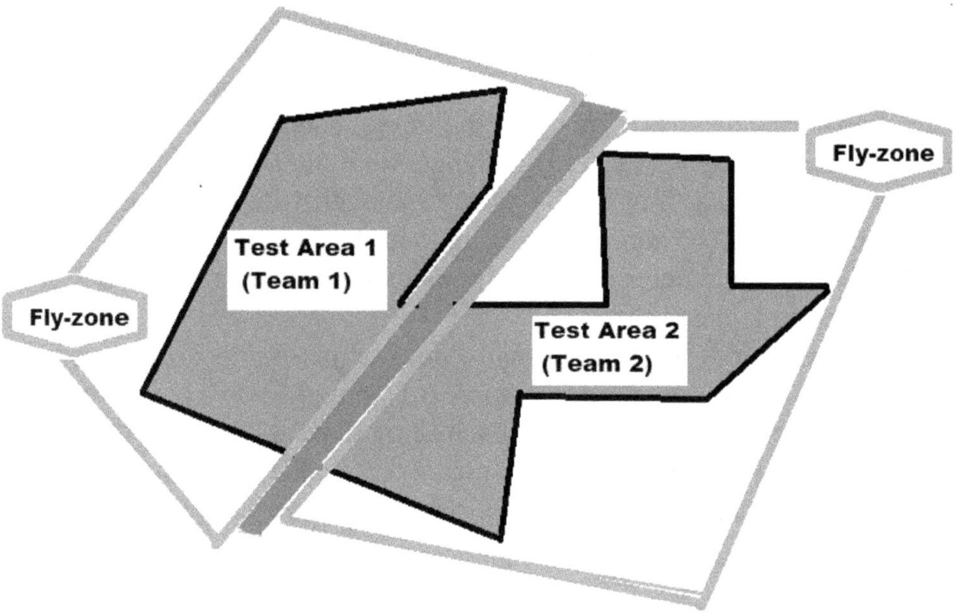

Which IoT communication protocols have to be considered? We have identified two classes of communication between the object within the smart system (IoHT): (i) near communication and (ii) distant communication. Protocols such as BLE (Bluetooth Low-energy), NB-IoT (NarrowBand-IoT), LoRa or Sigfox, ZigBee and other network protocols will be considered.

The proposed architecture refers to the 7 layers high-level IoT-architecture (i) the sensors (layer 1), (ii) fog/edge computing (layer 2), (iii) the cloud (layer 3), (iv) data ingestion (layer 4), (v) data analysis (layer 5), (vi) application (layer 6), and process (layer 7). A raspberry pi and a smartphone will be used to implement the layer 2. Protocols like CoAP, MQTT are selected for communication with the cloud or a web server. The functional architecture included protocols is represented in Figure 4. Figure 5 illustrates the seven and three layers architecture of the proposed system.

PROOF OF CONCEPT

Experimental

The global concept was experimentally verified for two (02) groups of individuals: (i) ill persons and (ii) healthy individuals. Appropriate architecture for optimizing data processing and covering energy consumption issues was also tested. We overfly a test crowd and measure individual temperature and thus detect any medical anomaly.

We overflew the part of the market where we placed some individuals, whereas three adults and three youths are suffering from malaria and their body temperatures were over the normal (normal body temperature is ≈ 37°C - cf. Table 1). According to NHS-UK (National Health Services), the normal human body temperature (HBT) is 37°C. NHS states that the HBT though depends on:

1. The person
2. His age
3. What He has been doing (Activity)
4. The time of day (ex. people, suffering from malaria, develop high temperature in the afternoon)
5. Which part of the body you take the temperature from (temperature taken from the mouth is more accurate than the other parts)

We then sensed the crowd and collect crowdsourced data. We evaluated the data. The results were conclusive, and the experiment has shown that our concept is feasible.

Table 1. Human body temperature range

Category	Age Range	Hypothermia (Low Temperature)	Normal	Hyperthermia (High Temperature)
Baby	Birth to 2 years	36° C	36 ° C - 37° C	37° - 38° C
Children	3 to 12 years	36° C	36° C - 36.77° C	38° C
Adult	13 to 40 years	36.1° C	36.1° C - 37.2° C	37.5° C
Elder	>40	35° C	35.77° C - 36.94° C	37.44° - 37.94° C

Source: (Ghosh & Chaudhary, 2016).

Test Infrastructure

For the test, we used a drone and had overflown a small market. The experiment was approved by the municipality and the local police responsible because of the drone, which will fly a public area.

We use a cat S60 smartphone as a gateway and as a temperature sensor since it features FLIR (Forward Looking Infra-Red) technology and can measure temperature variation. FLIR is a thermal imaging camera, components, and imaging sensors technology.

Drones Flight Authorization

Discussions we conducted with the aviation authorities reveal that most African countries lack stipulations and regulations on drone's flight.

Cohort Sampling

For the test purpose, we build two cohorts consisting of asymptomatic and ill individuals. We selected only people suffering from malaria-tropica since the disease cannot be transmitted by contact. Although malaria is an infectious disease, the transmission is only possible through its vector, the Anopheles.

To assure that the healthy would not be contaminated during the test, we worked with a clinic and medical laboratory which check the cohort population and thus eliminate any risk of contagion. Table 2 and Table 3 shows the structure of the testing cohort.

Table 2. Asymptomatic individuals involved in the test

Gender	Number of Adults	Number of Youth
Female	3	5
Male	3	2

Table 3. Individuals suffering from Malaria

Gender	Number of Adults	Number of Youth
Female	2	2
Male	1	1

Based on advice from the medical personnel which assisted the test we consider the genre aspect. Female temperature faces more variation than man body temperature. This variation is susceptible to bias the data.

Testing Methods

We build two testing teams which conducted the test without knowing where the test participants are placed in the market. Each team consists of 5 students: 2 drone-pilots and 3 assistants. The pilots are trained so that they may efficiently fly the drone within the delimited areas (Figure 6). The training took 2 days long. Additionally, the team's members learn how to use the application. They were provided with a list containing the assigned tasks and guidelines.

The first team collected the data in area 1 where all women involved in the test are placed. All involved men are placed in area 2 and team 2 collects their data.

A rapid prototype of the proposed system was implemented. The server site application was hosted on a Glassfish 4.0.1 on a laptop. A client application is used to visualize data received from the drone platform. The client application on the smartphone (Gateway, sensors) communicate directly with the server application.

Test Process

Table 4 indicates the test time and duration. Each team performed 2 times the data collection in the area assigned to it. Each test lasted 1 hour included 15 min preparation and 45 min net test time. During 45 min, each team flew assigned test area and collected data. The team 1 collects the first data between 11:00 and 12:00 h. The second test phase was 16:30 to 17:30 h. Team 2 performed its tests according to the timetable. These test periods are chosen based on the advice from the medical personnel. The reason is that

Table 4. Test time table

Test Duration		Test Time	
Total	**Net**	**Team 1**	**Team 2**
60 min	45 min	11:00 – 12:00	13:00 – 14:00
60 min	45 min	16:30 – 17:30	17:45 – 18:45

Figure 6. Illustration of the test-areas

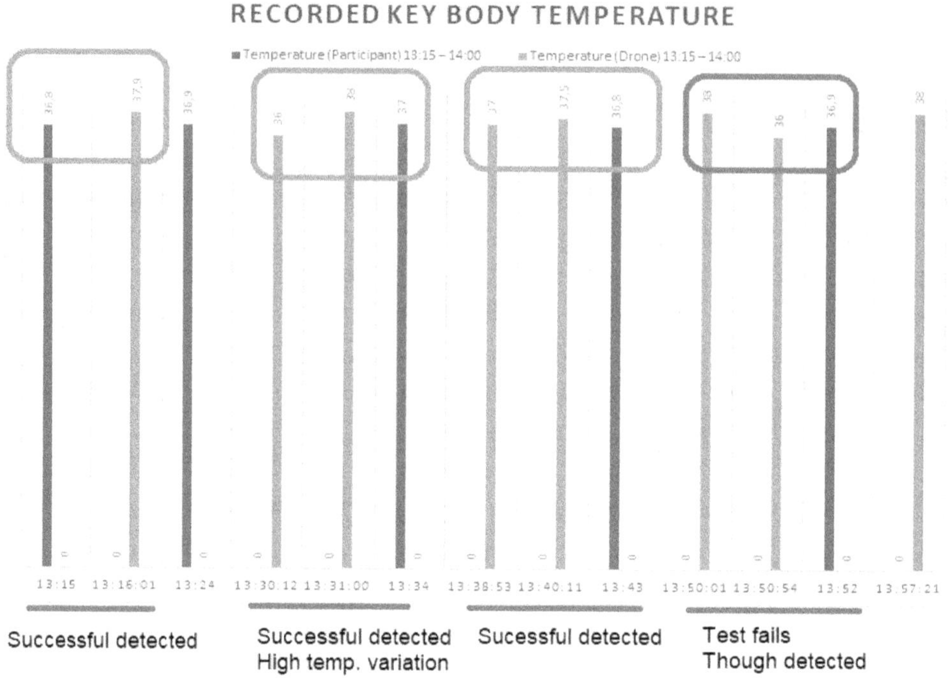

malaria patient develops high fever in the afternoon from 14:00 h. The data collected in the morning are intended to be compared with those collected in the afternoon, so to verify if the system detects any temperature variation.

Between the areas, we define a non-test zone. Any data collected in this area will not consider. Further, if a team collects in the non-assigned area, these collections will also be filtered and destroyed. Figure 6 illustrates the test areas. The brown areas shape the entire marketplace. Fly-zones are defined for each team. The participants are placed in brown areas. The red area is a no-fly-zone.

Each participant is provided with a mercury-type thermometer and is trained to measure his body temperature every 9 min. The illiterates are assisted. These data help to verify the reliability of the data collected with the drone.

Data Gathering

At the beginning and the end of the test, we measure the temperature of the cohort population, noted the geo-position of the members. We use purposely conventional methods the measure the parameter. We were advised to use a thermometer in the mouth. We use the information containing in Table 6 to classify the subject regarding their collected data.

At this stage of the project, we only collect body temperature, the geo-position of each sensing individual. measure the battery state. At end of the test, we compared the data collected at the beginning, in the test phase, and at the end of the test with each other. We thus detect the variation between the measures.

In the test phase, we were focused on finding the placed ill persons. They were asking to not move from the place (Geo-coordinates) so that we can determine them according to their geo-position if the system succeeds or fails. In the future, we plan to identify through their mobile phone GPS coordinates or the one of their neighbor.

We provide a mapping table in the application, that maps the Geo-position on participants names, so we can associate the collected data with the right person. Table 5 illustrates the application's output at the end of the test.

Table 5. Template of the structure of the collected data

Geo-Position/ Coordinates	Mapped Name	Time	Measured Temperature
35 51' 3.10"-78 53' 9.78	Person_x	2017.06.15 16:00:53	TT° C
		2017.06.15 16:03:54	TTT° C

Table 6. Human temperature and its impacts on the health

Temperature	Effect
44°C	Almost death. Sometimes patient is known to survive at up to 46.5°C
43°C	Normally death/brain damage/cardiorespiratory collapse
41-42°C	Fainting, confusion, very fast heart rate, convulsion, Low/high blood pressure
38-40°C	Severe sweating, dehydration, weakness, vomiting, headache, dizziness, fast heart rate, slightly hungry
37°C	Normal temperature
36°C	Mild or moderate shivering. Maybe normal temperature
34-35°C	Intensive shivering, numbness and bluish/grayness of the skin. Heart irritability. Confusion and Loss of movement of finger
29-33°C	Moderate to severe confusion or complete, sleepiness, progressive loss of shivering or stop, slow heartbeat, shallow breathing, unresponsive to stimulus and hallucinations
24-28°C	Breathing may stop. But mostly death. Sometimes patient is known to survive at 14.2°C

Source: (Ghosh & Chaudhary, 2016).

Data Analysis

Quantitative and qualitative analyses were undertaken on the number of target persons (ill persons) found in each test area as well as the quality of the collected data. The data were extracted from the system application.

The data we collected at the start and end of the test using a conventional thermometer is used together with the data collected by the testing team to perform qualitative analysis. The qualitative analysis is carried out using Microsoft Excel and focuses on two (02) points: (i) the variation between the data and (ii) the number of success and fails. Further, both test results have been compared with each other to determine the error rate and thus the quality of the test.

Ethical Consideration

Authorization and written informed participant consent are received from all major participants and parent of the young participants. We translate in a local tongue the participant consent for the illiterates. Their literate parents witness the translation and countersigned the consent. The consent allows the project to collect and process their epidemiological data and finally publish only anonymized data. Clinicians, laboratory personnel involved in this test have provided participant consent too.

An ad-hoc ethics committee at the involved clinics examined the request to conduct such a test involving patients. The participant consents were transmitted to the committee together with the request, the authorization from the municipality, and from the local police department. The committee has then approved the test.

Test Limitations

The few number of involved participants is one of the limitations of the proof-of-concept. Furthermore, we could not test the accuracy of optical fiber sensor. This project is an ongoing project, so the concept including the use of optical fiber sensors will be tested

RESULTS

Data Collected

The collected are processed and extracted. We filter the bad data out. Table 7 summarizes the test findings. As we can see, the results in both areas are similar. In area 1, 83,33% of the participants are sensed while in area 2, 100% of the participants are sensed.

Table 7. Participants detected through the test

Gender	Health Status	Age Category	Participant	Test Conducted by Team 1		Test Conducted by Team 2		Result/Comment
				1st Test	2nd Test	1st Test	2nd Test	
Female	Healthy	A	Paf1	ND	D	ND	ND	A participant in area 1 is sensed by the team 2. This reveals that the overflew a part of area 1. This result is not relevant to the test. Two other participants were neither detected in area 1 nor in area 2. The drone has collected no data on both. We investigate and found out that the drone did not overflow the part the participants were standing.
		A	Paf2	D	D	ND	ND	
		A	Paf3	D	D	ND	ND	
		Y	Paf4	D	ND	ND	ND	
		Y	Paf5	D	D	ND	ND	
		Y	Paf6	D	D	ND	ND	
		Y	Paf7	D	D	ND	ND	
		Y	Paf8	D	D	ND	ND	
	Malaria-Patient	A	Paf9	D	ND	ND	ND	
		A	Paf10	D	D	ND	ND	
		Y	Paf11	D	D	ND	ND	
		Y	Paf12	ND	D	ND	D	
Male	Malaria-Patient	A	Pam1	ND	ND	D	D	Test succeeded
		Y	Pam2	ND	ND	D	D	
	Healthy	A	Pam3	ND	ND	D	D	
		A	Pam4	ND	ND	D	D	
		A	Pam5	ND	ND	D	D	
		Y	Pam6	ND	ND	D	D	
		Y	Pam7	ND	ND	D	D	

Legend:
Paf = Participant female
Pam = Participant male
A = Adult
Y = Youth
ND = not sensed
D = Sensed

Table 8. Recorded data (participant Pam1 - male adult – malaria-patient)

Period	Times		Temperature		Data Source
	13:15 – 14:00	**18:00 – 18:45**	**13:15 – 14:00**	**18:00 – 18:45**	
Before the test	13:00	17:45	36,7	37,9	Research Team
During the test process	13:16:01	18:01:55	37,9	37	Drone
	13:30:12	18:12:13	36	35	
	13:31:00	18:20:07	38	34	
	13:38:53	18:33:16	37	38	
	13:40:11	18:35:10	37,5	36	
	13:50:01	18:40:01	38	36,9	
	13:50:54	18:43:58	36	38	
	13:57:21		38		
	13:15	18:00	36.8	38	Participant
	13:24	18:09	36.9	38,03	
	13:34	18:18	37	38,01	
	13:43	18:27	36,8	38	
	13:52	18:36	36,9	38,02	
After the test	14:05	18:50	37,01	38,6	Research Team

Table 9. Recorded data (participant Paf1 - female adult - malaria-patient)

Period	Times		Temperature		Data Source
	11:15 – 12:00	**16:45 – 17:30**	**11:15 – 12:00**	**16:45 – 17:30**	
Before the test	11:00	16:30	37,0	37,88	Research Team
During the test process		17:03		36,9	Drone
	11:20:55		36,80		
	11:55:33	17:29:23	37,01	36,01	
	11;15	16:45	37,00	37,90	Participant
	11:24	16:54	37,01	37,91	
	11:34	17:03	36,95	38,0	
	11:43	17:12	36,90	38,01	
	11:52	17:21	36,92	37,77	
After the test	12:05	17:35	37,02	37,58	Research Team

Table 10. Recorded data (participant Paf2 - female youth - malaria-patient)

Period	Times		Temperature		Data Source
	11:15 – 12:00	**16:45 – 17:30**	**11:15 – 12:00**	**16:45 – 17:30**	
Before the test	11:00	16:30	36,31	37,02	Research Team
During the test process	11:23:10	16:52:19	37	37,5	Drone
	11:28:12	17:14:01	36,06	37,8	
	11:38:03	17:23:13	37,9	39	
	11:50:57		37,1		
	11:52:00		37,05		
	11;15	16:45	36,8	37,72	Participant
	11:24	16:54	36,5	37,68	
	11:34	17:03	36,5	37,69	
	11:43	17:12	36,3	37.74	
	11:52	17:21	36,8	37,79	
After the test	12:05	17:35	36,7	38	Research Team

Table 11. Recorded data (participant Paf3 - female youth - malaria-patient)

Period	Times		Temperature		Data Source
	11:15 – 12:00	**16:45 – 17:30**	**11:15 – 12:00**	**16:45 – 17:30**	
Before the test	11:00	16:30	37,1	37,7	Research Team
During the test process	11:33:00	16:46:59	36,8	39	Drone
	11:48:12	17:10:11	35,01	36	
		17:29:03		36,93	
	11:15	16:45	37,8	37,72	Participant
	11:24	16:54	37,5	37,68	
	11:34	17:03	37,5	37,69	
	11:43	17:12	37,3	37.74	
	11:52	17:21	37,4	37,79	
After the test	12:05	17:35	37,8	38	Research Team

Data analyses in term of Temperature Variation is carried out and summarized in Table 8, Table 9, Table 10, Table 11. In the healthy groups, we figure out global temperature variations between ± 0.3°C to ± 0.8°C, where the temperature variation recorded with the mercury-type thermometer were between 0.1° and 0.25°C the entire day against 0.5°C – 1.2°C for the thermal camera.

The measurements in the malaria-patient groups were unsatisfactory. Although the participants were all detected and sensed, the recorded temperature values were very jumping. Two (02) participants data were excluded from the analysis due to biased data recorded through mercury-type thermometer.

Data Analysis

Based on extracted data, data analyses are carried out and findings are presented in this sub-section. Overall, the system detects and senses the key participants. The results reveal that smartphone embedded camera records are not accurate, though the system succeeds in detecting 88% on average. It worth to note that the drone flew constantly between 9 and 10 m to the ground. The distance to the object does not impact the value of the sensing data. We extract data sensed in different areas where the distance to object was similar, but the difference of body temperature was enormous. High-performance cameras and sensors are, therefore, mandatory for this system.

Adult Male Participant: 0.00 - 75% Success

Figure 7 presents the temperature variation between the data recorded using a mercury-type thermometer and those recorded through the drone. The participant was sensed 8 times. Two times, the test fails. The recorded values were very low (36° C against the real value:36, 9 and 37° C. 1 time the sensed value (37° C) was approximatively equal to the real value (36,8° C). 5 times, the recorded values were higher the real values.

Figure 8 presents similar results as the previous test (Figure 7). The test fails totally. The drone recorded wrong data (high temperature variation). The variations (37°, 38°, 34°, …) in the same person during 1 h demonstrate that the camera is not accurate and sensible enough to perform these tasks.

Adult Female Participant

- **First Young Female Participant:** 50 – 66% success rate
- **Second Young Female Participant:** 50% success rate

Figure 7. Key body temperature recorded in male participant Pam1 (11:15 to 12:00)

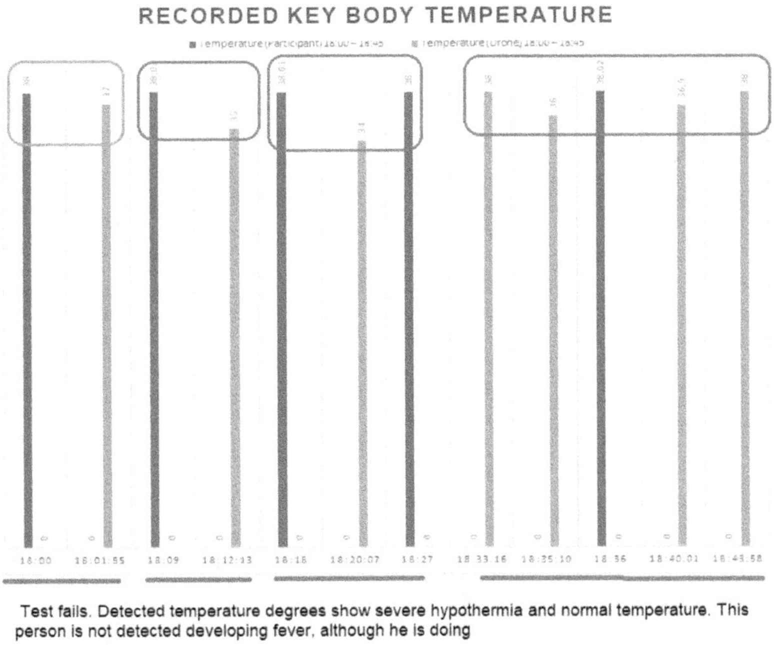

Figure 8. Key body temperature recorded in adult male participant Pam1 (16:45 to 17:30)

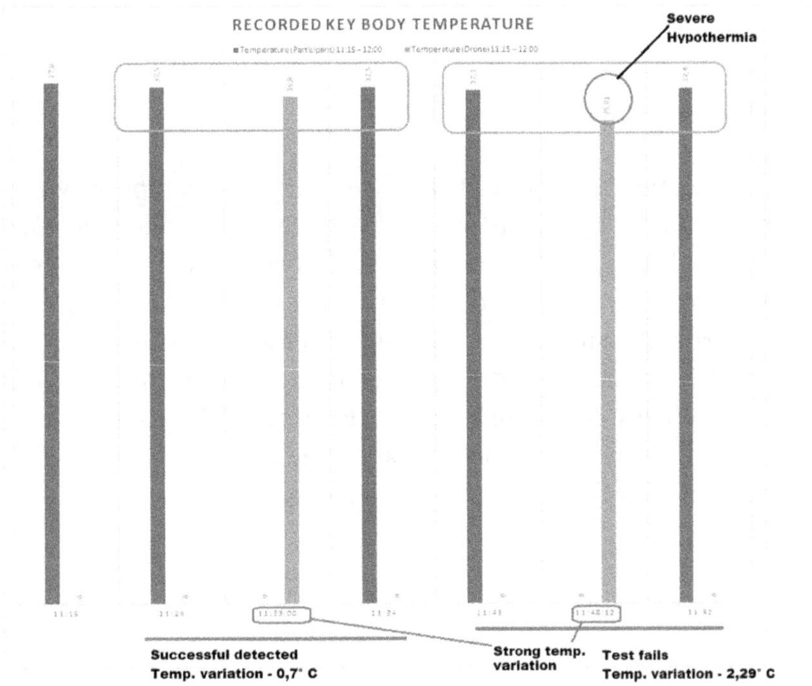

Figure 9. Key body temperature recorded in young female participant Paf2 (11:15 to 12:00)

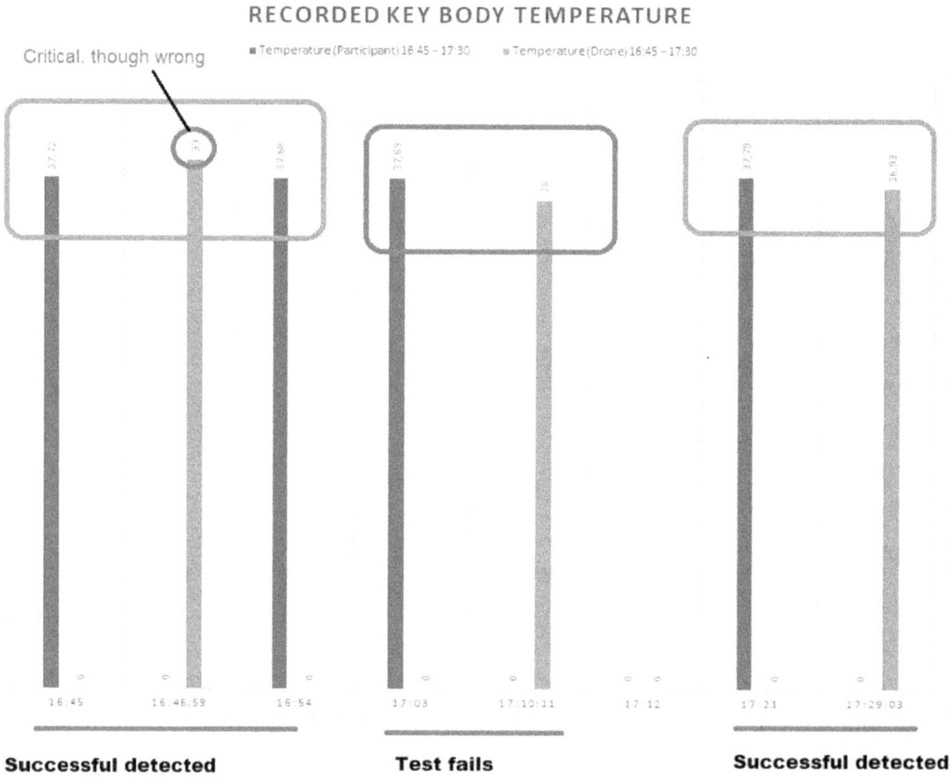

OVERALL RESULT

However, the Battery did not hold long. The energy consumption was very high. The thermal camera did not afford the assigned tasks, collected temperatures were jumping. We also face network issues. The main objectives were not to test this smartphone, though to test our concept.

This experiment shows that the system should be more non-invasive to not disturb the crowd. The drone we used requested the attention of everyone at the market. They felt observed and disturbed. This is an index that our sensing unit must be more non-invasive. The balloon is planned to overfly cities height at 25 – 50 km to the ground.

Figure 10. Key body temperature recorded in young female participant Paf2 (16:45 to 17:30)

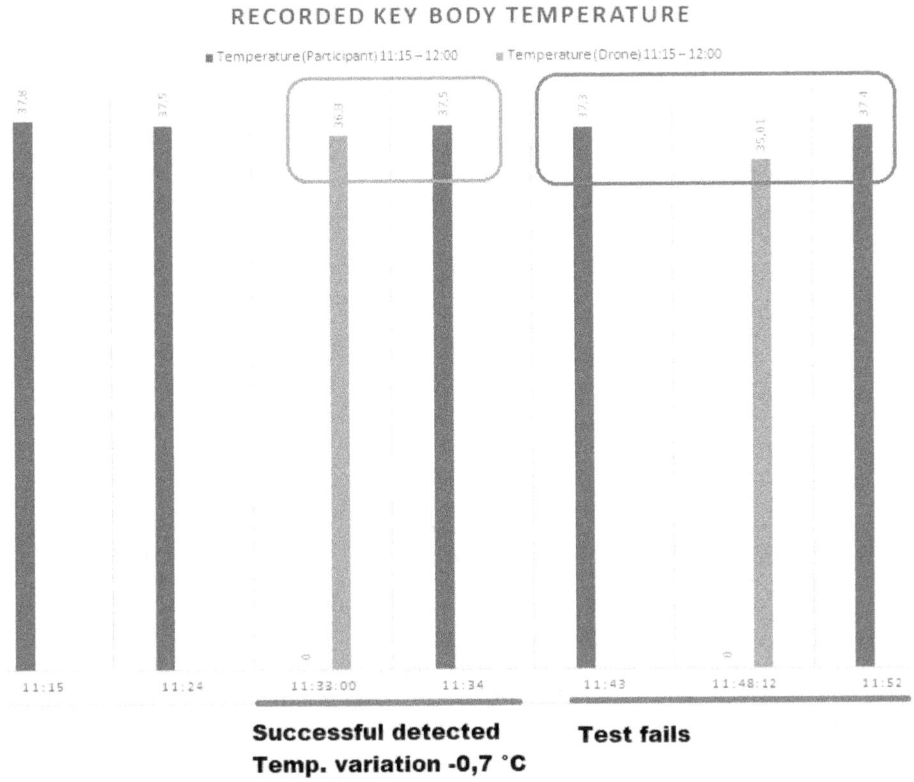

CHALLENGES AND FUTURE WORKS

In general, a person is considered developing a fever if his body temperature is over 37 °C. Though, each age group has different limits (see Table 1). The challenges we will tackle is to estimate, based on collected images, the age-range a sensing person belongs to so that the routine at the edges (sensors) could correctly pre-analyze the data and set the right alarm. For example, an adult sensed for 36,9°C would not be considered, though if it is a child the system would alert the operation center.

A further challenge is the optimization of the energy consumption for a high energy autonomy during each sensing phase.

The next steps in the project are to experiment the balloon, this requires collaborating with the aviation authorities to find the exact routes to use so to avoid any crash with airplanes.

Figure 11. Key body temperature recorded in young female participant Paf3 (11:15 to 12:00)

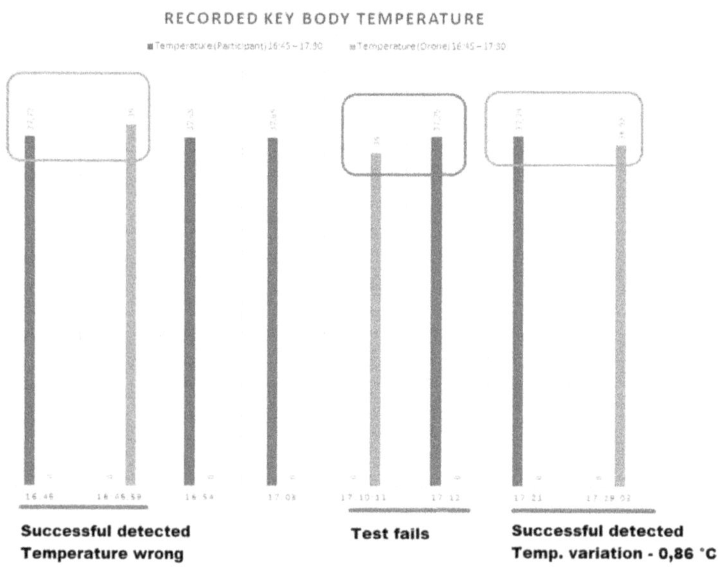

Figure 12. Key body temperature recorded in young female participant Paf3 (16:45 to 17:30)

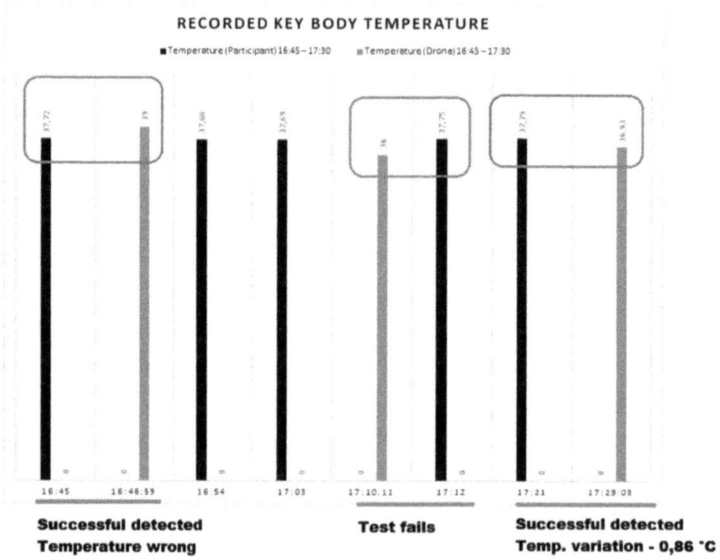

Big data analysis, memory and data storage optimization, real-time data processing, and data security, as well as reliability, would be also the focus of the next work-packages.

CONCLUSION

The test on site using a drone with cat s60 smartphone helps to refine the concept, to choose the right edge (devices, sensors), and research strategies.

The proposed system has the potential to prevent the spreads of diseases, monitor diseases epidemic risks. Though, we need to work with health authorities to implement strategies and policies on how to get people consent so that people would accept to be sensed.

The energy consumption and smartphone's batteries lifetime issues need to be resolved to give more energetical autonomy to the system and thus enable to keep the balloons for a while on air. The test has shown that the energy issues can be resolved through implementing an efficient architecture.

Our future work will consist of proving our concept in collecting data and processing the collected data with the proposed smart health system. Furthermore, we would use smartphone embedded sensors to collect crowdsourcing data and compare the quality and accuracy of sensing data from both systems. Our architecture would be tested, aspects such as scalability, data security, and privacy.

Several studies have been conducted to recognize congestion situation of indoor spaces in real-time. Based on the results of these studies, we would develop a method that combines indoor crowdsensing methods with our proposed system so that indoor crowd could also be monitored at risks of diseases spreads.

Finally, we would concentrate our effort on finding a solution to overcome the energy issues by using smartphones as a gateway.

REFERENCES

Aloi, G., Caliciuri, G., Fortino, G., Gravina, R., Pace, P., Russo, W., & Savaglio, C. (2017). Enabling IoT interoperability through opportunistic smartphone-based mobile gateways. *Journal of Network and Computer Applications*, *81*, 74–84. doi:10.1016/j.jnca.2016.10.013

Brownstein, J. S., Freifeld, C. C., Reis, B. Y., & Mandl, K. D. (2008). Surveillance sans frontières: Internet-based emerging infectious disease intelligence and the HealthMap project. *PLoS Medicine*, *5*(7), 1019–1024. doi:10.1371/journal.pmed.0050151 PMID:18613747

Carpenter, A., & Frontera, A. (2016). Smart-watches: A potential challenger to the implantable loop recorder? *Europace*, *18*(6), 791–793. doi:10.1093/europace/euv427 PMID:26847074

Chatzimilioudis, G., Konstantinidis, A., Laoudias, C., & Zeinalipour-yazti, D. (2012). *Crowdsourcing with Smartphones*. Academic Press.

Chessa, S., Corradi, A., Foschini, L., & Girolami, M. (2016). Empowering mobile crowdsensing through social and ad hoc networking. *IEEE Communications Magazine*, *54*(7), 108–114. doi:10.1109/MCOM.2016.7509387

Christaki, E. (2015). New technologies in predicting, preventing and controlling emerging infectious diseases. *Virulence*, *6*(6), 558–565. doi:10.1080/21505594.2015.1040975 PMID:26068569

Ghosh, A., & Chaudhary, A. (2016). Article. *Developments in Temperature Monitoring Systems*, *6*(4), 3596–3599. doi:10.4010/2016.833

Gong, Y., Fang, Y., & Guo, Y. (2016). Private Data Analytics on Biomedical Sensing Data via Distributed Computation. *IEEE/ACM Transactions on Computational Biology and Bioinformatics*, *13*(3), 431–444. doi:10.1109/TCBB.2016.2515610 PMID:26761861

Haddawy, P., Frommberger, L., Kauppinen, T., De Felice, G., Charkratpahu, P., Saengpao, S., & Kanchanakitsakul, P. (2015). Situation awareness in crowdsensing for disease surveillance in crisis situations. *Proceedings of the Seventh International Conference on Information and Communication Technologies and Development - ICTD '15*, 1–5. 10.1145/2737856.2737879

Kos, A., Tomazic, S., & Umek, A. (2016). Evaluation of smartphone inertial sensor performance for cross-platform mobile applications. *Sensors (Switzerland)*, *16*(4), 477. doi:10.339016040477 PMID:27049391

Liu, J., Shen, H., & Zhang, X. (2016). A survey of mobile crowdsensing techniques: A critical component for the internet of things. *2016 25th International Conference on Computer Communications and Networks, ICCCN 2016*. 10.1109/ICCCN.2016.7568484

Liu, S., Luo, Y., & Yang, S. (2007). Shape-based pedestrian detection in infrared images. *Journal of Information Science and Engineering*, *23*(1), 271–283.

Ma, H., Zhao, D., & Yuan, P. (2015). Opportunities in mobile crowd sensing. *Infocommunications Journal*, *7*(2), 32–38. doi:10.1109/MCOM.2014.6871666

Majethia, R., Mishra, V., Pathak, P., Lohani, D., Acharya, D., & Sehrawat, S. (2015). Contextual sensitivity of the ambient temperature sensor in Smartphones. *2015 7th International Conference on Communication Systems and Networks, COMSNETS 2015 - Proceedings*. 10.1109/COMSNETS.2015.7098674

Morón, M. J., Luque, R., & Casilari, E. (2014). On the capability of smartphones to perform as communication gateways in medical wireless personal area networks. *Sensors (Switzerland)*, *14*(1), 575–594. doi:10.3390140100575 PMID:24451456

Nanda, H., & Davis, L. (n.d.). Probabilistic template based pedestrian detection in infrared videos. In *Intelligent Vehicle Symposium* (Vol. 1, pp. 15–20). IEEE. 10.1109/IVS.2002.1187921

National Instruments. (2016). *Fundamentals of Fiber Bragg Grating (FBG) Optical Sensing*. Retrieved from http://www.ni.com/white-paper/11821/en/

Paolotti, D., Carnahan, A., Colizza, V., Eames, K., Edmunds, J., Gomes, G., ... Vespignani, A. (2014). Web-based participatory surveillance of infectious diseases: The Influenzanet participatory surveillance experience. *Clinical Microbiology and Infection*, *20*(1), 17–21. doi:10.1111/1469-0691.12477 PMID:24350723

Pesko, M., Smolnikar, M., Vucnik, M., & Javornic, T. (2014). Smartphone with Augmented Gateway Functionality as Opportunistic WSN Gateway Device. *Wireless Personal Communications*, *78*(3), 1811–1826. doi:10.100711277-014-1908-7

Soto, M. A., Bolognini, G., Di Pasquale, F., & Thévenaz, L. (2010). Simplex-coded BOTDA fiber sensor with 1 m spatial resolution over a 50 km range. *Optics Letters*, *35*(2), 259–261. doi:10.1364/OL.35.000259 PMID:20081987

Steinhubl, S. R., Marriott, M. P., & Wegerich, S. W. (2015). Remote Sensing of Vital Signs: A Wearable, Wireless "Band-Aid" Sensor With Personalized Analytics for Improved Ebola Patient Care and Worker Safety. *Global Health, Science and Practice*, *3*(3), 516–519. doi:10.9745/GHSP-D-15-00189 PMID:26374808

Van Hoe, B., Lee, G., Bosman, E., Missinne, J., Kalathimekkad, S., Maskery, O., ... Van Steenberge, G. (2012). Ultra small integrated optical fiber sensing system. *Sensors (Switzerland)*, *12*(9), 12052–12069. doi:10.3390120912052

ENDNOTES

1 www.foodbornechicago.org
2 https://flunearyou.org
3 www.foodbornechicago.org
4 https://flunearyou.org

Chapter 6
Early Detection Prediction and Prevention of Noncommunicable Diseases in People at High Risks of Communicable Diseases

ABSTRACT

The traditional screening for disease consists of medically testing individuals to detect diseases at an early stage. However, a screening or disease diagnosis is based on a patient-physician interview where patients answer the questions the physician asks him. It can be a direct (face-to-face) interview or an indirect communication by using a medium (video conference, phone, online web application, etc.). The traditional screening for NDCs presents certain limitations. Convergence of non-infectious and infectious diseases is not considered. This chapter proposes an innovative system and framework for pervasive/ubiquitous screening for early detection and prevention of NCDs in asymptomatic individuals at (tropical) infectious diseases risks. The proposed screening consists of pervasive sensing for physical, physiological, biochemical vital parameters, and quality of life by measuring the mental health, lifestyle, social, and climatic environmental modalities using the miniaturized wearable internet of things (IoT) systems and m-health application without activity restriction and behavior modification. It further determines the genetic/genomic predisposition and uses it for the prediction processing.

DOI: 10.4018/978-1-5225-5528-5.ch006

INTRODUCTION

Multimorbidities such as cardiovascular/heart diseases (CVD) associated with severe malaria; or other (tropical) infectious diseases associated with diabetics and/or CVD, HIV/Aids associated with tuberculosis, etc. are frequent in several patients. Some parasitic infections can be associated with significant morbidity and mortality in regions of high endemicity(Hidron et al., 2010). The concept of multimorbidity, developed and published in 1976 in Germany at the first time, is an extension of the concept of comorbidity, which is defined as the interaction between any disease or risk factors with one main disease with the effect of making it worse. According to World Health Organization (WHO), multimorbidity is defined as suffering of or affecting by two or more chronic health conditions (Le Reste et al., 2015).

Recently two cases of tropical infections have been reported causing cardiovascular diseases. A case of a fatal complication of myocardial infarction in individuals (patient) with delayed diagnosis of Plasmodium falciparum infection is reported in (Chandra & Chandra, 2011). Another case of a complication of acute coronary after an experimental test/case of Plasmodium falciparum infection is reported in (Nieman et al., 2009). The coronary syndrome was diagnosed after the successful treatment of the malaria infection. Considering these two reported cases above, a convergence of tropical infectious diseases such as malaria and CVD and/or other non-communicable diseases seems to exist. The convergence presents new challenges and new opportunities to enact responsive changes in policy and research (Remais, Zeng, Li, Tian, & Engelgau, 2013). The association of the infectious disease with the non-communicable disease will, therefore, be investigated in the scope of the present project.

Data Analytics, including machine learning and predictive analytics and modeling, leads to understand and mitigate the behavioral, genetic and environmental causes of disease and treatment's failure. Machine learning methods are being used for large datasets to set up different patient groups, healthy, asymptomatic or sick, as well as to perform early symptoms analyses for early detection of acute NCDs and infection. The data sets could consist of genetic material and information and/or biophysical and mental conditions information collected from the patient. The convergence of tropical infectious diseases, such as malaria, and non-communicable diseases is neither trivial nor transient; but represents a phase in the epidemiological transition (Remais et al., 2013), therefore, an improved early detection in asymptomatic or infected individuals is therefore highly motivated. Data analytics, including machine learning and predictive analytics and modeling, in form of predictive search (automated deduction or augmented reality), should be used, in early detecting, surveillance, and monitoring of non-communicable diseases risks factors in individuals/patients with tropical infectious diseases. Linking of wearable devices with big data analytics to provide feedback and a suggestion system for behavioral change is today well widespread (H. J. Wilson, 2013), the present study has used wearable IoT systems in determining causes of behavioral changes, to determine impacts of the behavioral changes on diseases treatment and vice-versa and also factors of non-communicable diseases risks.

The research work focuses on the improvement of early detection, prevention, monitoring, surveillance and treatment of medical conditions, particularly (tropical) infectious diseases and associated non-communicable diseases in individuals at high risk of tropical and other infectious diseases, such as malaria and AIDS/HIV. The study pursues the objectives of improving the traditional screening for disease using pervasive/ubiquitous sensing and thus, early detect and prevent multimorbidity, disability, the convergence of NCDs and CDs, and death. Individuals living and have sojourned in Tropical (Developing) Countries will be considered for in this study.

This study further focuses on quality of life assessment. Monitoring and detection of the physical state of a (chronic) patient are well advanced in comparison to the detection of mental and social state using wearable IoT systems (Roggen, Arnrich, Tröster, & Tr, 2006). Measuring the quality of life from the mental, social and climatic environmental parameters with wearable IoT systems is still an open question, which will be investigated because these modalities also could contribute to the improvement of screening for disease and consequently improve diseases prediction and early detection.

This chapter is organized as follows. In Section "*CONCEPT OF NOVEL SCREENING APPROACH*", we present the motivation to our proposal, the main problems to be overcome and how we address. The Section "*GUIDELINES TO IMPROVE THE COMMON SCREENING PROCESS*" presents the guidelines of the proposed best practice of our proposal for the improvement of the screening. In Section "*CONCEPT OF IOT BASED PERVASIVE/UBIQUITOUS SCREENING FOR NCDS*", we describe the concept underlying our system. We then describe the evaluation of the implemented prototype of the system in section "*PROOF OF CONCEPT AND RESULTS*". We finally outline the following-up works in "*FURTHER WORK*" and conclude the study.

CONCEPT OF NOVEL SCREENING APPROACH FOR DISEASES

Problem Statement

Limitation of the Traditional Screening for Diseases

The Traditional Screening and Assessment are strongly limited, then a screening is initiated by the healthcare services (HCS) and is holding among people who have not sought medical attention because they do not present any symptoms of the disease for which they are screened for (Strong, Wald, Miller, & Alwan, 2005). Due to the lack of symptoms and information paucity on one hand and due to medical fees (this is more relevant for health systems with weak health insurance systems); most people at risk of contracting or developing certain diseases do not take part in the screening programs offered. In Developing countries, most people have poor access to healthcare (see chapter 2) and thus to screening and assessment programs. Preventing a disease must not always include screening people at the high-risk factor, but can also propose or use the available resources for population education about risk factors (e.g. reduce tobacco consumption to reduce the heart disease risks).

In the globalized world, we are living nowadays, people are moving around the word and thus are limited to take part in a screening program. The global healthcare is facing a major challenge concerning the ubiquitous patient medical dossier. The units of the global care system are not connected at all. That means a patient traveling to a western country and coming from a developing country could access his medical data at the host country. If he takes part in a national screening at the host country maybe he can start eventual treatment and must bear the medical costs himself. A European in America or in another European cannot take part in national screening if he is not a permanent resident, then his health insurance at home would cover the medical cost. Also, the results of the screening will not store into his medical dossier at home.

People are easily traveling around the world nowadays and can quick attend regions, which were still a short time ago not reachable. Certain infectious diseases are endemic in these regions. Thus, the traveler can be infected and back home with infection. During a screening for NCDs at home, the infection carried from aboard would be considered. Only the infection control program will consider this infection.

What Are Non-Communicable Diseases (NCDs)?

Non-communicable diseases (NCDs) [Table 1], such as heart disease, stroke, cancer, chronic respiratory diseases, and diabetes, are the leading cause of mortality in the world. WHO figures the number of non-communicable diseases related deaths over 68%, in 2012, against 60%, in 2000. There is a rapid growth of the damage caused by these diseases. In 2012, 75% of deaths related to cardiovascular disease affected the low-income countries, particularly sub-Saharan Africans. These diseases remain an important factor for mortality worldwide and represent in developed countries 87% of mortalities against 37-57% in countries with low and middle incomes. Low- and middle-income countries, particularly Africa, bear the heavy burden of non- communicable diseases, such as cardiovascular, diabetes, etc.

Non-communicable diseases (NCDs) kill 38 million people each year. Almost three-quarters of NCD deaths - 28 million - occur in low- and middle-income countries. Sixteen million NCD deaths occur before the age of 70; 82% of these "premature" deaths occurred in low- and middle-income

Table 1. Common non-communicable diseases

Non-Communicable Diseases	Descriptions
Cancer	Cancer is a generic theme for a large group of diseases that can affect any part of the body. Other terms used are malignant tumors and neoplasms. One defining feature of cancer is the rapid creation of abnormal cells that grow beyond their usual boundaries, and which can then invade adjoining parts of the body and spread to other organs. This process is referred to as metastasis. Metastases are the major cause of death from cancer.
Diabetes	Diabetes is a chronic disease that occurs when the pancreas does not produce enough insulin, or when the body cannot effectively use the insulin it produces. Hyperglycemia, or raised blood sugar, is a common effect of uncontrolled diabetes and over time leads to serious damage to many of the body's systems, especially the nerves and blood vessels.
Cardiovascular diseases	Cardiovascular diseases are a group of disorders of the heart and blood vessels and include: • coronary heart disease: a disease of the blood vessels supplying the heart muscle; • cerebrovascular disease: a disease of the blood vessels supplying the brain; • peripheral arterial disease: a disease of blood vessels supplying the arms and legs; • rheumatic heart disease: damage to the heart muscle and heart valves from rheumatic fever, caused by streptococcal bacteria; • congenital heart disease: malformations of heart structure existing at birth; • deep vein thrombosis and pulmonary embolism: blood clots in the leg veins, which can dislodge and move to the heart and lungs. Heart attacks and strokes are usually acute events and are mainly caused by a blockage that prevents blood from flowing to the heart or brain. The most common reason is a build-up of fatty deposits on the inner walls of the blood vessels. Strokes can be caused by bleeding from a blood vessel in the brain or by blood clots
Digestive diseases	All diseases that pertain to the gastrointestinal tract are labeled as digestive diseases.

Source: http://www.who.int/.

countries. Thus, Cardiovascular diseases account for most NCD deaths, or 17.5 million people annually, followed by cancers (8.2 million), respiratory diseases (4 million), and diabetes (1.5 million) (WHO, 2013). NCDs are the most frequent causes of death in most countries in the Americas, the Eastern Mediterranean, Europe, South-East Asia, and the Western Pacific ((WHO), 2010)

Over the past decade, the prevalence of traditional risk factors for atherosclerotic cardiovascular diseases has been increasing in the major populous countries of the developing world, including China and India, with consequent increases in the rates of coronary and cerebrovascular events. Indeed, by 2020, cardiovascular diseases are predicted to be the major causes of morbidity and mortality in most developing nations around the world (Celermajer, Chow, Marijon, Anstey, & Woo, 2012).

Table 2. Lifestyle-related and metabolic risks factors

Related Risks Factors	Descriptions
Physical inactivity	Physical activity consists of body movements produced by skeletal muscles. Physical activity requires energy. Physical inactivity is the fourth leading risk factor for global mortality. Relating mortality is estimated at 3.2 million deaths. [WHO]
Tobacco use	Tobacco use is one of risk factors for many chronic diseases such as cancer, lung diseases, and cardiovascular diseases. [WHO]
Alcohol misuse	*Alcohol misuse means drinking excessively - more than the recommended limits of alcohol consumption.* [NHS]
Unhealthy diets (increased fat and sodium, with low fruit and vegetable intake).	*Unhealthy diets are linked to four of the world's top ten leading risk factors causing death: high blood pressure, high blood glucose, overweight and obesity and high cholesterol.* *Diets high in sugars, saturated and trans fats, low fiber foods, and high-sugar drinks contribute to non-communicable diseases (NCDs) and other health problems* (Smith S. et al, 2012).
Elevated glucose	Hyperglycemia is the technical theme for high blood glucose Also called blood sugar, it happens when the body has too little insulin or when the body can't use insulin properly. [American Diabetes Association]
Overweight and obesity	Overweight and obesity are defined as abnormal or excessive fat accumulation that may impair health. [WHO]
Raised blood pressure	Blood pressure is the force of blood pushing against the walls of the arteries as the heart pumps blood. High blood pressure, sometimes called hypertension, happens when this force is too high. Health care workers check blood pressure readings the same way for children, teens, and adults. [NIH National Heart, Lung, and Blood Institute]
Raised total cholesterol	Raised cholesterol increases the risks of heart disease and stroke. Globally, a third of ischemic heart disease is attributable to high cholesterol. Overall, raised cholesterol is estimated to cause 2.6 million deaths (4.5% of total) and 29.7 million disability-adjusted life years (DALYs), or 2.0% of total DALYs. Raised total cholesterol is a major cause of disease burden in both the developed and developing world as a risk factor for Ischemic heart disease and stroke. [WHO]

Lifestyle and Metabolic Risks Factors for NCDs

According to CDC, the lifestyle risks factors *(also called modifiable risks) causing NCDs are "An aspect of personal behavior or lifestyle, an environmental exposure, or a hereditary characteristic that is associated with an increase in the occurrence of a particular disease, injury, or other health condition." Metabolic risks factors are biochemical factors involved in the body's normal functioning. Lifestyles can lead to metabolic/physiologic changes. [Principles of Epidemiology, CDC, 2006/Overview of NCD's and Risk Factors]*

Table 2 summarizes the metabolic and lifestyle-related diseases risks factors. Almost three quarters occur in low- and middle-income countries, because of late diagnosis and poor knowledge of risk factors, such as unhealthy diets, physical inactivity, exposure to tobacco smoke or the effects of the harmful use of alcohol (WHO 2015).

Non-Modifiable Risks Factors for NCDs

Non-modifiable risks factors are factors that one cannot control or reduce. Various diseases are related to these factors. Table 3 summarizes some of the non-modifiable risks factors.

Infectious Diseases (Communicable Diseases) as NCD Risk Factor?

Among the (Tropical) Infectious Diseases [Table 4], tuberculosis, HIV, Trypanosomiasis, both American (Chagas' disease) and African (sleeping sickness), and Malaria (Plasmodium falciparum) reportedly are the most infectious diseases associated with non-communicable diseases such as

Table 3. Non-modifiable diseases risk factors

Related Risks Factors	Descriptions
Age	Certain NCDs (e. g. CVD) becomes increasingly common to elderly people.
Gender	A man is at greater risk of heart disease than a pre-menopausal woman. Once past the menopause, a woman's risk is like a man's. Risk of stroke, however, is similar for men and women.
Race Family history (genetics).	A family's history of NCDs (e. g. CVD) indicates a person's risk. If a first-degree blood relative has had coronary heart disease or stroke before the age of 55 years (for a male relative) or 65 years (for a female relative), the risk increases.

cardiovascular disease, diabetes (Le Reste et al., 2015) (Chandra & Chandra, 2011) (Remais et al., 2013). American (Chagas' disease) and African (sleeping sickness) constitute the most relevant parasitic infections involving the heart and lung affections. A case study (Roggen et al., 2006) conducted in Kenya has revealed that people living with HIV (PLHIV) may be at high risk of non-communicable diseases (NCDs).

(Tropical) Infectious Diseases

Tropical diseases are diseases that are prevalent in or unique to tropical and subtropical regions. The diseases are less prevalent in temperate climates, due in part to the occurrence of a cold season, which controls the insect population by forcing hibernation. Insects such as mosquitoes and flies are by far the most common disease carrier or vector. These insects may carry a parasite, bacterium or virus that is infectious to humans and animals. Most often the disease is transmitted by an insect "bite", which causes transmission of the infectious agent through subcutaneous blood exchange.

Infectious diseases are diseases that are prevalent not uniquely in tropical and subtropical regions but in the whole world. Infectious diseases such as hepatitis, HIV/AIDS, tuberculosis, and other sexually transmissible diseases are not only endemic in tropical and subtropical regions. They are also endemic in other regions of the world.

Migration and Infectious Diseases

Due to the growing migration, population displacement, and travel, tropical diseases are becoming available in non-endemic areas such as Europe. Thus, Chagas disease, a tropical infectious disease endemic in South America, Central America, and parts of North America (The Southern United States and Mexico) become available in Europe since the beginning of 2000. During the last century, Chagas disease cases were detected in non-endemic countries in North America (Canada and the United States) and the Western Pacific Region (mainly Australia and Japan), and only more recently in Europe (Celermajer et al., 2012)

In Italy, the available epidemiological data about the Chagas disease have been very limited up to now, although the country is second in Europe only to Spain in the number of residents from Latin American. Among 867 at-risk subjects screened between 1998 and 2010, the Center for Tropical Diseases in Negrar (Verona) and the Infectious and Tropical Diseases Unit, University of Florence found 4.2% patients with positive serology for Chagas (Angheben et al., 2011).

Migration from Latin America to the European Union has increased exponentially. Spain and Italy are more affected by this kind of migration. In 2008 101 Chagas' diseases cases were diagnosed among the Latin American's migrants. This quote is increasing with the number of migrants coming from the endemic areas. Although, tropical infectious diseases do not represent a risk for the European host populations since they are vaccinated against most of those infectious. Malaria, for example, cannot be transmitted in Europe or cold regions because the cold seasons control the insect population, the vectors (diseases carriers) by forcing hibernation. However, Chagas is an exception and can thus be transmitted in cold region like Europe. Migrant can transmit the diseases to the host population. Infections such as tuberculosis (TB), hepatitis, tuberculosis, and sexual diseases (e.g. HIV) can be transmitted to the host population too (Monge-Maillo et al., 2009) and are not only endemic in tropical regions.

Developing countries contribute to almost 90% of GBD worldwide. In comparison to the developed countries, the population in developing countries lags majorly behind in achieving ideal health situation. Most tropical infectious diseases are endemic in the developing countries and are one of the important causes of mortality in these regions of the world. Table 4 shows the certain infectious diseases and their causative agents.

STUDY MOTIVATION AND PURPOSES

Screening aims to detect specific or certain medical conditions in asymptomatic individuals at risk of or already latently suffering from certain medical conditions. These individuals mostly are not aware of their health state. The process of screening consists of asking or medically testing the concerned individual to identify diseases at an early stage. Disease diagnosis at an advanced stage can enable early detection and lead to early medical intervention to minimize the effect of the disease or avoid developing the disease. Early disease detection can prevent disability or death (Strong et al., 2005). *Childhood screening programs for conditions such as congenital*

Table 4. (Tropical) infectious diseases

Infectious Diseases	Causative Agent	Descriptions
Plasmodium Falciparum (Malaria)	Protozoan parasites	Transmitted by female Anopheles mosquitoes, as they are the blood feeders. The disease is caused by species of the genus Plasmodium. Malaria infects 300-500 million people each year, killing more than 1 million.
HIV/Aids	A human immunodeficiency Virus	The human immunodeficiency virus (HIV) is a retrovirus that infects cells of the immune system, destroying or impairing their function (Definition WHO).
Tuberculosis		A bacterial infection of the lungs or other tissues, which is highly prevalent in the world, with mortality over 50% if untreated. It is a communicable disease, transmitted by aerosol expectorant from a cough, sneeze, speak, kiss, or spit. Over one-third of the world's population has been infected with the TB bacterium.
Neurocysticercosis	Taenia solium	--
Schistosomiasis	Species of flatworm	Snail fever is a parasitic disease: The most common form of transmission is by wading or swimming in lakes, ponds and other bodies of water containing the snails and the parasite. More than 200 million people worldwide are infected by schistosomiasis
Onchocerciasis	Onchocerca volvulus, a parasitic worm.	A river blindness is the world's second leading infectious cause of blindness It is transmitted through the bite of a black fly. The worms spread throughout the body, and when they die, they cause intense itching and a strong immune system response that can destroy nearby tissue, such as the eye. About 18 million people are currently infected with this parasite. Approximately 300,000 have been irreversibly blinded by it.
Lymphatic filariasis	Thread-like parasitic filarial worms called nematode worms,	A parasitic disease transmitted by mosquitoes. Loa is another filarial parasite transmitted by the deer fly. 120 million people are infected worldwide. It is carried by over half the population in the most severe endemic areas. The most noticeable symptom is elephantiasis: a thickening of the skin and underlying tissues.
Leprosy	Mycobacterium leprae.	A chronic infectious disease. Leprosy is primarily a granulomatous disease of the peripheral nerves and mucosa of the upper respiratory tract; skin lesions are the primary external symptom. Left untreated, leprosy can be progressive, causing permanent damage to the skin, nerves, limbs, and eyes. Contrary to popular conception, leprosy does not cause body parts to simply fall off, and it differs from tzaraath.
Leishmaniasis	protozoan parasites of the genus Leishmania,	Transmissible by the bite of certain species of sand fly
African trypanosomiasis	Trypanosoma brucei, Trypanosoma gambiense	Sleeping sickness is a parasitic disease.
Chagas disease (American trypanosomiasis)	Trypanosoma cruzi (flagellate protozoan)	A parasitic disease, which occurs in the Americas, particularly in South America.

Source: http://www.news-medical.net/health/What-are-Tropical-Diseases.aspx.

hypothyroidism and phenylketonuria have proved extremely beneficial for early detection and intervention (Al-Qabandi, Gorter, & Rosenbaum, 2011)

Pervasive Diseases Screening for Early Detection of Medical Conditions

The purpose of pervasive screening using information and communication technology consists of pervasive and ubiquitous sensing bio-signals relating to a specific medical condition. Information about the concerned medical condition is automatically collected by using pervasive or ubiquitous devices (e.g. body sensor). Is ubiquitous something that is available anywhere, anytime, while is pervasive something that is permeated in the environment" (Varshney 2009, p. 39). However, traditional screening or disease diagnosis is based on a patient-physician interview where patients answer the questions the physician ask him. It can be a direct (face-to-face) interview or an indirect communication by using a medium (video conference, phone, online –web application -, etc.).

Pervasive diseases monitoring, and diseases surveillance are well spread, while pervasive screening is scarce. Disease monitoring intends to maintain the health of a given patient, while the goal of diseases surveillance is to provide health information about the prevalence of a specific disease or risk factor in the certain population. Screening consists of early detecting a medical condition in an asymptomatic individual at high risk of a disease or who is already affected by the medical condition. However, traditional screening has inherent limitations, then the patient needs to visit the doctor or the screening program center. Further, we cannot notice any infections related cause among the common causes of NCDs. That means infectious diseases as causes of developing NCDs is not yet recognized or admitted. This fact motivates the present work.

IoT opens new doors for the healthcare systems to better screening for NCDs. Pervasive/ubiquitous screening. using IoT enables anyone at anytime and anywhere to be (early) screened. So, the common cause factors of NCDs, as well as the impacts of infectious diseases on developing NCDs, could be continuously screening.

Several studies report that certain infectious diseases are associated with some non-communicable diseases. *The convergence of tropical infectious diseases, such as malaria, and non-communicable diseases is neither trivial nor transient; but represents a phase in the epidemiological transition* (Remais et al., 2013).

The importance of preventing infectious diseases (ID) and non-communicable diseases (NCDs) is to reduce risk factors. It is indicated that certain IDs could be associated with certain NCDs, a prevention of these IDs would increasingly reduce the risk of acute NCDs. Traditional prevention of NCDs focuses on reducing the risk factor such as tobacco, alcohol use, and weight. Due to the convergence of IDs and NCDs, prevention of NCDs has, therefore, to focus on major risks with relevance to IDs in addition to the traditional risks factors.

Overcome the Limitation of Traditional Screening

The proposed system is majorly aiming at overcoming the limitation of the traditional screening using modern information and communication technologies, then, it is today well known that screening's results can be false, thus people can wrongly be screened positive or negative and the subsequent treatment can be hazardous, or the disease would not be prevented.

Increase the Adherence to Screening for Diseases and Assessment of Diseases

Increasing the adherence to screening for disease among the population means to make the population aware of the importance of the screening programs. In developing countries, regarding the poor access to healthcare, increasing the adherence to screening programs means on one hand to improve access to healthcare and on other hand launch cost-effective and efficient pervasive/ubiquitous screening systems into the public health systems and make it accessible to the population so to increase the adherence to screening for disease among the population at high risk factors.

ICT becomes a global phenomenon, the technology base for introducing wearable and ubiquitous computing is already available to most of the population in both the developing and developed countries. The integration of wearable IoT technologies to satisfy unique needs of patients from these medical domains is a necessity of time. Wearable sensors hold the promise of early detection, diagnosis, and treatment of diseases.

Improve the Efficiency and Interoperability of Data Collection

Use novel Internet of Things technology to improve the efficiency and interoperability of data collection techniques for Emerging standards (e.g., IETF 6tisch) for Improving the Efficiency of data Gathering from (Wireless) Sensors in a Low Power Lossy Network (i.e., the sensor network) and a De-verticalized Middleware to expose the different data and services with a unique interface, on top of which vertical m-health applications can be created consists the technical novelty of the proposed system. We recently published the results of our work on low power consuming wireless sensors at MMHealth 2016 (https://www.mmhealth2016.uni-oldenburg.de/https://www.mmhealth2016.uni-oldenburg.de/page7/page7.html.)

Today, there are many players in the IoT fields with non-interoperable solutions which lead to complexity in communicating and interpreting their data and services. One interesting aspect of the system is to accept those differences and potential non-interoperability between two different systems and adapt on the fly (WHO, 2013). Such solutions use intelligent gateways and middleware. This can be called dynamic interoperability (WHO, 2013) and should be a continuous important research area with the growing complexity and heterogeneity of IoT environments. A middleware framework is the core element to be used for providing baseline sensor functionalities associated with registering and looking up Internet-connected objects, exchanging messages between objects, as well as fusing and reasoning data from multiple objects (WHO, 2013). That adaptation on the fly will be made easier if all actors agree on at least implementing the same standard to ease integration of their solutions. In scope of this study we would like to tackle some important challenges the Internet of Things is facing in relation to data include: (i) areas of the interoperability standard, (ii) consumption of the bandwidth, (iii) role of the standard, and (iv) importance of the interoperability ((WHO), 2010), since interoperability and standards still pose challenges and questions for the future of IoT devices. In addition, I would like to investigate on: (1) how to represent the data and standardize the data specifications, (2) if the data is correctly collected (trust and validity) and represented, and (3) if the information can be translated to a standard format (WHO, 2013).

Impact Analysis of (Tropical) Infectious Diseases on Non-Communicable Diseases

Impact Analysis is a technique designed to unearth the "unexpected" negative effects of a change in an organization. The convergence of infectious diseases and non-communicable disease is poorly investigated. The purpose of this study is to conduct an Impact analysis in examining in-depth the association of infectious diseases and NCDs as well as drafting a Diseases Association table, which will be included in a learning database and used by the proposed system to predict and prevent diseases. Following impacts should be analyzed.

Predictive Analytics and Modelling, in Form of Predictive Search (Automated Deduction or Augmented Reality)

Four areas would receive attention: person identification, surveillance/monitoring, 3D methods, and smart rooms/perceptual user interfaces.

Data Analytics, including machine learning and predictive analytics and modeling, can help to understand and mitigate the behavioral, genetic and environmental causes of disease and/or treatment's failure. Machine learning algorithms can learn from collected health-related data, use them to build pattern, and thus, can predict diseases.

We would also implement and test a machine-learning algorithm that could learn from and make predictions on collected health-related data. A comparative analysis of following learning algorithms will be conducted to determine the best suitable learning method for the system. We need an algorithm that can accurately predict disease in an asymptomatic individual at high risk.

We would design and implement an innovative technological solution approach for early detection and diagnosis of NCDs, using the Internet of Things system (IoTS). This system would be able to collect and process health-related data. A previous work had introduced a technical solution in the medical area by using wireless sensors networks, which responsibility is to acquire and process different signals that one finds in the medical area.

Genetic and Environmental Impacts Linking to Convergences of (Tropical) Infectious Diseases and Non-Communicable Diseases

The impact of the genetic and environmental on disease association in individuals should be investigated, then genetics and environment can impact the course of the disease. The genetic predisposition is getting more attention in diseases prediction. In (Christaki, 2015) the authors have presented the importance of considering genetic dimensions in predicting an infectious disease. They further state the advances realized in the genome sequencing and the new possibility the advancement in the microbiology offers to the predicting means. They start following:

... The rapid development and declining cost of new molecular techniques have provided the means for enhanced pathogen discovery. A shift has been taking place in microbiological surveillance, from diagnostic pathogen identification in humans and animals to wide screening for pathogens in samples collected at hotspots for emerging infectious diseases. The advancement of high throughput sequencing methods has made it possible to rapidly acquire detailed sequence data necessary for pathogen identification and analysis in large databases for the characterization of a new agent.

Association Non-Communicable Disease and Mental Health

How can mental health impact the development of non-communicable disease and vice-versa? Can mental health be associated with the lifestyle of individuals and their familiar and geographical environment? Sensing mental health is still poorly investigated and not all advanced in comparison with sensing physiologic modalities. Can the state of mental health and lifestyle boost the development of (associated) non-communicable diseases or multimorbidities? These questions should be answered in the scope of this study. Further, the study should focus on improvement of sensing mental health using wearable computing and management of life's quality for individuals at a high-risk factor of morbidities.

Individual Drug Metabolism and Convergence of Diseases or Multimorbidity

Studies (Smart, 2011) in Africa, especially in Kenya have shown the convergence of HIV/AIDS and myocardial function in people living with HIV. It is proved that some drugs used for curing affection can cause a non-communicable disease. For example, AZT and d4T (two medicines used for Anti-Viral- Therapy in HIV affected people) may affect myocardial function. The question that will be investigated here is whether some patients treated with some drugs face some drugs adverse and how those adverse can early be detected to prevent multimorbidity in the concerned patient? Together with medical partner and using the technology of pharmacogenomics/ pharmacogenetics, this question would be investigated. Additionally, the further objective of this project is to find a way to include pervasive sensing in the early detection of drug adverse.

Pharmacogenetics has been defined as the study of variability in drug response due to heredity (Nebert, 1999). Pharmacogenomics and pharmacogenetics are both interchangeable. Using this technology in determining individual drug metabolism will help to draw an adverse drug reaction map with regard to the genes determining the drug metabolism. Thus, individual at high risk of drug adverse can better be monitored, assessed, and treated.

STUDY QUESTIONS

How to improve the early detection of any associated non-communicable disease in individuals at high risk of or suffering from infectious diseases and thus prevent NCDs? To investigate the topic, this question should be broken down so that a complete chain of answers should be found.

1. Do Genetic and Environmental Impacts link to Convergences of (Tropical) Infectious Diseases and Non-Communicable Diseases?
2. Could Non-Communicable Disease be associated with Mental Health?
3. Could Individual Drug metabolism impact Convergence of Diseases or Multimorbidity?

4. How considering the genetic dimension could improve the traditional screening for diseases so that to reduce the wrong negative or positive screened? How the genetic impacts this effect?
5. How to sense sufficient risk of a specific disease using wearable IoT systems? How to measure the risk through the bio-signals?
6. Can Pervasive sensing of NCDs improve the traditional screening methods for disease?
7. Can Measuring health-related quality-of-life and sensing mental health may contribute to the early detection and diagnosis of NCD?
8. are beyond the most known and well-investigated NCDs risk factors, infectious diseases also causing NCDs?
9. Can monitor infectious diseases in infected individuals contribute to predicting and thus early detect NCDs?

To answers the questions above, we will follow the stepwise approach we proposed to solve key problems of medicine delivery and medical consultation for the patients living in rural regions of Benin (T. O. Edoh & Teege, 2011). Additionally, technological approach from recent works on wireless sensors networks (T. O. C. Edoh, Atchome, Alahassa, & Pawar, 2016), remote care delivery systems (T. O. Edoh & Pravin Amrut Pawar, Bernd Brügge, 2016), and Off-Label-Use drugs would also be considered. The key steps in the proposed approach are as follows:

1. Identification of basic health care problems in the implementation region and conduct a long-term cohort study;
2. Identification and analysis of prevalent non-communicable and infectious diseases and risk factors in the implementation region;
3. Impact Analysis of (Tropical) Infectious Diseases on Non-Communicable Diseases and Drafting a Disease Association Table in the implementation region;
4. Feasibility analysis of ICT implementation of the IoT supporting early detection technology and identification of relevant ICT implementation obstacles in the implementation region;
5. Researching scientific and technical architecture for Improving the Early Detection of Non-Communicable Diseases (NCD)
6. Use Predictive Analytics and Modelling, in Form of Predictive Search (Automated Deduction or Augmented Reality) to understand and mitigate the behavioral, genetic and environmental causes of disease and/or treatment's failure.

7. Implementation of proposed system architecture, pervasive/wearable sensing applications and adaptations to alleviate ICT implementation obstacles;
8. For remote sensing of disease, similar technics as these used in (Cheng, n.d.; H. Qu, Q. Cheng, 2006) for remote monitoring will be taken to account
9. Setup necessary technical and organizational environment to offer system to the patient population and healthcare professionals;
10. Online offering of the system and patient empowerment applications to people in the implementation region aiming to adhere to disease sensing using their smart and adapted sensors kits (will be implemented); and
11. Investigate further challenges and suitable business model(s) in the mass implementation of a system to positively affect the health of the population and generate employment in the eHealth sector.
12. Drafting a universally valid Screening's methodology
13. Each public health system defines its own program for screening for diseases.

STUDY RISK ASSESSMENT

The risky and challenging nature of the proposed objectives requires special attention during the cohort study and terminal testing phase of the study. The main risks arise from the recruitment of adequate people and quality of the data. The quality of the data is the central piece of this work, then the learning algorithm should learn from accurate data and thus build correct partner for future recognition. Table 5 summarizes the risks level and how to mitigate them.

GUIDELINES TO IMPROVE THE COMMON SCREENING PROCESS

This section presents the guidelines of a proposed best practice for improving the screening process. Following steps can improve the screening and overcome the major limitations the common screening methods present.

The concept is to define universal screening guidelines for disease and additionally improve the methods of screening for diseases using ICT systems.

Table 5. Risk management plan

Risk and Barriers	Impact on Study Success	Mitigation/Management Plan
Recruitment sufficient cohort population at the study regions for long-term study	High	To prevent any issue at this stage, a collaboration with healthcare centers will be made, selected people will be informed on the importance of the study as well as the expected outcomes. Incentives would be offered about and respecting the local anti-corruption law.
Collection of sufficient data from asymptomatic and infected patient for significant data analysis for investigating the link between infectious diseases and NCDs	High	Due to data protection law, it can be difficult to access certain medical data or collect them. Enrolled people would be informed about how their data will be processed. Data will be anonymously collected and processed.
Possible interference between patient medical device such cardiac pacemaker and the proposed IoTS	Medium	Only asymptomatic and people suffering from (tropical) infectious diseases will be enrolled. NCDs patient at advanced stage won't be enrolled at cohort study phase. At the testing phase, they will be enrolled to test the IoTS only under permanent medical surveillance
Quality of collected data	High	The data collector can intentionally falsify the data. The same data will be collected by 3 different persons so that they can be compared to detect any manipulation. A Quality assurance will be implemented and should be strictly followed by the data collectors

Considering the Genetic Dimension

The genetic dimension should be considered during a screening process, then it is well known that the genetic predisposition can contribute to early detect or predict certain diseases in an individual.

WHO had determined the criteria of screening for diseases since 1968. These criteria are well spread and widely used till today(J. M. Wilson & Jungner, 1968). Those criteria do not take into consideration the genetic diversities among the population. It is now well known that intermittent ART therapy increases the cardiovascular disease risk in certain people living with HIV (PLWH). The question to investigate here: does intermittent ART therapy have the same effects in all PLWH? How the genetic impacts this effect?

Pervasive Sensing Physical Bio-Signals

In general, sensing physical/physiological values is well advanced. This technology is to be used to improve the traditional screening, increasing the adherence to screening among the population and finally reducing and/or bringing down to zero the number of wrongly positive or negative screened individual. Certain disease modalities could be sensed at early stage of the disorder

A fundamental question is still open. How to sense sufficient risk of a specific disease using wearable IoT systems? How to measure the risk through the bio-signals?

Pervasive Sensing Mental Modalities

Most common solution approaches for sensing mental health are using video and web conferencing in mental health delivery (Kinley, Zibrik, Cordeiro, Lauscher, & Ho, 2012), also for facial gestures recognition. However, facial gestures cannot 100% reveal the mental health of an individual, therefore, it is mandatory to analyze, in-depth, the brain activities as well as other physiological modalities in individuals suffering from any mental disorder and thus, design an innovative solution for sensing mental health. Harris Georgiou has recently evaluated the number of active CPU cores in the human brain during the human brain is performing a simple task using a functional Magnetic Resonance Imaging (fMRI) (H. Haddadi, P. Healey, R. McCabe, 2014). This result is a fundament on which we can build further research for an innovative method of sensing mental health. Our hypothesis is that the number of parallel active processes in the human brain may determine the mental health of an individual.

Use Non-Invasive Screening

There exist today many non-invasive sensors on the market, which we advise to use such sensors and miniaturized devices so that the individual is not restricted in his daily activities. People carry pervasively their smartphone. The smartphone can play the role of the gateway and will be connected to the cloud to forward all useful data. We recommend using IoT infrastructure such as raspberry pi, which will be assigned to pre-processing tasks at the edge.

Provide a National Screening Database With Integration of Patient Dossiers

Data collected from the population should be stored somewhere and call for analytics and decision tasks. This database can be a cloud (public or private)

CONCEPT OF IOT BASED PERVASIVE/ UBIQUITOUS SCREENING FOR NCDS

This section presents our IT concept for an improved screening process. The proposal is an interdisciplinary effort that combines two major domains – healthcare and ICT, whereas each objective is focused on using advanced ICT techniques to solve problems in health data collection, analysis and interpretation as well as improve existing health systems – especially in developing countries. The objectives of pervasive disease screening for early detection of medical conditions are using pervasive devices such as body sensor to automatically and autonomously screen an individual (patient or asymptomatic), overcome the limitation of tools and methods related to traditional screening, rise the development of innovative ICT tools to increase patient's adherence to screening programs, and the creation of less invasive tools. Furthermore, improving the efficiency and interoperability of health data collection will make use of novel power-saving Internet of Things technology based on emerging standards and will create vertical m-health applications on top of a de-verticalized middleware

The system proposal consists, therefore, of a cloud and a web server, a client (intended for physicians and control/data centers), a smartphone as a gateway (patient own device), raspberry pi.

MQTT (Message Queue Telemetry Transport), CoAP (Constrained Application Protocol), are the candidate data protocols. MQTT and CoAP are data protocols, which are suitable to the constrained environment. They support asynchronous communication via IP.

For the communication layers, Bluetooth (short range, and low energy), ZigBee (low Energy, higher range), WIFI are selected to enable communication between the end-devices (for ex. sensors), system and Internet.

We propose to use noninvasive sensors to collect vital parameters during a medication and infection period. The collected data are pre-processed at the edge (edge/fog computing) and useful data are sent to the gateway, which in turn sends the data to the cloud for depth data analysis.

The system aims at detecting any abnormal vital parameter value that would analyze and controlled by a physician to check if the abnormal values are temporary and related to the infectious disease or a dysfunction that lead to an NCD.

At the cloud, the analytics application will consider the results of the genome sequencing as well the patient dossier entries.

The system features a patient dossier (EMR – electronic medical record), where all patient medical data are recorded.

Figure 1. Proposed platform

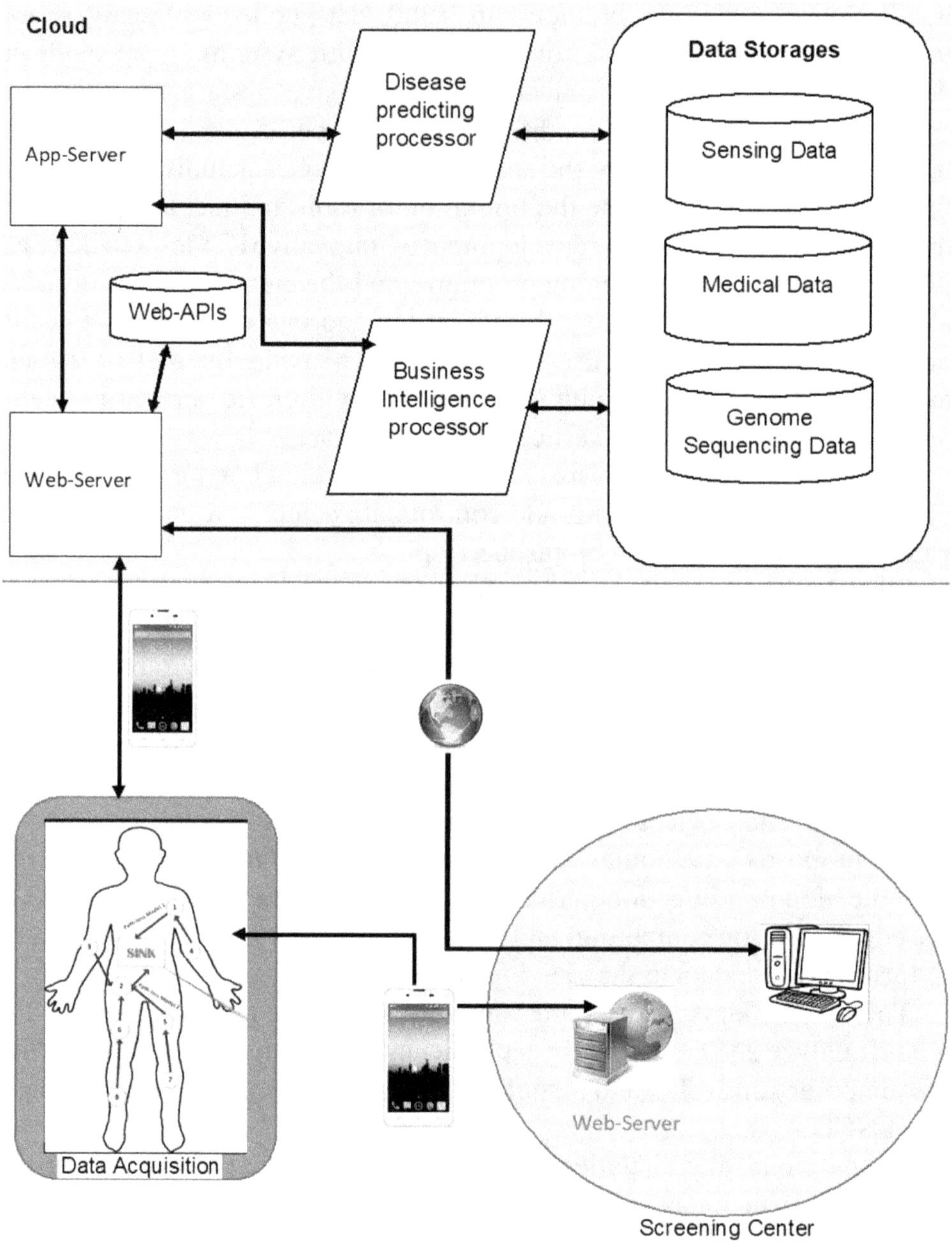

As platform (Figure 1), we propose a wireless sensor network based Body Area Network (BAN), that is connected to the patient smartphone (the IoT gateway) through a raspberry pi playing the role of edge gateway. Data are collected by the sensors and sent to the raspberry, which sends them to the smartphone. The smartphone receives only useful data, then the data protocol used here is MQTT (subscribe/Publish). The smartphone sends (publishes) in turn the data to the cloud for further analysis. The smartphone can also send the data to a web-server using the CoAP protocol.

The Cloud platform consists of disease prediction processor (input: collected data and genome sequencing results, medical data), business intelligence processor, data storage: medical data, Genome data, collected/sensing data. illustrates the overview architecture of the proposed system.

- **Data Acquisition:** Individuals are provided with different kind of medical sensors to pervasively collect the vital sign anywhere anytime. We consider non-invasive sensors that are connected to a gateway. The gateway pre-processes all collect data and sends only useful data to the cloud for further data analysis and disease prediction.
- **Screening Center:** The screening center is the central place where epidemiologists analyze the collected data. They access the data through the cloud. They can also send a command to the collection unit (balloon or drone) to proceed with special tasks. Additionally, they can directly contact the potential patient, he owns a mobile phone, otherwise, an emergency team would be sent to him for further measurement.
- **Cloud:** The cloud is used for data storage (persistent) and processing. At the cloud, the web-application, as well as prediction and business intelligence processor, are hosted. Disease predicting processor extracts the provided data and determine patterns that are used to predict diseases outbreak at the individual. The business intelligence processor provides the control center with necessary data to help for taking an adequate decision. The cloud enables remote access to the collected data.

The security (data etc.) is to assure by the provider of the cloud.

PROOF OF CONCEPT AND RESULTS

The proposed screening system for diseases prevention is an IoT based information system using biomedical sensors to collect bio signal and smartphone as a gateway, where lightweight data processing is taken place. The smartphone can then inform the patient and transfer the filtered data (pre-processed data) to the cloud. At the cloud, genetic data are associated with the received data to perform global data analytics as well as impact analytics with the objective to predict potential risk level to develop the certain disease as well as to early detect eventual non-communicable diseases in the patient. Disease prevention can then be triggered to avoid developing the detected disease.

We performed a test, which still ongoing. At this stage of the test, we conducted a causal research to explore certain study questions, e.g. the convergence of NDCs and CDs.

In (T. O. C. Edoh et al., 2016), we had already tested the biosignal collection using information system (wireless sensor network.).

Rapid Prototype

We implemented a rapid prototype of a bio-signal collector like the system described in (T. O. C. Edoh et al., 2016). We use eclipse an IDE running Java 1.8 (Java ME 8) to implement a Java IoT using Bluetooth (BLE) as a

Table 6. Test infrastructure

Infrastructure	Description
Data collection (Sensors)	We use following sensors to collect vital parameters, which is sent to the cloud. 1. Respiratory, 2. Heart/ECG, 3. Blood pressure/pulse and oxygen, 4. Temperature, (v) air humidity, and 5. Accelerometer/position sensor.
Web server	Web-Apache 2.4 with a backend Glassfish 4
Cloud	Cloud (Amazon AWS)
IoT	Edge/fog computing • Raspberry pi
IoT Gateway	• Smartphone
Data protocols And Communication/Transport Layer	• MQTT (Message Queuing Telemetry Transport) • CoAP • NB-IoT (NarrowBand-IoT) • Bluetooth Low Energy (BLE)

communication protocol between the raspberry pi and the smartphone which sends the data to the cloud. The raspberry pi is connected to the different sensors.

Infrastructure

The devices needed and used for the test are summarized in Table 6.

Cohort

We build a cohort of 251 persons (see Table 8). The cohort members were judiciously selected according to certain criteria: (i) age, (ii) gender, (iii) NCDs predisposition, access to healthcare [we consider the financial capacity to purchase any prescription], and social aspect.

With this cohort, we like to investigate the convergence of ID and NCDs as well as the impacts of socialization, mental health (stress, financial and emotional problems, ...) on developing NCDs. For this purpose, we selected the candidates using a snowball approach and meeting defined requirements (see Test design and methods). Table 7 indicates the sampling criteria.

TEST DESIGN AND METHODS

This section presents the test scenarios. Our requirements were to select people free of malaria infection long time before the rainy season and who do not present any of the indices present by WHO in (Gachot & Ringwald, 1998) (Table 1) [see Table 9]. The rain season is May to July. In this period, according to the data presented by the MOH on the DHIS/SNIGS an AVG of 60% tested people are a position[1] (Figure 2).

We worked together with medical doctors and laboratory personnel who medically check the candidate fitting the criteria. We eliminated every people

Table 7. Sampling criteria

Categories	Age Ranges
1. Female, good access to health 2. Male, good access to healthcare 3. Female, poor access to health 4. Male, poor access to healthcare	1. Children: 1 -5 y 2. Teenager: 6 -19 y 3. Youth: 20 -25 y 4. Adult: 26 – 49 y 5. Elderly: 50 + y

Table 8. Structure and characteristics of the study/test cohort

Age Range	Disease Predisposition/ or Suffering From Acute NDS	Social Connected	Mental Health	Access to Healthcare	Number per Gender F	M	Description
1 – 5	X	Y	Y	Y	3	4	Children
6 – 19	Y	Y	Y	Y	5	5	School boys and girls
	N	Y	Y	Y	5	5	
20 – 25	N	Y	Y	Y	2	2	Students, Workers, Jobless
				N	2	2	
			N	Y	2	2	
				N	2	2	
		N	Y	Y	2	2	Students, Workers, Jobless
				N	2	2	
			N	Y	2	2	
				N	2	2	
	Y	Y	Y	N	2	2	Students, Workers, Jobless
				Y	2	2	
			N	Y	2	2	
				N	2	2	
		N	Y	Y	2	2	Students, Workers, Jobless
				N	2	2	
			N	N	2	2	
				Y	2	2	
26 – 49	N	Y	Y	Y	2	2	Workers, Jobless
				N	2	2	
			N	Y	2	2	
				N	2	2	
		N	Y	Y	2	2	Workers, Jobless
				N	2	2	
			N	Y	2	2	
				N	2	2	
	Y	Y	Y	N	2	2	Workers, Jobless
				Y	2	2	
			N	Y	2	2	
				N	2	2	
		N	Y	Y	2	2	Workers, Jobless
				N	2	2	
			N	N	2	2	
				Y	2	2	

continued on following page

Table 8. Continued

Age Range	Disease Predisposition/ or Suffering From Acute NDS	Social Connected	Mental Health	Access to Healthcare	Number per Gender		Description
					F	M	
50+	N	Y	Y	Y	3	3	Workers, Jobless, Retired
				N	3	3	
			N	Y	3	3	
				N	3	3	
		N	Y	Y	3	3	
				N	3	3	
			N	Y	3	3	
				N	3	3	
	Y	Y	Y	N	3	3	Workers, Jobless, Retired
				Y	3	3	
			N	Y	3	3	
				N	3	3	
		N	Y	Y	3	3	Workers, Jobless, Retired
				N	3	3	
			N	N	3	3	
				Y	3	3	
Total					125	126	
					251		

Legend:
Y = Yes
N = No
X = Unknown
F = Female
M = Male

who present any risk factors described in Table 2 since we are investigating the impacts of developing NCDs. Including any other risk factors will complicate the test and can bias the results. In the malaria high season, we selected only those who malaria-infected. So, we selected 251 people who were enrolled in the test program.

Presently, we screened the family medical history of each enrolled people to determine if they are predisposed to develop NCDs, this is the common method used today. In the future, we like to use the genome sequencing to determine any disease predisposition.

People enrolled give written consent to use their anonymized data.

Figure 2. Population tested malaria positive in 2017
Source: SNIGS/Ministry of Health in Benin.

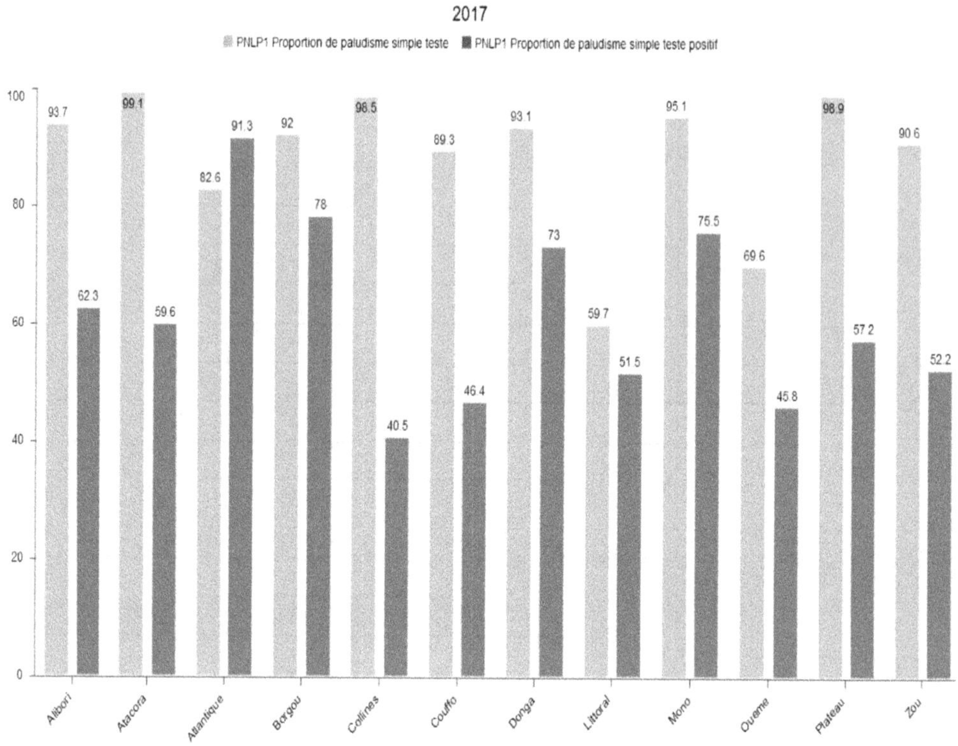

Table 9. Laboratory indices in case of severe malaria

Table 1 Severe manifestations of *Plasmodium falciparum* malaria in adults and children

Prognostic value (+ to +++)			Frequency (+ to +++)	
Children	Adults	Clinical manifestations	Children	Adults
+++	+++	Impaired consciousness	+++	++
+++	+++	Respiratory distress (acidotic breathing)	+++	++
+	++	Multiple convulsions	+++	+
+	+	Prostration	+++	+++
+++	+++	Shock	+	+
+++	+++	Pulmonary oedema (radiological)	+/–*	+
+++	++	Abnormal bleeding	+/–*	+
++	+	Jaundice	+	+++
		Laboratory indices		
+	+	Severe anaemia	+++	+
+++	+++	Hypoglycaemia	+++	++
+++	+++	Acidosis	+++	++
+++	+++	Hyperlactataemia	+++	++
++	++	Renal impairment†	+	+++
+/–	++	Hyperparasitaemia	++	+

*Infrequent.
†Acute kidney injury.

Source: WHO/(Gachot & Ringwald, 1998).

Our test and research are ongoing. We are using the action study approach to refine the system proposal.

Scenario 1: Individual suffering from malaria-tropica, socially isolated, no NCDs pre-detected, no mental disorder
Scenario 2: Individual suffering from malaria-tropica, social well connected, no NCDs pre-detected, no mental disorder
Scenario 3: Individual suffering from malaria-tropica, socially isolated, NCDs pre-detected, no mental disorder
Scenario 4: Individual suffering from malaria-tropica, social well connected, NCDs pre-detected, no mental disorder
Test Duration: 3 months (June –August) Rain Period
Endemic Infection: Malaria-tropica

RESULTS

Our results relating to the indices () are similar to the results carried out by WHO in Africa and illustrated with Figure 3. We, therefore, concentrate our investigation and data analysis on (i) heart disease, (ii) hyperglycemia, and (iii) digestive diseases.

Figure 3. Detected lab indices in a study carried out by WHO
Source WHO/(Gachot & Ringwald, 1998).

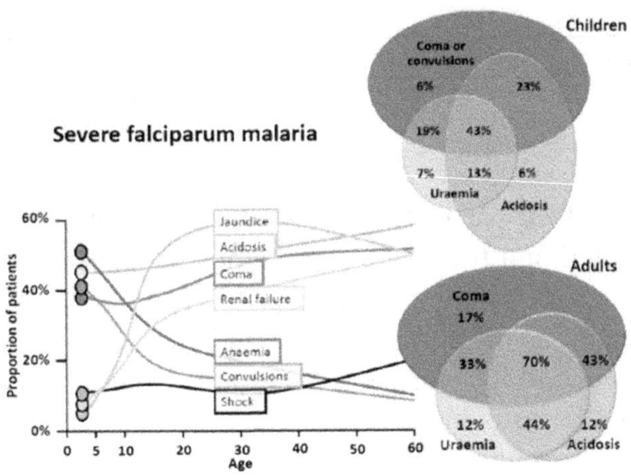

Figure 1 Data compiled from prospective series of severe falciparum malaria in 6189 children in studies conducted in Africa and 2605 adults in studies conducted in South-East Asia. Left side shows the prevalence of different features of severe falciparum malaria by age, and Venn diagrams on the right show the mortality in children and adults associated with manifestations of cerebral and renal impairment and metabolic acidosis alone or in combination. The sizes of the ovals are proportional to number of cases.

Figure 4. Comparison of symptoms and diseases development among females and males without NCDs predisposition

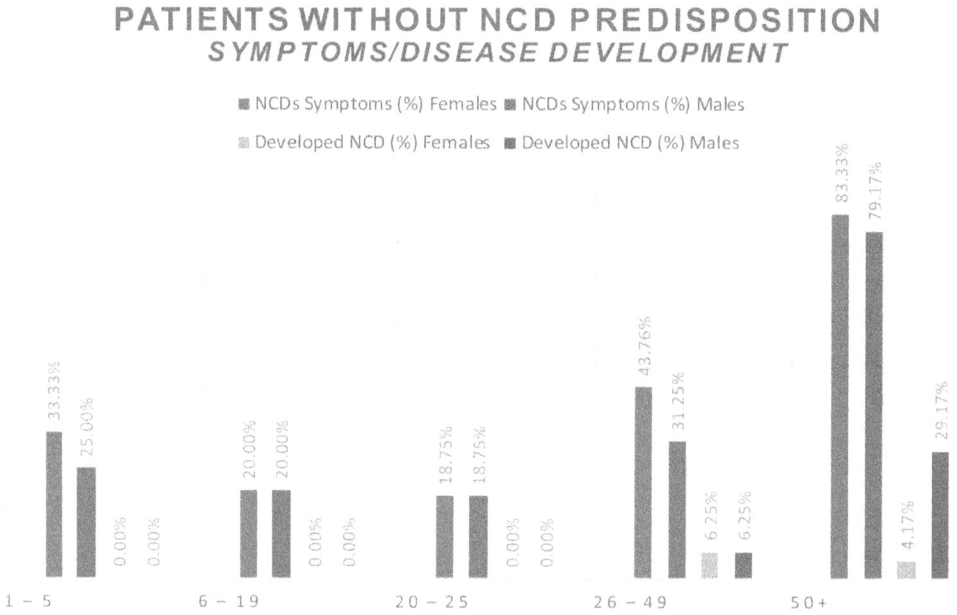

Table 10. Symptoms and diseases development among female participants (without NCDs predisposition)

Age Range	Number	Infection Duration (AVG Day) and Severity	Predisposition NCDs	NCDs Symptoms (%)	Developed NCD (%)
1 – 5	3	30 days	No	33,33%	0,0%
6 – 19	5	43 days	No	20,00%	0,0%
20 – 25	16	25 days	No	18,75%	0,0%
26 – 49	16	32 days	No	43,755%	6,25%
50+	24	35 days	No	83,33%	4,17%

The test reveals that all involved participants present symptoms of the digestive disorder. They vomited and have stomach cramps. According to the project medical assistant, these symptoms are relating to the malaria-tropica. Though, we did not examine the participants to find out if they have developed digestive disorders due to the short test duration. In contrast, we examine the participant of heart diseases and hyperglycemia. The participants are provided with "Akku-Check" a device to measure and control the glucose

Table 11. Symptoms and diseases development among male participants (without NCDs predisposition)

Age Range	Number	Infection Duration (AVG Day) and Severity	Predisposition NCDs	NCDs Symptoms (%)	Developed NCD (%)
1 – 5	4	28 days	No	25,00%	0,00%
6 – 19	5	40 days	No	20,00%	0,00%
20 – 25	16	23 days	No	18,75%	0,00%
26 – 49	16	27 days	No	31,25%	6,25%
50+	24	30 days	No	79,17%	29,17%

Table 12. Symptoms and diseases development among female participants (with NCDs predisposition)

Age Range	Number	Infection Duration (AVG Day) and Severity	Predisposition NCDs	NCDs Symptoms (%)	Developed NCD (%)
6 – 19	5	43 days	Yes	80,00%	20,00%
20 – 25	16	25 days	Yes	62,50%	6,25%
26 – 49	16	32 days	Yes	50,00%	6,250%
50+	24	35 days	Yes	87,50%	8,33%

Table 13. Symptoms and diseases development among male participants (with NCDs predisposition)

Age Range	Number	Infection Duration (AVG Day) and Severity	Predisposition NCDs	NCDs Symptoms (%)	Developed NCD (%)
6 – 19	5	40 days	Yes	60,00%	0,00%
20 – 25	16	23 days	Yes	56,25%	0,00%
26 – 49	16	27 days	Yes	37,50%	0,00%
50+	24	30 days	Yes	83,33%	4,17%

level. The data thus collected reveal that certain participants have developed the tendency to diabetes type II. Once a week, we examine the participants to figure out if they are developing any heart disease.

We analyze the collected data and present the results with respect to the gender in 10, Table 11, Table 12, and Table 13.

Participant Without NDCs Predisposition

Comparing females with males, who are not predisposed to develop NCDs has pointed out that females have more shown symptoms and more developed the NCDs than the males. It is worth to note that this results only show a tendency. The study duration was too short and the cohort size too small. Figure 4 illustrates the results.

Participants With NDCs Predisposition

We further compare females with males with a predisposition to NCDs. The results present the same tendency as within-participant without NCDs predisposition. We can then prudently conclude that females are more tendency to develop acute NCDs after a malaria infection. Figure 5 demonstrates the tendency participants predisposed to NCDs have to develop acute NCDs after suffering from malaria infection.

Figure 5. Comparison of symptoms and diseases development among females and males without NCDs predisposition

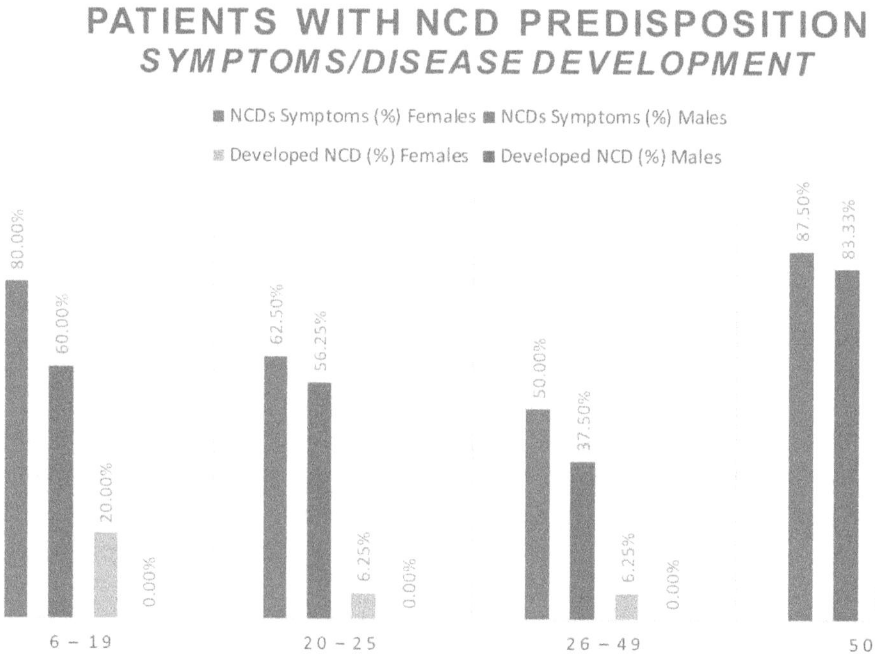

Figure 6. Comparison of the female ability to develop NCDs regarding their predisposition to develop NCDs

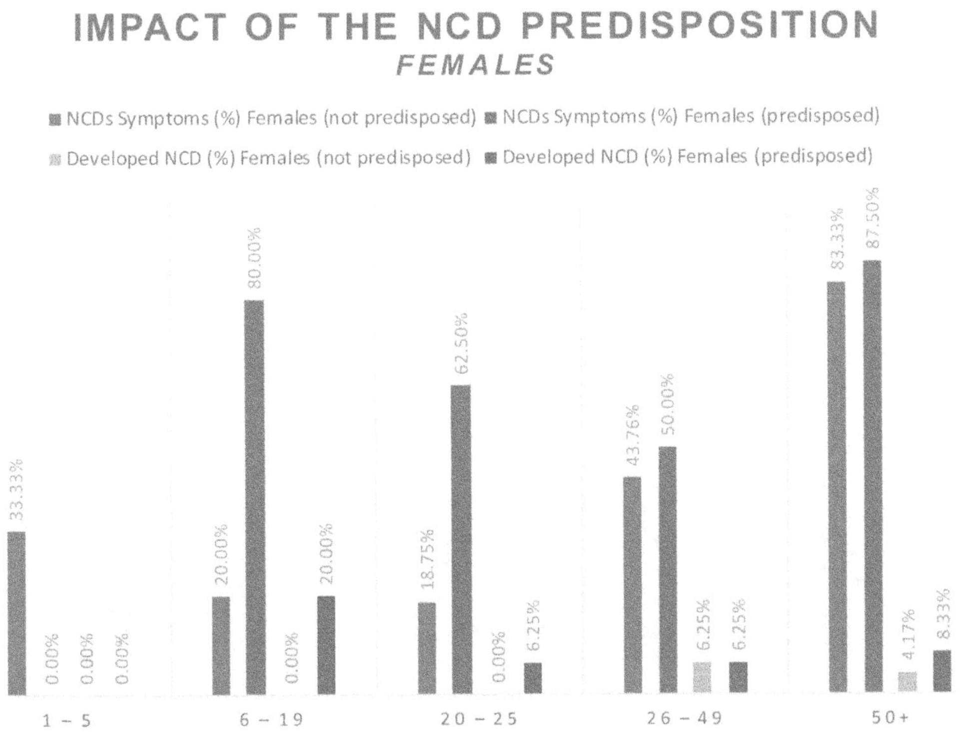

Impacts of the NCDs Predisposition on Developing NCDs During or After a Malaria Infection

We have also analyzed the impact of NCDs predisposition among each gender group. We, therefore, compare non-predisposed females with predisposed females and the same for the males.

We can figure out in female's cohort that age is also a factor in developing NCDs after suffering from malaria infection. We only detected in the group of 50+ years participants with acute NCDs. The analysis also reveals that the NCDs predisposed participants develop more NCDs than the other. Figure 6 presents the comparison of both groups of female participants.

We also conduct the same analysis in the male's cohort. We detect in two age groups (26 to 49 and 50+) that participants non-predisposed to NCDs have more developed NCDs than those predisposed to developed NCDs. Figure 7 shows the comparison of both groups of male participants.

Figure 7. Comparison of the male ability to develop NCDs regarding their predisposition to develop NCDs

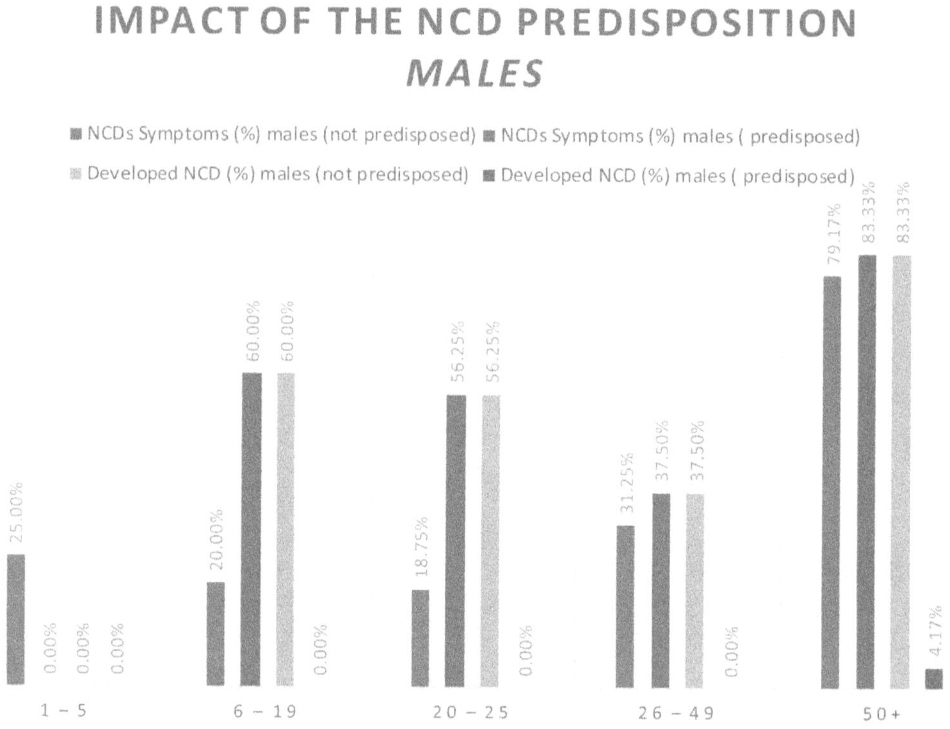

Females and males present different diseases development picture. We need a long-term test to confirm these results.

Though, our concept, to consider genomics parameters, gender, and pervasively screening/sensing individuals at high risk to contract (tropical) infections to predict an early detect the risk of developing acute and/or chronic NCDs, is demonstrated to be an improved method to prevent NCDs.

TEST LIMITATION AND DISCUSSION

The test was conducted for 3 months. This period is too short to obtain useful results. Another limitation of the test was the few number of participants involved. Though, this test demonstrates the feasibility of the concept and shows a certain tendency on the correlation between infectious diseases and non-communicable diseases.

FURTHER WORK

Our future work would consist to investigate following questions:

1. Could an infectious disease provoke an NCD in an individual without a genetic predisposition for NCDs?
2. Do infectious diseases accelerate the NCDs outbreak in an individual with genetic predisposition?
3. What is the impact of pharmacogenomics on the outbreak of NCDs in individuals at high risks of infectious diseases?
4. How to, efficiently and cost-effectively, pervasively sense the evidence of NCDs outbreak in an individual without genetic predisposition?
5. How to pervasively measure if ID affects the acceleration of NCDs outbreak if our study reveals that ID can accelerate the NCDs outbreak?
6. Monitor the adverse drug reactions that could provoke the NCDs outbreak.

Furthermore, we would implement an efficient IoT architecture to de-verticalize the data collection. Additionally, we will extend our system with a business intelligence feature that will help the physician to give appropriate treatment to prevent NCDs.

IoT systems are facing the interoperability problem. It is well known that web services could help to overcome this problem.

It matters to conduct a long-term test to obtain useful data for a definitive statement.

CONCLUSION

The chapter discusses the limitation of the conventional screening and proposes a new way for improved screening. It proposes guidelines for improving the conventional screening process.

The chapter proposes an IoT-based solution for pervasive screening combined with genome sequencing. Data gained from genome sequencing, pharmacogenomics, mental health-related data, social and life quality, and environmental (climate, air pollution) are the input data for the system. A cloud performs data analytics on a large dataset and determines certain patterns, which are used for prediction and thus prevent the disease.

This tendency demonstrates the need to conduct depth a long-term test with a large size cohort. The results also show the feasibility of the concept.

REFERENCES

Al-Qabandi, M., Gorter, J. W., & Rosenbaum, P. (2011). Early Autism Detection: Are We Ready for Routine Screening? *Pediatrics*, *128*(1), e211–e217. doi:10.1542/peds.2010-1881 PMID:21669896

Angheben, A., Anselmi, M., Gobbi, F., Marocco, S., Monteiro, G., Buonfrate, D., ... Bartoloni, A. (2011). Chagas disease in Italy: Breaking an epidemiological silence. *Eurosurveillance*, *16*(37), 1. PMID:21944554

Celermajer, D. S., Chow, C. K., Marijon, E., Anstey, N. M., & Woo, K. S. (2012). Cardiovascular disease in the developing world: Prevalences, patterns, and the potential of early disease detection. *Journal of the American College of Cardiology*, *60*(14), 1207–1216. doi:10.1016/j.jacc.2012.03.074 PMID:22858388

Chandra, S., & Chandra, H. (2011). *Myocardial Infarction Associated with Plasmodium Falciparum Malarial Infection*. Academic Press.

Cheng, X. L. (n.d.). Unconfined mobile Bluetooth nursing and daily data collection. In *IEEE Consumer Communications and Networking Conf. (CCNC '04)*. IEEE.

Christaki, E. (2015). New technologies in predicting, preventing and controlling emerging infectious diseases. *Virulence*, *6*(6), 558–565. doi:10.1080/21505594.2015.1040975 PMID:26068569

Edoh, T. O., Pawar, P. A., Brügge, B., & Teege, G. (2016). A Multidisciplinary Remote Healthcare Delivery System to Increase Health Care Access, Pathology Screening, and Treatment in Developing Countries. *International Journal of Healthcare Information Systems and Informatics*, *11*(4), 1–31. doi:10.4018/IJHISI.2016100101

Edoh, T. O., & Teege, G. (2011). Using information technology for an improved pharmaceutical care delivery in developing countries. Study case: Benin. *Journal of Medical Systems*, *35*(5), 1123–1134. doi:10.100710916-011-9717-y PMID:21519942

Edoh, T. O. C., Atchome, A., Alahassa, B. R. U., & Pawar, P. (2016). Evaluation of a Multi-Tier Heterogeneous Sensor Network for Patient Monitoring – The Case of Benin. In *MMHealth '16 Proceedings of the 2016 ACM Workshop on Multimedia for Personal Health and Health Care* (pp. 23–29). Amsterdam, The Netherlands: ACM Digital Library. 10.1145/2985766.2985772

Gachot, B., & Ringwald, P. (1998). Severe malaria. *La Revue du Praticien, 48*(5), 273–278. doi:10.1111/tmi.12313 PMID:9781074

Haddadi, Healey, McCabe, & M. P. (2014). *Healthcare informatics for mental health: recent advances and the outlook for the future*. Ment. Health Found.

Hidron, A., Vogenthaler, N., Santos-Preciado, J. I., Rodriguez-Morales, A. J., Franco-Paredes, C., & Rassi, A. (2010). Cardiac involvement with parasitic infections. *Clinical Microbiology Reviews, 23*(2), 324–349. doi:10.1128/CMR.00054-09 PMID:20375355

Kinley, A., Zibrik, L., Cordeiro, J., Lauscher, H. N., & Ho, K. (2012). *TeleHealth for Mental Health and Substance Use*. Academic Press.

Le Reste, J. Y., Nabbe, P., Rivet, C., Lygidakis, C., Doerr, C., Czachowski, S., ... Van Royen, P. (2015). The European general practice research network presents the translations of its comprehensive definition of multimorbidity in family medicine in ten European languages. *PLoS One, 10*(1), 1–13. doi:10.1371/journal.pone.0115796 PMID:25607642

Monge-Maillo, B., Jiménez, B. C., Pérez-Molina, J. A., Norman, F., Navarro, M., Pérez-Ayala, A., ... López-Vélez, R. (2009). Imported infectious diseases in mobile populations, Spain. *Emerging Infectious Diseases, 15*(11), 1745–1752. doi:10.3201/eid1511.090718 PMID:19891861

Nebert, D. W. (1999). Pharmacogenetics and pharmacogenomics: Why is this relevant to the clinical geneticist? *Clinical Genetics, 56*(4), 247–258. doi:10.1034/j.1399-0004.1999.560401.x PMID:10636440

Nieman, A.-E., de Mast, Q., Roestenberg, M., Wiersma, J., Pop, G., Stalenhoef, A., ... van der Ven, A. (2015, November). Cardiac complication after experimental human malaria infection: A case report. *Malaria Journal, 8*(1), 277. doi:10.1186/1475-2875-8-277 PMID:19958549

Qu, H., Cheng, Q., & Yaprak, E. (2006). Unconfined e-healthcare system using UMTS-WLAN. *Int. Journal of Modeling and Simulation, 26*(3), 261–270. doi:10.1080/02286203.2006.11442376

Remais, J. V., Zeng, G., Li, G., Tian, L., & Engelgau, M. M. (2013). Convergence of non-communicable and infectious diseases in low- and middle-income countries. *International Journal of Epidemiology, 42*(1), 221–227. doi:10.1093/ije/dys135 PMID:23064501

Roggen, D., Arnrich, B., Tröster, G., & Tr, G. (2006). Life Style Management using Wearable Computer. *International Workshop on Ubiquitous Computing for Pervasive Healthcare Applications.*

Smart, T. (2011). HIV and non-communicable diseases (NCDs). *HIV & AIDS Information/HATIP, 182.*

Smith, S. (2012). *Urbanization and Cardiovascular Disease Fact Sheet.* Retrieved from http://www.world-heart-federation.org/press/fact-sheets/urbanization-and-cardiovascular-disease/

Strong, K., Wald, N., Miller, A., & Alwan, A. (2005). Current concepts in screening for noncommunicable disease: World Health Organ .... *The Library, 12*(1), 12–19.

WHO. (2013). *Cardiovascular diseases (CVDs).* Retrieved from http://www.who.int/mediacentre/factsheets/fs317/en/

WHO. (2010). *Global status report on noncommunicable diseases.* Retrieved from http://www.who.int/about/licensing/copyright_form/en/index.html

Wilson, H. J. (2013). Wearables in the Workplace. *Harvard Business Review,* 1–6.

Wilson, J. M., & Jungner, Y. G. (1968). Principles and practice of screening for disease. *Boletin de La Oficina Sanitaria Panamericana, 65*(4), 281–393. doi:10.1001/archinte.1969.00300130131020

ENDNOTE

1 https://dhis-bj.org/dhis-web-visualizer/

Conclusion

OVERALL CONCLUSION AND RESEARCH QUESTIONS

The Preface introduced this book; where the supporting technologies (those used to implement the different solutions presented along this book) are defined and described; the overall goal of the book as well as the target audience have been presented.

The challenges facing the global (public and private) health care services delivery have been discussed in the first chapter entitled "Challenges Facing Health Care Delivery Systems in Low-, Middle-, and High-Income Countries". The chapter has compared the medical structures and infrastructures available in low-, middle-, and high-income countries with each other. It has resulted structural and infrastructural gap between the health care services in both developing and developed countries. The challenges facing these different health care systems are at certain level and somehow common, though have different severity degree. It is worth to notice that developing countries are facing severe lack of ICT-infrastructure, budget shortage (lack of health insurances), undertrained healthcare professionals, and massive brain drain. Poor health and pharmaceutical care services delivery and accessibility characterize the global health care system in den developing countries. In contrary to developing countries, developed countries mostly possess excellent and well-structured health care systems, as well as disposing of excellent medical infrastructure. Almost health care systems in the high-income countries are relied on statutory and private individual health insurances as well as on states subsidies. The health care services delivery is well organized and thus health care services accessibility is higher than that in den developing countries. Despite this fact, the chapter reveals that high-income countries also are facing poor access to health care services, particularly in their rural areas. Certain groups of individuals are mostly facing this challenge, for example, elderly people, poor people or minorities (for example in USA). It has been shown that patients use to wait longtime until to get an appointment with medical experts. This phenomenon leads to weak care accessibility.

Overall, the chapter presents the challenges the global health care system is facing and discusses and analyzes the causes with the objective to design and implement solution approaches that can meet these challenges.

Most challenges can be met by implementing and deploying ICT-based solution approaches. The chapter presents a multidisciplinary remote health care services delivery system that's aiming to overcome care accessibility issues in both developing and developed countries. The novelty of the proposed solution is that traditional practitioners have been involved in the proposed system. The proposed system is composed of a multidisciplinary medical team and a set of ICT-systems. The multidisciplinary team is composed of healthcare professionals, traditional practitioners, and para-medical professionals. Involved traditional practitioners are intended for developing countries, where rural populations are more confident in traditional practitioners regarding their health means. Admittedly, involving traditional practitioners in the proposed system has promise to increase access to care services delivery in developing countries. Though, this is not sufficient. Therefore, the chapter proposes ICT-based solution to meet structural and infrastructural limitations and educational as well as training approach for involved traditional practitioners in order to help them to improve their diagnostic and treatment methods.

The proposed system is adaptable and can thus be used for health care system in high-income countries.

Solution approaches have been made in the following chapters. Certain solutions aim to overcome the limitations of existing methodologies regarding diseases early detection, prevention, and treatment. The chapter has answered the research questions like:

- What are the causes of the poor health care services accessibility?
- How to increase the accessibility to the health care services, particularly in medically underserved regions?
- Why exist disparities between health care services delivery in the same health care system, ex. USA public health care system?
- Can the health care services delivery get improved by involving traditional practitioners (TP) into those health care systems, where people are more confident in TP?
- How to then get involved the TP in those health care systems?

Chapter 2, entitled "Scale the Agility in a Multidisciplinary Remote Care Services Delivery System", has dealt with scaling the agility in remote care system proposed in Chapter 1. As proposed in Chapter 1, the system is an agile health care involving traditional practitioners. The second chapter, therefore, dealt with the research question like:

- How to scale the medical treatment in the case the same multidisciplinary team is involved in several medical treatments with several patients

The chapter discusses different aspects of the agile healthcare and how to manage medical treatment processes using scale agile methodic. This chapter has presented the background of the agile development methodology. The chapter figure out an important issue regarding the scrum board. The issue is to provide a multimodal digital scrum board to permit to traditional practitioners (TPs) to adhere to the scrum process. Illiterates TPs can use their voice to manage a scrum board. Future work will present this novel scrum board.

As discussed in Chapter 1, the global health care is facing enormous challenges. Chapter 3, entitled "Towards Secure Off-Label Drug Prescribing and Improved Drug Supply", has issued the off-label use problematics the global health care system is facing. It presents a case study, where the off-label use leading causes have been investigated. Off-Labe use, in developing countries, is a subsequent of drugs shortage since these countries do not produce drugs or other pharmaceutical products. In contrary to developing countries, off-label use in high-income countries is due to lack of adequate drugs for certain therapies, thus, off-label use is becoming an essential part of therapies in oncology, neurology, and pediatrics. Pediatrics oncology lacks drugs, which are produced and specially intended for children treatment. Therefore, off-label use is a medical treatment approach.

The chapter presents interesting solution approaches for secure off-label use, since these drugs used for off-label use are not tested in prior. Thus, this practice presents certain risks for the patient health. The chapter proposes an evidence-based system in term of big/large knowledge database to collect evidence information to be provide to healthcare professionals willing to practice off-label use.

A direct consequence of using drugs (also in the case off-label use) is the adverse drug reactions (ADR). The global health care system is facing ADR issues since the last century. The chapter has especially investigated and answered the question:

- Why the global public health care is facing the off-label use of drugs, although the developed countries have a well-developed pharmaceutical industry and produce sufficient medicine for each medical condition?
- Do the off-label use leading causes worldwide the same?
- The term of off-label use is facing a definition issue in the medical world; is this the main cause of the observed uncertainty among the healthcare professionals?
- There exist several definitions of the term of off-label use; which one could be the most accepted and which regulatory and medical aspects should be considered?
- To what extent could the information and communication technology help to decrease the existing uncertainty among the healthcare professionals?

Chapter 4 deals with "Pharmacovigilance and Drug Monitoring". The chapter presents the history of the pharmacovigilance, defines the topic. It further presents the data collection methodology regarding the ADRs. The yellow card is being used to collect ADR related data. The yellow card is presented, and the data collection process and methodology are discussed. The chapter issues challenges facing the data collection regarding ADRs. The chapter proposes an approach to improve ADR related data collection methodology and process. The chapter has discussed a topic similar to the one discussed in the previous one. It has investigated:

Why the adherence to pharmacovigilance is so poor in the developing countries and to what extent the information and communication technology can help to increase the adherence.

Chapter 5 entitled "Novel Approach to Anticipate Emerging Infectious Diseases Spreading and Epidemics" and the Chapter 6, "Early Detection Prediction and Prevention of Noncommunicable Diseases in People at High Risks of Communicable Diseases", proposes some approaches to improve diseases monitoring and prediction.

Chapter 5 presented a novel approach to prevent disease spreading and epidemics. The recent Ebola epidemics in Afrika has shown the limitations of existing epidemiological data collection. The risk of spreading diseases within (ad-hoc) crowds and the need to pervasively screen asymptomatic individuals to protect the population against emerging infectious diseases, request permanent crowd surveillance, particularly in high-risk regions. The case of Ebola epidemic in West Africa in recent years has shown the need for pervasive screening.

Chapter 5 has proposed a concept of a novel hybrid crowdsensing where optical sensors would be used to sense bio-signals of individuals within (ad-hoc) crowd with the objectives to monitor risks of emerging infectious diseases.

The proposed hybrid crowdsensing Framework uses large-distance non-contact sensors based on Fiber Bragg Grating and participants smartphone for opportunistic crowd sensing. Emergency team members devices are also used for participatory crowdsensing.

A proof-of-concept has been performed using a drone armed with a cat s60 smartphone featuring a Forward Looking Infra-Red (FLIR) camera. The concept has the potential to improve the conventional epidemiological data collection.

The test on site helps to refine the concept and to choose the right edge (devices, sensors), and research strategies.

The proposed system has the potential to prevent the spreads of diseases, monitor diseases epidemic risks. However, there is the need to work with health authorities to implement strategies and policies on how to get people consent so that people would accept to be sensed.

The main question this chapter has investigated was how to improve the existing the methodology of epidemiological data collection, particularly in developing countries with poor ICT infrastructure.

Since diseases spreads rapidly in crowds, this chapter specially investigation how to better monitor crowds and quickly prevent disease spreading and epidemics.

Chapter 6, "Early Detection Prediction and Prevention of Noncommunicable Diseases in People at High Risks of Communicable Diseases", has discussed a novel approach of screening for diseases, that is consisting in pervasively sensing vital/bio, environmental, and social parameters of an individual in order to earlier detect any eventual disease in the person. The proposed method is called pre-screening, that happens before the traditional screening. The main objective of this methodology is to collect enough data on the health of the concerning individual for many reasons such as:

1. Overcome the limitations of the traditional screening methodology
2. Accommodate to the people modern life requirements in changing the paradigm. The healthcare systems have to follow the data producer and collect the data at any time and everywhere without disturbing the potential patient.

The chapter has presented a set of recommendations and guidelines in order to improve the traditional and common screening methodology. It has further presented a concept of an IoT-based innovative system for a so so-called pre-screening.

MAIN FINDINGS OF THE STUDY

The important finding of the different studies presented in this book is that modern information and communication technology can contribute to improve existing disease prevention, systems promotion, and detection methodologies. The provided solutions are simple and reduce the ICT infrastructure gap existing between the low- as well as middle-income and the high-income countries.

This series of studies presents the benefits of the reverse innovation, then several simple IT-based solutions that are designed, implemented, and intended for developing countries have shown the potential to be adapted for similar problems occurred in developed countries.

LIMITATION OF THE RESEARCH

The studies discussed in this book present some limitation regarding the size of the testing cohort and the duration of certain tests.

The snowball research methodology was the research approach used to build the different research cohort. This way of building cohorts gives us a few room free to really select the cohort members accordingly. It was sometimes very difficult to build the cohort in respect to the gender quota. It further was difficult to recruit the cohort on time. This aspect has led to delays in the research planning and running phases.

During the implementation, deployment, and testing of the proposed multidisciplinary remote health care services delivery system, several technical and technological issues were faced. For example, most areas are not covered by the internet although mobile communication (SMS, telephony) are possible there. Data upload and download streams are very low, less than 1 MB/sec. This fact represents a major limitation we had faced.

Additionally, the analphabetism and the lack of a voice driven scrum board had shown the limitation of certain solutions in the context of developing countries. Agile healthcare is thus limited in the framework of the designed solution if a voice driven or multimodal electronic scrum board is not provided.

Other minor limitations are not discussed here.

OPEN ISSUES AND PERSPECTIVES (FUTURE WORKS)

The studies described in this book are ongoing studies. Several systems will be improved, extended, and tested.

Following works are planed:

Chapter 2

Design and implement a multimodal scrum board in order to prevent the exclusion of illiterate traditional practitioners from taking part in the remote care services delivery system and thus practicing the agile healthcare.

Chapter 5

The challenges that will be tackled are to estimate, based on collected images, the age-range a sensing person belongs to so that the routine at the edges (sensors) could correctly pre-analyze the data and set the right alarm. For example, an adult sensed for 36.9°C would not be considered ill, though if it is a child the system would alert the operation center. Additionally, it will be important to make difference between a body of an ill individual and the body expiration of a person after having physical activities like sport, since people get hotter after sport.

Overall, the follow-up of this book will deeply present the implementation of the proposed solution as well as give some tutorial on designing and implementing telehealthcare/telemedicine solutions.

Appendix

ACRONYMS

ADR: Adverse Drug Reaction
AR: Augmented reality
CD/ID: Communicable Diseases or Infectious Diseases
CDC: Center for Diseases Control and Prevention
D2D: Device-to-Device
EMA: European Medicines Agency
FDA: Federal Drug and Foods Administration
HCP: Health Care Professionals
ICT: Information and Communication Technology
IoHT: Internet of the Health Things
IoT: Internet of Things
IT: Information Technology
M2M: Machine-to-Machine
NCD: Non-Communicable Diseases
NEPAD: New Partnership for Africa's Development
PV: Pharmacovigilance
SNIGS: Strengthening of the National Information and Health Management System
USA: The United States of America
WHO: World Health Organization

Glossary

Adverse Drug Reaction: Adverse Drug Reactions are colloquially also called side effects. The World Health Organization (WHO) defines an adverse drug reaction as a response to a drug which is noxious and unintended, and which occurs at doses normally used in man for the prophylaxis, diagnosis, or therapy of disease, or for the modification of physiological function. According to this definition, medication errors, overdose, or abuse are not considered as ADRs. Pharmaceutical entrepreneurs are obligated to collect and assess all adverse drug reactions that become known and to list these in the package leaflet. In the interest of improving therapeutic safety, healthcare professionals are also legally bound to report ADRs. BfArM (The German Federal Institute for Drugs and Medical Devices) offers online access to its database with suspected cases of adverse drug reactions. The new internet presence offers physicians and patients a further possibility for accessing in-depth information on drug risks (https://www.bfarm.de/SharedDocs/Glossareintraege/EN/A/AdverseDrugReactions-ADR.html).

Augmented Reality: Augmented reality (AR) is a technology in which a computer-generated image is superimposed onto the user's vision of the real world, giving the user additional information generated from the computer model. This technology is different from virtual reality, in which the user is immersed in a virtual world generated by the computer.

Internet of Things: Internet of Things (IoT) is a scenario in which objects, animals or people are provided with unique identifiers and the ability to transfer data over a network without requiring human-to-human or human-to-computer interaction (http://whatis.techtarget.com).

Multimorbidities: The concept of multimorbidity, developed and published in 1976 in Germany at the first time, is an extension of the concept of comorbidity, which is defined as the interaction between any disease or risk factors with one main disease with the effect of making it worse. According to World Health Organization (WHO), multimorbidity is defined as suffering of or affecting by two or more chronic health conditions.

Pervasive Healthcare: Pervasive healthcare can be defined as healthcare to anyone, anytime, and anywhere by removing locational, time and other restraints while increasing both its coverage and quality. The broad definition includes prevention, healthcare maintenance and checkups, short-term monitoring (or home healthcare monitoring), long-term monitoring (nursing home), personalized healthcare monitoring, incidence detection and management, and, emergency intervention, transportation, and treatment.

Related Readings

To continue IGI Global's long-standing tradition of advancing innovation through emerging research, please find below a compiled list of recommended IGI Global book chapters and journal articles in the areas of healthcare systems, disease prevention, and public healthcare. These related readings will provide additional information and guidance to further enrich your knowledge and assist you with your own research.

Abugabah, A., Afarraj, O., & Sansogni, L. (2015). Information Systems in Healthcare with a Special Focus on Developing Countries. In M. Sheikh, A. Mahamoud, & M. Househ (Eds.), *Transforming Public Health in Developing Nations* (pp. 309–327). Hershey, PA: IGI Global. doi:10.4018/978-1-4666-8702-8.ch014

Al Saleem, N., & Sheikh, M. (2015). Approaches to Evidence-Based Management and Decision-Making in Healthcare Organizations: Lessons for Developing Nations. In M. Sheikh, A. Mahamoud, & M. Househ (Eds.), *Transforming Public Health in Developing Nations* (pp. 69–89). Hershey, PA: IGI Global. doi:10.4018/978-1-4666-8702-8.ch003

Al-Zahrani, W., & Sheikh, M. (2015). Detection of Pre-Analytical Laboratory Testing Errors: Leads and Lessons for Patient Safety. In M. Sheikh, A. Mahamoud, & M. Househ (Eds.), *Transforming Public Health in Developing Nations* (pp. 241–263). Hershey, PA: IGI Global. doi:10.4018/978-1-4666-8702-8.ch011

Alajmi, D., Khalifa, M., Jamal, A., Zakaria, N., Alomran, S., El-Metwally, A., ... Househ, M. (2015). The Role and Use of Telemedicine by Physicians in Developing Countries: A Case Report from Saudi Arabia. In M. Sheikh, A. Mahamoud, & M. Househ (Eds.), *Transforming Public Health in Developing Nations* (pp. 293–308). Hershey, PA: IGI Global. doi:10.4018/978-1-4666-8702-8.ch013

Albawardi, N. M. (2015). Harnessing Non-Communicable Diseases: Lessons for Health Professionals in the Middle Eastern Gulf. In M. Sheikh, A. Mahamoud, & M. Househ (Eds.), *Transforming Public Health in Developing Nations* (pp. 103–120). Hershey, PA: IGI Global. doi:10.4018/978-1-4666-8702-8.ch005

Alghodaier, H., Al-Nasser, L., Al-Shehri, A., Khalifa, M., Househ, M., Alsalamah, M., & El-Metwally, A. (2015). Barriers to Accessing Healthcare Services in Developing Nations: Reflective Lessons for the Gulf Cooperation Council Countries. In M. Sheikh, A. Mahamoud, & M. Househ (Eds.), *Transforming Public Health in Developing Nations* (pp. 121–132). Hershey, PA: IGI Global. doi:10.4018/978-1-4666-8702-8.ch006

Allison, K., & Allison, C. (2017). Mental Illness, Youth, and Lessons from Residential Treatment Centers. In V. Bryan & J. Bird (Eds.), *Healthcare Community Synergism between Patients, Practitioners, and Researchers* (pp. 126–151). Hershey, PA: IGI Global. doi:10.4018/978-1-5225-0640-9.ch007

Alsalamah, S., Alsalamah, H., Gray, A. W., & Hilton, J. (2016). Information Security Threats in Patient-Centred Healthcare. In A. Moumtzoglou (Ed.), *M-Health Innovations for Patient-Centered Care* (pp. 298–318). Hershey, PA: IGI Global. doi:10.4018/978-1-4666-9861-1.ch015

Altinpulluk, H., & Kurubacak, G. (2016). MoBip Project: To Raise Awareness about Bipolar Disorder through an 3D Pop-Up Book. In A. Moumtzoglou (Ed.), *M-Health Innovations for Patient-Centered Care* (pp. 147–169). Hershey, PA: IGI Global. doi:10.4018/978-1-4666-9861-1.ch008

Amira, A., Ramzan, N., Grecos, C., Wang, Q., Casaseca-de-la-Higuera, P., Pervez, Z., ... Luo, C. (2015). A Reconfigurable Supporting Connected Health Environment for People with Chronic Diseases. In M. Tavana, A. Ghapanchi, & A. Talaei-Khoei (Eds.), *Healthcare Informatics and Analytics: Emerging Issues and Trends* (pp. 332–352). Hershey, PA: IGI Global. doi:10.4018/978-1-4666-6316-9.ch017

Anastasiou, A., Giokas, K., Koutsouri, G., & Iliopoulou, D. (2017). Intelligent Medication Adherence Monitoring System. In A. Moumtzoglou (Ed.), *Design, Development, and Integration of Reliable Electronic Healthcare Platforms* (pp. 72–85). Hershey, PA: IGI Global. doi:10.4018/978-1-5225-1724-5.ch004

Anderson, S. (2015). Publicness, Goal Ambiguity and Patient Safety: Exploring Organizational Factors in Hospital Practice. *International Journal of Privacy and Health Information Management*, *3*(2), 1–26. doi:10.4018/IJPHIM.2015070101

Anwar, J. (2015). Reproductive and Mental Health during Natural Disaster: Implications and Issues for Women in Developing Nations – A Case Example. In M. Sheikh, A. Mahamoud, & M. Househ (Eds.), *Transforming Public Health in Developing Nations* (pp. 265–291). Hershey, PA: IGI Global. doi:10.4018/978-1-4666-8702-8.ch012

Arling, P. A., Miech, E. J., & Arling, G. W. (2017). Improving Quality Improvement Collaboratives: Mixing Communication Media to Attain Multiple Measures of Success. In A. Moumtzoglou (Ed.), *Design, Development, and Integration of Reliable Electronic Healthcare Platforms* (pp. 243–254). Hershey, PA: IGI Global. doi:10.4018/978-1-5225-1724-5.ch014

Arnan, P., & Adugu, E. (2016). Individual, Institutional, and Environmental Factors Promoting Patient Retention and Dropout. In G. Graffigna (Ed.), *Promoting Patient Engagement and Participation for Effective Healthcare Reform* (pp. 41–57). Hershey, PA: IGI Global. doi:10.4018/978-1-4666-9992-2.ch003

Arshad, F., Nnamoko, N., Wilson, J., Roy, B., & Taylor, M. (2015). Improving Healthcare System Usability Without Real Users: A Semi-Parallel Design Approach. *International Journal of Healthcare Information Systems and Informatics*, *10*(1), 67–81. doi:10.4018/IJHISI.2015010104

Bahkali, S., Househ, M., Bawazir, A., Khalifa, M., & Sheikh, M. (2015). The Role of Primary Health Care in Prevention, Early Detection, and Control of Cancer. In M. Sheikh, A. Mahamoud, & M. Househ (Eds.), *Transforming Public Health in Developing Nations* (pp. 52–67). Hershey, PA: IGI Global. doi:10.4018/978-1-4666-8702-8.ch002

Barazandeh, I., & Gholamian, M. R. (2015). Knowledge Discovery and Data Mining Applications in the Healthcare Industry: A Comprehensive Study. In M. Tavana, A. Ghapanchi, & A. Talaei-Khoei (Eds.), *Healthcare Informatics and Analytics: Emerging Issues and Trends* (pp. 241–262). Hershey, PA: IGI Global. doi:10.4018/978-1-4666-6316-9.ch013

Becker, L. C. (2016). Habilitation, Healthy Agency, and Patient-Participation. In G. Graffigna (Ed.), *Promoting Patient Engagement and Participation for Effective Healthcare Reform* (pp. 1–24). Hershey, PA: IGI Global. doi:10.4018/978-1-4666-9992-2.ch001

Bello-Bravo, J., Lutomia, A. N., Songu, T., & Pittendrigh, B. R. (2017). Viral Education via Mobile Phone: Virtual International Networks and Ebola Prevention in Sierra Leone. In K. Moahi, K. Bwalya, & P. Sebina (Eds.), *Health Information Systems and the Advancement of Medical Practice in Developing Countries* (pp. 78–92). Hershey, PA: IGI Global. doi:10.4018/978-1-5225-2262-1.ch005

Binhadyan, B., & Wickramasinghe, N. (2016). An Investigation of the Role of Using IS/IT in the Delivery of Treatments for ADHD in University Students. In T. Iyamu & A. Tatnall (Eds.), *Maximizing Healthcare Delivery and Management through Technology Integration* (pp. 58–75). Hershey, PA: IGI Global. doi:10.4018/978-1-4666-9446-0.ch005

Bird, J. L. (2017). Writing Healing Narratives. In V. Bryan & J. Bird (Eds.), *Healthcare Community Synergism between Patients, Practitioners, and Researchers* (pp. 1–28). Hershey, PA: IGI Global. doi:10.4018/978-1-5225-0640-9.ch001

Blake, J., & Kerr, D. (2015). Sleep Disorder Diagnosis: An Analytical Approach. In M. Tavana, A. Ghapanchi, & A. Talaei-Khoei (Eds.), *Healthcare Informatics and Analytics: Emerging Issues and Trends* (pp. 145–164). Hershey, PA: IGI Global. doi:10.4018/978-1-4666-6316-9.ch008

Bougoulias, K., Kouris, I., Prasinos, M., Giokas, K., & Koutsouris, D. (2017). Ob/Gyn EMR Software: A Solution for Obstetricians and Gynecologists. In A. Moumtzoglou (Ed.), *Design, Development, and Integration of Reliable Electronic Healthcare Platforms* (pp. 101–111). Hershey, PA: IGI Global. doi:10.4018/978-1-5225-1724-5.ch006

Bourek, A. (2017). How to Make Your Work Really Influence Future Healthcare: From Projects through Policies to Integration into Health Systems. In A. Moumtzoglou (Ed.), *Design, Development, and Integration of Reliable Electronic Healthcare Platforms* (pp. 271–296). Hershey, PA: IGI Global. doi:10.4018/978-1-5225-1724-5.ch016

Bruscaglioni, L. (2016). No Entry: Prohibitions and Violations in Organizational Spaces across the Patient-Staff Interface in Hospital. In G. Graffigna (Ed.), *Promoting Patient Engagement and Participation for Effective Healthcare Reform* (pp. 171–191). Hershey, PA: IGI Global. doi:10.4018/978-1-4666-9992-2.ch009

Bwalya, K. J. (2017). Next Wave of Tele-Medicine: Virtual Presence of Medical Personnel. In K. Moahi, K. Bwalya, & P. Sebina (Eds.), *Health Information Systems and the Advancement of Medical Practice in Developing Countries* (pp. 168–180). Hershey, PA: IGI Global. doi:10.4018/978-1-5225-2262-1.ch010

Calogero, A., Longo, F., Nicoletti, L., & Padovano, A. (2017). Evaluating the Impacts of Lean Management Practices in Healthcare via Simulation. *International Journal of Privacy and Health Information Management*, *5*(1), 1–22. doi:10.4018/IJPHIM.2017010101

Ceruti, M., Geninatti, S., & Siliquini, R. (2015). Use and Reuse of Electronic Health Records: Building Information Systems for Improvement of Health Services. In M. Tavana, A. Ghapanchi, & A. Talaei-Khoei (Eds.), *Healthcare Informatics and Analytics: Emerging Issues and Trends* (pp. 212–226). Hershey, PA: IGI Global. doi:10.4018/978-1-4666-6316-9.ch011

Chakraborty, C., Gupta, B., & Ghosh, S. K. (2016). Mobile Telemedicine Systems for Remote Patient's Chronic Wound Monitoring. In A. Moumtzoglou (Ed.), *M-Health Innovations for Patient-Centered Care* (pp. 213–239). Hershey, PA: IGI Global. doi:10.4018/978-1-4666-9861-1.ch011

Chavez, A., & Kovarik, C. (2017). Open Source Technology for Medical Practice in Developing Countries. In K. Moahi, K. Bwalya, & P. Sebina (Eds.), *Health Information Systems and the Advancement of Medical Practice in Developing Countries* (pp. 33–59). Hershey, PA: IGI Global. doi:10.4018/978-1-5225-2262-1.ch003

Costarides, V., Zygomalas, A., Giokas, K., & Koutsouris, D. (2017). Robotics in Surgical Techniques: Present and Future Trends. In A. Moumtzoglou (Ed.), *Design, Development, and Integration of Reliable Electronic Healthcare Platforms* (pp. 86–100). Hershey, PA: IGI Global. doi:10.4018/978-1-5225-1724-5.ch005

Darcy, N., Perera, S., Stanley, G., Rumisha, S., Assenga, K., Polycarp, F., ... Teesdale, S. (2017). Case Study: The Tanzania Health Facility Registry. In K. Moahi, K. Bwalya, & P. Sebina (Eds.), *Health Information Systems and the Advancement of Medical Practice in Developing Countries* (pp. 208–236). Hershey, PA: IGI Global. doi:10.4018/978-1-5225-2262-1.ch013

Donato, S., & Bertoni, A. (2016). A Relational Perspective on Patient Engagement: Suggestions from Couple-Based Research and Intervention. In G. Graffigna (Ed.), *Promoting Patient Engagement and Participation for Effective Healthcare Reform* (pp. 83–106). Hershey, PA: IGI Global. doi:10.4018/978-1-4666-9992-2.ch005

Dotson, E., Hibbler, D. K., & Scott, L. (2017). Culture of Learning Cities: Connecting Leisure and Health for Lifelong Learning Communities. In V. Bryan & J. Bird (Eds.), *Healthcare Community Synergism between Patients, Practitioners, and Researchers* (pp. 152–175). Hershey, PA: IGI Global. doi:10.4018/978-1-5225-0640-9.ch008

Drowos, J. L., & Wood, S. K. (2017). Preparing Future Physicians to Adapt to the Changing Health Care System: Promoting Humanism through Curricular Design. In V. Bryan & J. Bird (Eds.), *Healthcare Community Synergism between Patients, Practitioners, and Researchers* (pp. 106–125). Hershey, PA: IGI Global. doi:10.4018/978-1-5225-0640-9.ch006

Dumbrell, D., & Steele, R. (2015). Privacy Perceptions of Older Adults when Using Social Media Technologies. In M. Tavana, A. Ghapanchi, & A. Talaei-Khoei (Eds.), *Healthcare Informatics and Analytics: Emerging Issues and Trends* (pp. 67–82). Hershey, PA: IGI Global. doi:10.4018/978-1-4666-6316-9.ch004

Dumbrell, D., & Steele, R. (2015). Twitter and Its Role in Health Information Dissemination: Analysis of the Micro-Blog Posts of Health-Related Organisations. In M. Tavana, A. Ghapanchi, & A. Talaei-Khoei (Eds.), *Healthcare Informatics and Analytics: Emerging Issues and Trends* (pp. 1–17). Hershey, PA: IGI Global. doi:10.4018/978-1-4666-6316-9.ch001

Edoh, T. O., Pawar, P. A., Brügge, B., & Teege, G. (2016). A Multidisciplinary Remote Healthcare Delivery System to Increase Health Care Access, Pathology Screening, and Treatment in Developing Countries: The Case of Benin. *International Journal of Healthcare Information Systems and Informatics*, *11*(4), 1–31. doi:10.4018/IJHISI.2016100101

Ellington, L., & Bryan, V. C. (2017). Incognito: The Neuroscience of Grief and Grieving. In V. Bryan & J. Bird (Eds.), *Healthcare Community Synergism between Patients, Practitioners, and Researchers* (pp. 272–291). Hershey, PA: IGI Global. doi:10.4018/978-1-5225-0640-9.ch012

Estrella, P., & Tsourakis, N. (2017). Migrating from ISO/IEC 9126 to SQUARE: A Case Study on the Evaluation of Medical Speech Translation Systems. In A. Moumtzoglou (Ed.), *Design, Development, and Integration of Reliable Electronic Healthcare Platforms* (pp. 160–178). Hershey, PA: IGI Global. doi:10.4018/978-1-5225-1724-5.ch010

Faruq, Q. O. (2016). General Practitioners' Adoption and Use of ICT. In T. Iyamu & A. Tatnall (Eds.), *Maximizing Healthcare Delivery and Management through Technology Integration* (pp. 152–168). Hershey, PA: IGI Global. doi:10.4018/978-1-4666-9446-0.ch010

Fatima-Zohra, Y., Djamila, H., & Omar, B. (2015). A Surveillance and Spatiotemporal Visualization Model for Infectious Diseases using Social Network. *International Journal of Decision Support System Technology*, *7*(4), 1–19. doi:10.4018/IJDSST.2015100101

Gaspar, R., Domingos, S., Diniz, A. M., & Falanga, R. (2016). Barriers to and Facilitators of Older Adult's Adherence to Health Recommendations: Towards an Engaging Two-way Health Communication. In G. Graffigna (Ed.), *Promoting Patient Engagement and Participation for Effective Healthcare Reform* (pp. 58–82). Hershey, PA: IGI Global. doi:10.4018/978-1-4666-9992-2.ch004

Giokas, K., Costarides, V., & Koutsouris, D. (2016). Integrated Platform for the Lifestyle Change and Holistic Approach to Personalized Prevention and Self-Management of Patients with High Blood Pressure. In A. Moumtzoglou (Ed.), *M-Health Innovations for Patient-Centered Care* (pp. 72–90). Hershey, PA: IGI Global. doi:10.4018/978-1-4666-9861-1.ch004

Giokas, K., Katrakazas, P., & Koutsouris, D. (2016). A Collaborative m-Health Platform for Evidence-Based Self-Management and Detection of Chronic Multimorbidity Development and Progression. In A. Moumtzoglou (Ed.), *M-Health Innovations for Patient-Centered Care* (pp. 52–71). Hershey, PA: IGI Global. doi:10.4018/978-1-4666-9861-1.ch003

Gorli, M., Liberati, E. G., Galuppo, L., & Scaratti, G. (2016). The Patient Centered Organizational Model in Italian Hospitals: Practical Challenges for Patient Engagement. In G. Graffigna (Ed.), *Promoting Patient Engagement and Participation for Effective Healthcare Reform* (pp. 152–170). Hershey, PA: IGI Global. doi:10.4018/978-1-4666-9992-2.ch008

Graffigna, G., & Barello, S. (2016). The Value of Measuring Patient Engagement in Healthcare: New Frontiers for Healthcare Quality. In G. Graffigna (Ed.), *Promoting Patient Engagement and Participation for Effective Healthcare Reform* (pp. 192–214). Hershey, PA: IGI Global. doi:10.4018/978-1-4666-9992-2.ch010

Gure, S. M. (2015). Nomadic Clinics as Innovative Concept that Transforms Health Care Services in Mobile Population: Case Example from North Eastern Kenya. In M. Sheikh, A. Mahamoud, & M. Househ (Eds.), *Transforming Public Health in Developing Nations* (pp. 90–102). Hershey, PA: IGI Global. doi:10.4018/978-1-4666-8702-8.ch004

Gürsel, G. (2015). Perceived Importance of User Expectations from Healthcare Information Systems. In M. Tavana, A. Ghapanchi, & A. Talaei-Khoei (Eds.), *Healthcare Informatics and Analytics: Emerging Issues and Trends* (pp. 84–95). Hershey, PA: IGI Global. doi:10.4018/978-1-4666-6316-9.ch005

Haider, M., Makrinos, T., & Sarkar, M. (2015). Improving the Effects of Global Health Initiatives through FOMENT: An Enhancement to the Diffusion Process. In M. Sheikh, A. Mahamoud, & M. Househ (Eds.), *Transforming Public Health in Developing Nations* (pp. 134–152). Hershey, PA: IGI Global. doi:10.4018/978-1-4666-8702-8.ch007

Hamunyela, S., & Iyamu, T. (2016). Healthcare Services for Nomadics through a Mobile Framework. In T. Iyamu & A. Tatnall (Eds.), *Maximizing Healthcare Delivery and Management through Technology Integration* (pp. 46–57). Hershey, PA: IGI Global. doi:10.4018/978-1-4666-9446-0.ch004

Han-Lin, C., Yang, A. W., Pittayachawan, S., & Wickramasinghe, N. (2016). An Analysis on the Utilisation of Health Information Technology to Support Clinical Operation of Chinese Medicine. In T. Iyamu & A. Tatnall (Eds.), *Maximizing Healthcare Delivery and Management through Technology Integration* (pp. 113–132). Hershey, PA: IGI Global. doi:10.4018/978-1-4666-9446-0.ch008

Handayani, P. W., Sandhyaduhita, P. I., Hidayanto, A. N., Pinem, A. A., Fajrina, H. R., Junus, K. M., ... Ayuningtyas, D. (2016). Integrated Hospital Information System Architecture Design in Indonesia. In T. Iyamu & A. Tatnall (Eds.), *Maximizing Healthcare Delivery and Management through Technology Integration* (pp. 207–236). Hershey, PA: IGI Global. doi:10.4018/978-1-4666-9446-0.ch013

Hartman, A., & Brown, S. (2017). Synergism through Therapeutic Visual Arts. In V. Bryan & J. Bird (Eds.), *Healthcare Community Synergism between Patients, Practitioners, and Researchers* (pp. 29–48). Hershey, PA: IGI Global. doi:10.4018/978-1-5225-0640-9.ch002

Horner, V., & Coleman, A. (2016). Strengthening Implementation of Guidelines at Primary Health Care. In T. Iyamu & A. Tatnall (Eds.), *Maximizing Healthcare Delivery and Management through Technology Integration* (pp. 133–151). Hershey, PA: IGI Global. doi:10.4018/978-1-4666-9446-0.ch009

Høstgaard, A. M. (2016). Constructive eHealth Evaluation: Involving the End-User. In A. Dwivedi (Ed.), *Reshaping Medical Practice and Care with Health Information Systems* (pp. 44–86). Hershey, PA: IGI Global. doi:10.4018/978-1-4666-9870-3.ch003

Hume, M., Hume, C., Johnston, P., Soar, J., & Whitty, J. (2015). The Role of Knowledge Management (KM) in Aged Care Informatics: Crafting the Knowledge Organization. In M. Tavana, A. Ghapanchi, & A. Talaei-Khoei (Eds.), *Healthcare Informatics and Analytics: Emerging Issues and Trends* (pp. 284–302). Hershey, PA: IGI Global. doi:10.4018/978-1-4666-6316-9.ch015

Iltchev, P., Śliwczyński, A., Szynkiewicz, P., & Marczak, M. (2016). Mobile Health Applications Assisting Patients with Chronic Diseases: Examples from Asthma Care. In A. Moumtzoglou (Ed.), *M-Health Innovations for Patient-Centered Care* (pp. 170–196). Hershey, PA: IGI Global. doi:10.4018/978-1-4666-9861-1.ch009

Iyamu, T., & Mkhomazi, S. S. (2016). Managing Knowledge towards Enabling Healthcare Service Delivery. In T. Iyamu & A. Tatnall (Eds.), *Maximizing Healthcare Delivery and Management through Technology Integration* (pp. 15–26). Hershey, PA: IGI Global. doi:10.4018/978-1-4666-9446-0.ch002

Jabri, F. F. (2015). Antimicrobial Consumption and Multidrug Resistant Organisms in Intensive Care Units: Lessons from Saudi Arabia. In M. Sheikh, A. Mahamoud, & M. Househ (Eds.), *Transforming Public Health in Developing Nations* (pp. 209–240). Hershey, PA: IGI Global. doi:10.4018/978-1-4666-8702-8.ch010

Kaissi, A. (2015). *Flipping Health Care through Retail Clinics and Convenient Care Models* (pp. 1–306). Hershey, PA: IGI Global. doi:10.4018/978-1-4666-6355-8

Karon, R. (2016). Utilisation of Health Information Systems for Service Delivery in the Namibian Environment. In T. Iyamu & A. Tatnall (Eds.), *Maximizing Healthcare Delivery and Management through Technology Integration* (pp. 169–183). Hershey, PA: IGI Global. doi:10.4018/978-1-4666-9446-0.ch011

Kasemsap, K. (2017). Telemedicine and Electronic Health: Issues and Implications in Developing Countries. In K. Moahi, K. Bwalya, & P. Sebina (Eds.), *Health Information Systems and the Advancement of Medical Practice in Developing Countries* (pp. 149–167). Hershey, PA: IGI Global. doi:10.4018/978-1-5225-2262-1.ch009

Katuu, S. (2017). Health Information Systems, eHealth Strategy, and the Management of Health Records: The Quest to Transform South Africa's Public Health Sector. In K. Moahi, K. Bwalya, & P. Sebina (Eds.), *Health Information Systems and the Advancement of Medical Practice in Developing Countries* (pp. 237–261). Hershey, PA: IGI Global. doi:10.4018/978-1-5225-2262-1.ch014

Kazandjian, V. A. (2017). We Can Trust without Data, But We Are Accountable Only through Measurement. In A. Moumtzoglou (Ed.), *Design, Development, and Integration of Reliable Electronic Healthcare Platforms* (pp. 255–270). Hershey, PA: IGI Global. doi:10.4018/978-1-5225-1724-5.ch015

Keikhosrokiani, P., Mustaffa, N., Zakaria, N., & Baharudin, A. S. (2015). User Behavioral Intention toward Using Mobile Healthcare System. In M. Tavana, A. Ghapanchi, & A. Talaei-Khoei (Eds.), *Healthcare Informatics and Analytics: Emerging Issues and Trends* (pp. 128–143). Hershey, PA: IGI Global. doi:10.4018/978-1-4666-6316-9.ch007

Kenski, C. M., & Falcone, J. N. (2017). Humane Education: A Call to Action for Elementary School Students. In V. Bryan & J. Bird (Eds.), *Healthcare Community Synergism between Patients, Practitioners, and Researchers* (pp. 88–105). Hershey, PA: IGI Global. doi:10.4018/978-1-5225-0640-9.ch005

Khumalo, N. B. (2017). "It Has Been Quite a Journey": Experiences and Evolution in Health Information Systems in Zimbabwe. In K. Moahi, K. Bwalya, & P. Sebina (Eds.), *Health Information Systems and the Advancement of Medical Practice in Developing Countries* (pp. 193–207). Hershey, PA: IGI Global. doi:10.4018/978-1-5225-2262-1.ch012

King, B. M., Barry, C. D., Bamdas, J. A., Bronner, K., & Edwards, K. A. (2017). HeartMath®: A University Initiative. In V. Bryan & J. Bird (Eds.), *Healthcare Community Synergism between Patients, Practitioners, and Researchers* (pp. 49–64). Hershey, PA: IGI Global. doi:10.4018/978-1-5225-0640-9.ch003

Kipanyula, M. J., Sanga, C. A., Geofrey, A. M., & Fue, K. G. (2016). On Piloting Web-Based Rabies Surveillance System for Humans and Animals: Web-Based Rabies Surveillance System. In T. Iyamu & A. Tatnall (Eds.), *Maximizing Healthcare Delivery and Management through Technology Integration* (pp. 305–323). Hershey, PA: IGI Global. doi:10.4018/978-1-4666-9446-0.ch017

Koumaditis, K., & Themistocleous, M. (2016). SOA Governance in Healthcare: Beyond Early Ideas to a Structured Framework. In A. Dwivedi (Ed.), *Reshaping Medical Practice and Care with Health Information Systems* (pp. 266–286). Hershey, PA: IGI Global. doi:10.4018/978-1-4666-9870-3.ch009

Koumpouros, Y., & Georgoulas, A. (2016). mHealth R&D Activities in Europe. In A. Moumtzoglou (Ed.), M-Health Innovations for Patient-Centered Care (pp. 20-51). Hershey, PA: IGI Global. doi:10.4018/978-1-4666-9861-1.ch002

Kuusisto-Niemi, S., Saranto, K., & Rissanen, S. (2015). Informatics in Social Services: Research, Developments, and Outcomes from the Finnish Perspective. In M. Tavana, A. Ghapanchi, & A. Talaei-Khoei (Eds.), *Healthcare Informatics and Analytics: Emerging Issues and Trends* (pp. 18–43). Hershey, PA: IGI Global. doi:10.4018/978-1-4666-6316-9.ch002

Lembachar, I., Diouny, S., Serhier, Z., & Othmani, M. B. (2015). The E-Learning Experience in Medical School of Casablanca. In M. Tavana, A. Ghapanchi, & A. Talaei-Khoei (Eds.), *Healthcare Informatics and Analytics: Emerging Issues and Trends* (pp. 227–240). Hershey, PA: IGI Global. doi:10.4018/978-1-4666-6316-9.ch012

Lewis, L. (2015). Using Narrative with Avatars and Robots to Enhance Elder Care. In M. Tavana, A. Ghapanchi, & A. Talaei-Khoei (Eds.), *Healthcare Informatics and Analytics: Emerging Issues and Trends* (pp. 264–283). Hershey, PA: IGI Global. doi:10.4018/978-1-4666-6316-9.ch014

Lidia, B., Federica, G., & Maria, V. E. (2016). The Patient-Centered Medicine as the Theoretical Framework for Patient Engagement. In G. Graffigna (Ed.), *Promoting Patient Engagement and Participation for Effective Healthcare Reform* (pp. 25–39). Hershey, PA: IGI Global. doi:10.4018/978-1-4666-9992-2.ch002

Lin, C., Jalleh, G., & Huang, Y. (2016). Evaluating and Managing Electronic Commerce and Outsourcing Projects in Hospitals. In A. Dwivedi (Ed.), *Reshaping Medical Practice and Care with Health Information Systems* (pp. 132–172). Hershey, PA: IGI Global. doi:10.4018/978-1-4666-9870-3.ch005

Lindberg-Repo, K., & Dube, A. (2015). Customer Value Dimensions in E-Healthcare Services: Lessons from Finland. *International Journal of E-Services and Mobile Applications*, *7*(4), 17–29. doi:10.4018/IJESMA.2015100102

Magnavita, N. (2016). Engagement in Health and Safety at the Workplace: A New Role for the Occupational Health Physician. In G. Graffigna (Ed.), *Promoting Patient Engagement and Participation for Effective Healthcare Reform* (pp. 265–289). Hershey, PA: IGI Global. doi:10.4018/978-1-4666-9992-2.ch013

Malanga, D. F. (2017). Implementation of Mobile Health Initiatives in Malawi: Current Status, Issues, and Challenges. In K. Moahi, K. Bwalya, & P. Sebina (Eds.), *Health Information Systems and the Advancement of Medical Practice in Developing Countries* (pp. 115–128). Hershey, PA: IGI Global. doi:10.4018/978-1-5225-2262-1.ch007

Manzoor, A. (2016). RFID Applications in Healthcare-State-of-the-Art and Future Trends. In T. Iyamu & A. Tatnall (Eds.), *Maximizing Healthcare Delivery and Management through Technology Integration* (pp. 184–206). Hershey, PA: IGI Global. doi:10.4018/978-1-4666-9446-0.ch012

Mazzoni, D., & Alberici, A. I. (2016). Why do Patients Protest? Collective Action Processes in People with Chronic Illnesses: A Psychosocial Perspective. In G. Graffigna (Ed.), *Promoting Patient Engagement and Participation for Effective Healthcare Reform* (pp. 128–150). Hershey, PA: IGI Global. doi:10.4018/978-1-4666-9992-2.ch007

McCormack, J., Rawstorne, P., & Sheikh, M. (2015). Seeking Solutions to the Challenges in Health Services in Developing Nations: Primary Health Care Revisited. In M. Sheikh, A. Mahamoud, & M. Househ (Eds.), *Transforming Public Health in Developing Nations* (pp. 1–51). Hershey, PA: IGI Global. doi:10.4018/978-1-4666-8702-8.ch001

Mehta, P. (2017). Framework of Indian Healthcare System and its Challenges: An Insight. In V. Bryan & J. Bird (Eds.), *Healthcare Community Synergism between Patients, Practitioners, and Researchers* (pp. 247–271). Hershey, PA: IGI Global. doi:10.4018/978-1-5225-0640-9.ch011

Mendes, D., Lopes, M., Romão, A., & Rodrigues, I. P. (2017). Healthcare Computer Reasoning Addressing Chronically Ill Societies Using IoT: Deep Learning AI to the Rescue of Home-Based Healthcare. In A. Moumtzoglou (Ed.), *Design, Development, and Integration of Reliable Electronic Healthcare Platforms* (pp. 32–48). Hershey, PA: IGI Global. doi:10.4018/978-1-5225-1724-5.ch002

Metelmann, B., & Metelmann, C. (2016). M-Health in Prehospital Emergency Medicine: Experiences from the EU funded Project LiveCity. In A. Moumtzoglou (Ed.), *M-Health Innovations for Patient-Centered Care* (pp. 197–212). Hershey, PA: IGI Global. doi:10.4018/978-1-4666-9861-1.ch010

Miglioretti, M., Mariani, F., & Vecchio, L. (2016). Could Patient Engagement Promote a Health System Free From Malpractice Litigation Risk? In G. Graffigna (Ed.), *Promoting Patient Engagement and Participation for Effective Healthcare Reform* (pp. 240–264). Hershey, PA: IGI Global. doi:10.4018/978-1-4666-9992-2.ch012

Misra, R. (2016). The Benefits and Challenges of Using Mobile-Based Tools in Self-Management and Care. In A. Dwivedi (Ed.), *Reshaping Medical Practice and Care with Health Information Systems* (pp. 1–13). Hershey, PA: IGI Global. doi:10.4018/978-1-4666-9870-3.ch001

Moahi, K. H. (2017). Big Data and Healthcare: Implications for Medical and Health Care in Low Resource Countries. In K. Moahi, K. Bwalya, & P. Sebina (Eds.), *Health Information Systems and the Advancement of Medical Practice in Developing Countries* (pp. 14–32). Hershey, PA: IGI Global. doi:10.4018/978-1-5225-2262-1.ch002

Moahi, K. H., & Bwalya, K. J. (2017). Knowledge Sharing for Healthcare and Medicine in Developing Countries: Opportunities, Issues, and Experiences. In K. Moahi, K. Bwalya, & P. Sebina (Eds.), *Health Information Systems and the Advancement of Medical Practice in Developing Countries* (pp. 60–77). Hershey, PA: IGI Global. doi:10.4018/978-1-5225-2262-1.ch004

Moghimi, H., Wickramasinghe, N., & Schaffer, J. L. (2016). Intelligent Risk Detection in Healthcare Contexts of Hip and Knee Athroplasty and Paediatric Congenital Heart Disease. In T. Iyamu & A. Tatnall (Eds.), *Maximizing Healthcare Delivery and Management through Technology Integration* (pp. 1–14). Hershey, PA: IGI Global. doi:10.4018/978-1-4666-9446-0.ch001

Moumtzoglou, A. (2017). Digital Medicine: The Quality Standpoint. In A. Moumtzoglou (Ed.), *Design, Development, and Integration of Reliable Electronic Healthcare Platforms* (pp. 179–195). Hershey, PA: IGI Global. doi:10.4018/978-1-5225-1724-5.ch011

Moumtzoglou, A., & Pouliakis, A. (2017). Population Health Management and Cervical Cancer Screening Programs: Roadmap, Design, and Implementation of a Supporting IT System. In A. Moumtzoglou (Ed.), *Design, Development, and Integration of Reliable Electronic Healthcare Platforms* (pp. 1–31). Hershey, PA: IGI Global. doi:10.4018/978-1-5225-1724-5.ch001

Moumtzoglou, A. S. (2016). Tailored M-Health Communication in Patient-Centered Care. In A. Moumtzoglou (Ed.), *M-Health Innovations for Patient-Centered Care* (pp. 319–340). Hershey, PA: IGI Global. doi:10.4018/978-1-4666-9861-1.ch016

Moumtzoglou, A. S. (2016). The Nexus of M-Health and Self-Efficacy. In A. Moumtzoglou (Ed.), *M-Health Innovations for Patient-Centered Care* (pp. 341–365). Hershey, PA: IGI Global. doi:10.4018/978-1-4666-9861-1.ch017

Ndlovu, K., Mauco, K. L., & Littman-Quinn, R. (2017). Telemedicine in Low Resource Settings: A Case for Botswana. In K. Moahi, K. Bwalya, & P. Sebina (Eds.), *Health Information Systems and the Advancement of Medical Practice in Developing Countries* (pp. 129–148). Hershey, PA: IGI Global. doi:10.4018/978-1-5225-2262-1.ch008

Nemutanzhela, P., & Iyamu, T. (2016). Introducing Mobile Device for Health Services: The Semantics of Language Translation. In T. Iyamu & A. Tatnall (Eds.), *Maximizing Healthcare Delivery and Management through Technology Integration* (pp. 101–112). Hershey, PA: IGI Global. doi:10.4018/978-1-4666-9446-0.ch007

Nishimura, S., & Scott, D. J. (2016). Waseda University's E-School: 10 Years of E-Education in Japan. In A. Dwivedi (Ed.), *Reshaping Medical Practice and Care with Health Information Systems* (pp. 173–204). Hershey, PA: IGI Global. doi:10.4018/978-1-4666-9870-3.ch006

Noordin, M. F., Arshad, A., & Othman, R. (2017). KIIPF - An Integrated Inter-Operable Knowledge Management Process Framework for Healthcare: Implementation in Pakistani Healthcare Industry. *Journal of Cases on Information Technology*, *19*(3), 24–41. doi:10.4018/JCIT.2017070103

Ola, O., Buchel, O., & Sedig, K. (2015). Interactive Visualizations as "Decision Support Tools" in Developing Nations: The Case of Vector-Borne Diseases. In M. Sheikh, A. Mahamoud, & M. Househ (Eds.), *Transforming Public Health in Developing Nations* (pp. 328–352). Hershey, PA: IGI Global. doi:10.4018/978-1-4666-8702-8.ch015

Osman, A. D., Robinson, P., Lin, V., Jackson, D., & Mwanthi, M. (2015). Water and Sanitation: A Case Study for Policy Implication to Reaching Global Development Goals in Developing Nations. In M. Sheikh, A. Mahamoud, & M. Househ (Eds.), *Transforming Public Health in Developing Nations* (pp. 153–171). Hershey, PA: IGI Global. doi:10.4018/978-1-4666-8702-8.ch008

Patil, H. G., Babu, A. N., & Ramkumar, P. S. (2016). Non-Invasive Data Acquisition and Measurement in Bio-Medical Technology: An Overview. In T. Iyamu & A. Tatnall (Eds.), *Maximizing Healthcare Delivery and Management through Technology Integration* (pp. 27–45). Hershey, PA: IGI Global. doi:10.4018/978-1-4666-9446-0.ch003

Pedell, S., Lopez-Lorca, A. A., Miller, T., & Sterling, L. (2015). Don't Leave Me Untouched: Considering Emotions in Personal Alarm Use and Development. In M. Tavana, A. Ghapanchi, & A. Talaei-Khoei (Eds.), *Healthcare Informatics and Analytics: Emerging Issues and Trends* (pp. 96–127). Hershey, PA: IGI Global. doi:10.4018/978-1-4666-6316-9.ch006

Piovesan, L., Molino, G., & Terenziani, P. (2015). Supporting Physicians in the Detection of the Interactions between Treatments of Co-Morbid Patients. In M. Tavana, A. Ghapanchi, & A. Talaei-Khoei (Eds.), *Healthcare Informatics and Analytics: Emerging Issues and Trends* (pp. 165–193). Hershey, PA: IGI Global. doi:10.4018/978-1-4666-6316-9.ch009

Pomares-Quimbaya, A., González, R. A., Sierra, A., Daza, J. C., Muñoz, O., García, A., ... Bohórquez, W. R. (2017). ICT for Enabling the Quality Evaluation of Health Care Services: A Case Study in a General Hospital. In A. Moumtzoglou (Ed.), *Design, Development, and Integration of Reliable Electronic Healthcare Platforms* (pp. 196–210). Hershey, PA: IGI Global. doi:10.4018/978-1-5225-1724-5.ch012

Pouliakis, A., Archondakis, S., Margari, N., & Karakitsos, P. (2016). From Telecytology to Mobile Cytopathology: Past, Present, and Future. In A. Moumtzoglou (Ed.), *M-Health Innovations for Patient-Centered Care* (pp. 240–261). Hershey, PA: IGI Global. doi:10.4018/978-1-4666-9861-1.ch012

Provenzi, L., Borgatti, R., & Montirosso, R. (2016). The Light Side of Preterm Behavioral Epigenetics: An Epigenetic Perspective on Caregiver Engagement. In G. Graffigna (Ed.), *Promoting Patient Engagement and Participation for Effective Healthcare Reform* (pp. 107–127). Hershey, PA: IGI Global. doi:10.4018/978-1-4666-9992-2.ch006

Rahimi, A., Liaw, S., Ray, P. K., Taggart, J., & Yu, H. (2015). Ontology for Data Quality and Chronic Disease Management: A Literature Review. In M. Tavana, A. Ghapanchi, & A. Talaei-Khoei (Eds.), *Healthcare Informatics and Analytics: Emerging Issues and Trends* (pp. 303–331). Hershey, PA: IGI Global. doi:10.4018/978-1-4666-6316-9.ch016

Rodrigues, P. M., Freitas, D., Teixeira, J. P., Alves, D., & Garrett, C. (2017). Early Detection of Electroencephalogram Temporal Events in Alzheimer's Disease. In A. Moumtzoglou (Ed.), *Design, Development, and Integration of Reliable Electronic Healthcare Platforms* (pp. 112–131). Hershey, PA: IGI Global. doi:10.4018/978-1-5225-1724-5.ch007

Ross, D. B., Exposito, J. A., & Kennedy, T. (2017). Stress and Its Relationship to Leadership and a Healthy Workplace Culture. In V. Bryan & J. Bird (Eds.), *Healthcare Community Synergism between Patients, Practitioners, and Researchers* (pp. 213–246). Hershey, PA: IGI Global. doi:10.4018/978-1-5225-0640-9.ch010

Sagahyroon, A. (2016). mHealth: Sleeping Disorders Diagnosis. In A. Moumtzoglou (Ed.), M-Health Innovations for Patient-Centered Care (pp. 115-125). Hershey, PA: IGI Global. doi:10.4018/978-1-4666-9861-1.ch006

Sam, S. (2017). Mobile Phones and Expanding Human Capabilities in Plural Health Systems. In K. Moahi, K. Bwalya, & P. Sebina (Eds.), *Health Information Systems and the Advancement of Medical Practice in Developing Countries* (pp. 93–114). Hershey, PA: IGI Global. doi:10.4018/978-1-5225-2262-1.ch006

Sarkar, B. K. (2017). Big Data and Healthcare Data: A Survey. *International Journal of Knowledge-Based Organizations, 7*(4), 50–77. doi:10.4018/IJKBO.2017100104

Sarwar, K., & Shah, M. A. (2015). Cost Effective Design of an RFID Based Healthcare Service System. *International Journal of Privacy and Health Information Management, 3*(2), 51–65. doi:10.4018/IJPHIM.2015070103

Sebina, P. M., & Grand, B. (2017). Records Management and Open Data in Healthcare Provision in Africa: Reflections and Lessons for Botswana. In K. Moahi, K. Bwalya, & P. Sebina (Eds.), *Health Information Systems and the Advancement of Medical Practice in Developing Countries* (pp. 1–13). Hershey, PA: IGI Global. doi:10.4018/978-1-5225-2262-1.ch001

Shaanika, I. N. (2016). Human Interaction in the Use of Health Information Systems: A Case of a Developing Country. In T. Iyamu & A. Tatnall (Eds.), *Maximizing Healthcare Delivery and Management through Technology Integration* (pp. 257–269). Hershey, PA: IGI Global. doi:10.4018/978-1-4666-9446-0.ch015

Shi, J., Erdem, E., & Liu, H. (2016). Expanding Role of Telephone Systems in Healthcare: Developments and Opportunities. In A. Dwivedi (Ed.), *Reshaping Medical Practice and Care with Health Information Systems* (pp. 87–131). Hershey, PA: IGI Global. doi:10.4018/978-1-4666-9870-3.ch004

Sourial, M., Bamdas, J. A., Constanzo, A., & Ishak, M. E. (2017). A Need for Greater Collaboration: Initiatives to Improve Transitions of Care. In V. Bryan & J. Bird (Eds.), *Healthcare Community Synergism between Patients, Practitioners, and Researchers* (pp. 65–87). Hershey, PA: IGI Global. doi:10.4018/978-1-5225-0640-9.ch004

Spinelli, R., & Benevolo, C. (2016). From Healthcare Services to E-Health Applications: A Delivery System-Based Taxonomy. In A. Dwivedi (Ed.), *Reshaping Medical Practice and Care with Health Information Systems* (pp. 205–245). Hershey, PA: IGI Global. doi:10.4018/978-1-4666-9870-3.ch007

Srinivasan, U., & Uddin, S. (2015). A Social Network Framework to Explore Healthcare Collaboration. In M. Tavana, A. Ghapanchi, & A. Talaei-Khoei (Eds.), *Healthcare Informatics and Analytics: Emerging Issues and Trends* (pp. 44–66). Hershey, PA: IGI Global. doi:10.4018/978-1-4666-6316-9.ch003

Stavros, A., Vavoulidis, E., & Nasioutziki, M. (2016). The Use of Mobile Health Applications for Quality Control and Accreditational Purposes in a Cytopathology Laboratory. In A. Moumtzoglou (Ed.), *M-Health Innovations for Patient-Centered Care* (pp. 262–283). Hershey, PA: IGI Global. doi:10.4018/978-1-4666-9861-1.ch013

Tamposis, I., Pouliakis, A., Fezoulidis, I., & Karakitsos, P. (2016). Mobile Platforms Supporting Health Professionals: Need, Technical Requirements, and Applications. In A. Moumtzoglou (Ed.), *M-Health Innovations for Patient-Centered Care* (pp. 91–114). Hershey, PA: IGI Global. doi:10.4018/978-1-4666-9861-1.ch005

Tanzariello, M., Bucci, S., Ricciardi, W., & Giulio de Belvis, A. (2016). Accountability and Public Reporting: Publication of Performance to Improve Quality. In G. Graffigna (Ed.), *Promoting Patient Engagement and Participation for Effective Healthcare Reform* (pp. 215–239). Hershey, PA: IGI Global. doi:10.4018/978-1-4666-9992-2.ch011

Taweel, A. (2016). Semantic Interoperability-Enabled Architecture for Connected Health Services. In A. Dwivedi (Ed.), *Reshaping Medical Practice and Care with Health Information Systems* (pp. 246–265). Hershey, PA: IGI Global. doi:10.4018/978-1-4666-9870-3.ch008

Teixeira, J. P., Fernandes, M. G., & Costa, R. A. (2017). Automatic Determination of Pauses in Speech for Classification of Stuttering Disorder. In A. Moumtzoglou (Ed.), *Design, Development, and Integration of Reliable Electronic Healthcare Platforms* (pp. 132–149). Hershey, PA: IGI Global. doi:10.4018/978-1-5225-1724-5.ch008

Tiago, M. T., Tiago, F., Amaral, F. E., & Silva, S. (2016). Healthy 3.0: Healthcare Digital Dimensions. In A. Dwivedi (Ed.), *Reshaping Medical Practice and Care with Health Information Systems* (pp. 287–322). Hershey, PA: IGI Global. doi:10.4018/978-1-4666-9870-3.ch010

Tshiamo, W. B., Kgositau, M., & Magowe, M. (2017). Use of Information and Communication Technology by Health Care Providers for Continuing Professional Development in Botswana. In K. Moahi, K. Bwalya, & P. Sebina (Eds.), *Health Information Systems and the Advancement of Medical Practice in Developing Countries* (pp. 181–192). Hershey, PA: IGI Global. doi:10.4018/978-1-5225-2262-1.ch011

Unnithan, C., & Fraunholz, B. (2015). Radio Frequency Identification Technology as an Analytical Lens and Solution in Hospitals: A Novel Approach in BPR/BPM. In M. Tavana, A. Ghapanchi, & A. Talaei-Khoei (Eds.), *Healthcare Informatics and Analytics: Emerging Issues and Trends* (pp. 194–211). Hershey, PA: IGI Global. doi:10.4018/978-1-4666-6316-9.ch010

Unnithan, C., & Tatnall, A. (2016). Radio Frequency Identification Technology in an Australian Regional Hospital: An Innovation Translation Experience with ANT. In T. Iyamu & A. Tatnall (Eds.), *Maximizing Healthcare Delivery and Management through Technology Integration* (pp. 76–100). Hershey, PA: IGI Global. doi:10.4018/978-1-4666-9446-0.ch006

Unwin, D. W., Sanzogni, L., & Sandhu, K. (2017). Developing and Measuring the Business Case for Health Information Technology. In K. Moahi, K. Bwalya, & P. Sebina (Eds.), *Health Information Systems and the Advancement of Medical Practice in Developing Countries* (pp. 262–290). Hershey, PA: IGI Global. doi:10.4018/978-1-5225-2262-1.ch015

Usher, W. (2017). E-Health: Modern Communication Technology Platforms for Accessing Health Information. In A. Moumtzoglou (Ed.), *Design, Development, and Integration of Reliable Electronic Healthcare Platforms* (pp. 49–71). Hershey, PA: IGI Global. doi:10.4018/978-1-5225-1724-5.ch003

Vezyridis, P., Timmons, S., & Wharrad, H. (2016). Lessons Learned from the Implementation of an Emergency Department Information System. In T. Iyamu & A. Tatnall (Eds.), *Maximizing Healthcare Delivery and Management through Technology Integration* (pp. 237–256). Hershey, PA: IGI Global. doi:10.4018/978-1-4666-9446-0.ch014

Vlachopapadopoulou, E., & Fotiadis, D. I. (2016). The Contribution of mHealth in the Care of Obese Pediatric Patients. In A. Moumtzoglou (Ed.), *M-Health Innovations for Patient-Centered Care* (pp. 126–146). Hershey, PA: IGI Global. doi:10.4018/978-1-4666-9861-1.ch007

Waegemann, C. P. (2016). mHealth: History, Analysis, and Implementation. In A. Moumtzoglou (Ed.), M-Health Innovations for Patient-Centered Care (pp. 1-19). Hershey, PA: IGI Global. doi:10.4018/978-1-4666-9861-1.ch001

Wei, D., & Rubino, L. (2015). Public Hospitals in China: The Next Priority for Meaningful Health Care Reform. *International Journal of Public and Private Healthcare Management and Economics*, *4*(1), 53–72. doi:10.4018/IJPPHME.2015010104

Weiss-Randall, D. N. (2017). The Role of Self-Efficacy and Aging in Managing Disease. In V. Bryan & J. Bird (Eds.), *Healthcare Community Synergism between Patients, Practitioners, and Researchers* (pp. 176–212). Hershey, PA: IGI Global. doi:10.4018/978-1-5225-0640-9.ch009

Wickramasinghe, N., Troshani, I., & Goldberg, S. (2016). A Transaction Cost Economics Perspective for Pervasive Technology. In A. Dwivedi (Ed.), *Reshaping Medical Practice and Care with Health Information Systems* (pp. 14–43). Hershey, PA: IGI Global. doi:10.4018/978-1-4666-9870-3.ch002

Wrightman, S. (2015). Community Development and Faith-Based Organizations: Lessons for Global Health. In M. Sheikh, A. Mahamoud, & M. Househ (Eds.), *Transforming Public Health in Developing Nations* (pp. 172–207). Hershey, PA: IGI Global. doi:10.4018/978-1-4666-8702-8.ch009

Yu, B., Wijesekera, D., & Costa, P. C. (2017). Informed Consent in Healthcare: A Study Case of Genetic Services. In A. Moumtzoglou (Ed.), *Design, Development, and Integration of Reliable Electronic Healthcare Platforms* (pp. 211–242). Hershey, PA: IGI Global. doi:10.4018/978-1-5225-1724-5.ch013

Zimeras, S. (2016). Computer Virus Models and Analysis in M-Health IT Systems: Computer Virus Models. In A. Moumtzoglou (Ed.), *M-Health Innovations for Patient-Centered Care* (pp. 284–297). Hershey, PA: IGI Global. doi:10.4018/978-1-4666-9861-1.ch014

Zimeras, S. (2017). Surface Segmentation: The Case of Bronchus Anatomical Structure. In A. Moumtzoglou (Ed.), *Design, Development, and Integration of Reliable Electronic Healthcare Platforms* (pp. 150–159). Hershey, PA: IGI Global. doi:10.4018/978-1-5225-1724-5.ch009

Ziminski, T. B., Demurjian, S. A., Sanzi, E., & Agresta, T. (2016). Toward Integrating Healthcare Data and Systems: A Study of Architectural Alternatives. In T. Iyamu & A. Tatnall (Eds.), *Maximizing Healthcare Delivery and Management through Technology Integration* (pp. 270–304). Hershey, PA: IGI Global. doi:10.4018/978-1-4666-9446-0.ch016

About the Author

Thierry Edoh is an associate researcher at the University of Bonn (Germany)/department of pharmacy, visiting associate lecturer at the Institute of Mathematics and Physics (IMSP)/University Abomey-Calavi, (Benin-Africa), visiting lecturer at IUT Lokossa (Benin-Africa), and an associate researcher at Technical University of Munich/department of Applied Software Engineering (Germany). He received Diploma in computer sciences from the Technical University of Munich in Germany and hold a Ph.D. at the German Federal Army University, where he worked for several years on the improvement of rural health care provision and access to healthcare in developing countries using ITC systems. He was award-winner at the 1st International Health Informatics Conference IHI ACM in Washington in 2010 and in 2013 at Afrinic conference in Indonesia. He performed Postdoctoral research works at the University of Bonn (Germany)/department of pharmacy. His research interests are mobile computing, pervasive health and health informatics, telehealth and IoT in medical applications. He is an expert in telemedicine, bio-Informatics and Drug Regulatory Affairs. He has led several telemedicine projects in Africa, Ireland, and Germany. He works with many European, American, African and Asian universities. He is editorial board member at Internet Technology Letters (Willey journal) [http://onlinelibrary.wiley.com/journal/10.1002/(ISSN)2476-1508] and advisory board member and speaker at Internet Of Things Community (IOTC) [http://healthcare.iotslam.com/, http://healthcare.iotslam.com/2016-speakers, http://iotslam.com/session/sessionpanel-healthcare-iot-a-physicians-view-point/].

Index

I

L

M

O

P

R

S

U

Y

www.ingramcontent.com/pod-product-compliance
Lightning Source LLC
LaVergne TN
LVHW061538290926
849162LV00004B/829